Straight A's
in
Nursing
Pharmacology

Second Edition

 Wolters Kluwer | Lippincott Williams & Wilkins
Health

Philadelphia · Baltimore · New York · London
Buenos Aires · Hong Kong · Sydney · Tokyo

STAFF

Executive Publisher
Judith A. Schilling McCann, RN, MSN

Editorial Director
David Moreau

Clinical Director
Joan M. Robinson, RN, MSN

Art Director
Mary Ludwicki

Senior Managing Editor
Jaime Stockslager Buss, MSPH, ELS

Editorial Project Manager
Liz Schaeffer

Clinical Project Manager
Jennifer Meyering, RN, BSN, MS, CCRN

Producer, Electronic Products
John Macalino

Editors
Sharon R. Cole, Sid Karpoff,
Diane M. Labus, Gale Thompson,
Beth Wegerbauer, Susan Williams

Copy Editors
Kimberly Bilotta (supervisor),
Carol Brown, Scotti Cohn,
Amy Furman, Shana Harrington

Designer
Linda Franklin

Digital Composition Services
Diane Paluba (manager),
Joyce Rossi Biletz, Donald Knauss,
Donna S. Morris

Associate Manufacturing Manager
Beth J. Welsh

Editorial Assistants
Karen J. Kirk, Jeri O'Shea,
Linda K. Ruhf

Design Assistant
George W. Purvis IV

Indexer
Barbara Hodgson

STRPHM011107

**Library of Congress
Cataloging-in-Publication Data**

Straight A's in nursing pharmacology.—2nd ed.
   p. ; cm.
   Includes bibliographical references and index.
   1. Pharmacology—Examinations, questions, etc. 2. Nursing—Examinations, questions, etc. I. Lippincott Williams & Wilkins.
   [DNLM: 1. Pharmaceutical Preparations—Examination Questions. 2. Pharmaceutical Preparations—Nurses' Instruction. 3. Pharmacology, Clinical—Examination Questions. 4. Pharmacology, Clinical—Nurses' Instruction. QV 18.2 S896 2008]
   RM301.14.S75 2008
   615'.1076—dc22
   ISBN-13: 978-1-58255-696-3 (alk. paper)
   ISBN-10: 1-58255-696-2 (alk. paper)   2007030614

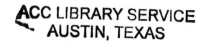

Contents

Advisory board

Contributors and consultants

Dana Bartlett, RN, BS, MS, MA
Poison Information Specialist; Philadelphia (Pa.) Poison Control Center

Virginia Birnie, RN, BSc(N), MN
Nursing Faculty; Camosun College; Victoria, British Columbia

Cheryl Brady, RN, MSN
Adjunct Faculty; Youngstown (Ohio) State University

Nancy E. Dunn, RN, MSN
Nursing Faculty; Gateway Community College; Phoenix, Ariz.

Shelba Durston, RN, MSN, CCRN
Nursing Faculty; San Joaquin Delta College; Stockton, Calif.; Staff Nurse, Intensive Care Unit; San Joaquin General Hospital; French Camp, Calif.

Linda Fuhrman, RN, MS, ANP
Nurse Practitioner; Department of Veterans Affairs Medical Center; San Francisco

Julia A. Isen, RN, MS, FNP-C
Family Nurse Practitioner; University of California, San Francisco Medical Center; Assistant Clinical Professor; University of California, San Francisco School of Nursing

Mary T. Kowalski, RN, BA, MSN
Director, Health Career Programs; Cerro Coso Community College; Ridgecrest, Calif.

Bernadette Madara, APRN, BC, EdD
Associate Professor of Nursing; Southern Connecticut State University; New Haven

N. Darlene Rainwater, RN, MSN
Associate Faculty in Nursing; St. Joseph's College; Rensselaer, Ind.; Assistant Professor of Nursing; St. Elizabeth School of Nursing; Lafayette, Ind.

Monica Narvaez Ramirez, RN, MSN
Nursing Instructor; University of the Incarnate Word School of Nursing & Health Professions; San Antonio, Tex.

Lori Riden, RN, MSN
Nursing Faculty; Gateway Community College; Phoenix, Ariz.

Sheryl Thomas, RN, MSN
Nursing Instructor; Wayne County Community College; Detroit

Donna L. Van Houten, RN, BSN, MS
Nursing Faculty; Gateway Community College; Phoenix, Ariz.

How to use this book

Straight A's is a multivolume study guide series developed especially for nursing students. Each volume provides essential course material in a unique two-column design. The easy-to-read interior outline format offers a succinct review of key facts as presented in leading textbooks on the subject. The bulleted exterior columns provide only the most crucial information, allowing for quick, efficient review right before an important quiz or test.

Special features appear in every chapter to make information accessible and easy to remember. The **Pretest** helps the student identify topic areas that may require more study. **Learning objectives** encourage the student to evaluate knowledge before and after study. The **Chapter overview** highlights the chapter's major concepts. The **NCLEX checks** at the end of each chapter offer additional opportunities to review material and assess knowledge gained before moving on to new information.

Other features appear throughout the book to facilitate learning. **Clinical alerts** appear in color to bring the reader's attention to important, potentially life-threatening considerations that could affect patient care. **Time-out for teaching** highlights key areas to address when teaching patients. **Go with the flow** charts promote critical thinking. Finally, a Windows-based software program (see CD-ROM on inside back cover) poses more than 250 multiple-choice and alternate-format NCLEX-style questions to assess student knowledge.

The *Straight A's* volumes are designed as learning tools, not as primary information sources. When read conscientiously as a supplement to class attendance and textbook reading, *Straight A's* can enhance understanding and help improve test scores and final grades.

Foreword

Welcome to *Straight A's in Nursing Pharmacology*, Second Edition! As you well know, nursing is a profession that requires lifelong learning, especially in the areas of pharmacology and safe medication administration. Although it's impossible for a nurse to know every little thing about every drug out there, it *is* possible to learn about broad groups of drugs and apply that core knowledge throughout your nursing practice. You have in your hands a valuable resource for mastering this complex topic. Whether you're a student who's working toward the goal of an "A" grade in a pharmacology class or a nurse returning to work who needs a refresher before taking a pre-employment competency test, *Straight A's in Nursing Pharmacology*, Second Edition can help you review and master nursing pharmacology.

Straight A's in Nursing Pharmacology offers two ways to study. For a quick review of the most crucial information, scan the outer columns of each chapter. For more in-depth review, read the interior columns, which provide detailed information in an easy-to-read outline format. The first chapter reviews the fundamentals of nursing pharmacology, including drug legislation and the nursing process as it applies to drug administration. Subsequent chapters cover drugs and their uses in specific body systems or conditions. From the autonomic nervous system to the sensory system, pain to cancer, this book provides quick access to the mechanism of action, pharmacokinetics, indications, contraindications and precautions, adverse reactions, and interactions of various drug types. Nursing responsibilities and teaching points for various drug types are also included in each chapter. The main text is enhanced by appendices on herbal drugs and commonly abused drugs. A handy glossary of the terms is also provided.

Had enough of studying? Then apply your knowledge and critical thinking skills to the many practice questions. Each chapter has a pretest and an NCLEX®-style posttest. For more practice, check out the accompanying CD-ROM with more than 250 NCLEX-style questions, including those pesky alternate format questions!

As an educator, I would be remiss if I didn't remind you of your professional obligation to provide safe, effective and knowledgeable nursing care. *Straight A's in Nursing Pharmacology*, Second Edition can assist you in meeting this obligation. Wishing you all the best in your nursing career!

Patricia Lange-Otsuka, EdD, APRN, BC, CNE
Interim Dean and Professor of Nursing
Hawaii Pacific University
Kaneohe

1

Fundamentals of nursing pharmacology

PRETEST

1. Which phase of pharmacokinetics refers to a drug's movement from systemic circulation into the tissues?

☐ 1. Absorption
☐ 2. Distribution
☐ 3. Metabolism
☐ 4. Secretion

CORRECT ANSWER: 2

2. How many classes are in the schedule of controlled substances?

☐ 1. Two
☐ 2. Three
☐ 3. Four
☐ 4. Five

CORRECT ANSWER: 4

3. The assessment phase of the nursing process includes which action in relation to drug administration?

☐ 1. Determining if the client has food or drug allergies
☐ 2. Developing a nursing diagnosis
☐ 3. Developing outcomes with input from the client and his family
☐ 4. Putting the developed care plan into action

CORRECT ANSWER: 1

4. The I.M. injection site most commonly used in children is the:
   ☐ 1. deltoid muscle.
   ☐ 2. ventrogluteal muscle.
   ☐ 3. vastus lateralis muscle.
   ☐ 4. dorsogluteal muscle.

CORRECT ANSWER: 3

5. What's the best action to take if a drug order is unreadable?
   ☐ 1. Guess what the drug should be.
   ☐ 2. Call the physician and clarify the order.
   ☐ 3. Ask the client what drug he normally takes.
   ☐ 4. Ask the charge nurse to read the order.

CORRECT ANSWER: 2

LEARNING OBJECTIVES

After studying this chapter, you should be able to:

- Identify the pharmacodynamic and pharmacokinetic phases of drug action.
- Discuss legislation of drug standards, controlled substances, and the schedule of controlled substances.
- Describe how to apply the nursing process when administering medications.
- Discuss measures to avoid or reduce the risk of medication errors.
- Describe techniques for administering I.M., subcutaneous, and intradermal medications.
- Describe special drug considerations in pregnant women, children, and elderly patients.

CHAPTER OVERVIEW

This chapter begins by exploring two major concepts in pharmacology: pharmacodynamics—the mechanism by which drugs produce chemical and physiologic changes in the body—and pharmacokinetics—the movement of drugs into systemic circulation. Key concepts regarding adverse reactions and drug interactions are also discussed. In addition, this chapter provides a review of federal legislation and regulations governing the manufacture and sale of drugs and laws governing administration of controlled substances. The chapter also provides guidelines for using the nursing process as a framework for administering medications, teaching patients and families about their drug therapy, and evaluating pharmacologic effects. Considerations for special populations are included.

PHARMACODYNAMICS

● **Definition**
  • Refers to the mechanisms by which drugs produce biochemical and physiologic changes in the body
● **Pharmacodynamic events** (what a drug does to the body.)
  • A drug may modify cell function or the rate of cell function
  • A drug may interact with specific receptor sites
    – Agonist drugs stimulate receptors to produce an effect
    – Antagonist drugs inhibit receptors and prevent a response from occurring
  • A drug may work on various receptors (nonselectivity) and produce multiple, widespread effects

PHARMACOKINETICS

● **General information**
  • Refers to movement of a drug across body membranes to reach its target organ
  • Involves four stages of drug movement: absorption, distribution, metabolism, and excretion
● **Absorption**
  • Refers to movement of a drug from its administration site through or across tissue into the systemic circulation
  • Degree and rate of drug absorption depend on:
    – Administration route
    – Patient's age and physical condition
    – Lipid or water solubility of the drug
    – Potential interactions with other drugs or food
    – Mechanism of absorption, such as passive transport (diffusion, passive diffusion, carrier-mediated diffusion), active transport, or pinocytosis

Key definitions

● Pharmacodynamics: mechanisms by which drugs produce biochemical and physiologic changes in the body
● Pharmacokinetics: movement of a drug across body membranes to reach its target organ
● Pharmacotherapeutics: use of drugs to treat specific disease or produce a desired effect
● Adverse reactions: unwanted or potentially harmful effects of a drug
● Interactions: alterations of pharmacokinetic, pharmacodynamic, or pharmacotherapeutic characteristics of drugs

Stages of drug movement

● Absorption
● Distribution
● Metabolism
● Excretion

Key facts about absorption

● Refers to a drug's movement from its administration site into systemic circulation
● Can vary depending on factors such as administration route, patient's age and condition, drug's solubility, interactions, and mechanism of absorption

Key facts about distribution

- Refers to movement of a drug from the systemic circulation into tissues
- May be affected by several physiologic factors

Key facts about metabolism

- Refers to alteration of a drug to a water-soluble form for excretion
- Usually occurs in the liver
- May be affected by genetics, age, physical condition, or the drug itself

Key facts about excretion

- Refers to elimination of drug from circulation
- Occurs:
  - by the kidneys via urine
  - by the liver via bile and into feces
  - by the lungs via exhaled air
  - into breast milk
  - through saliva, tears, and sweat

Key facts about dosing schedules

- Route of administration: area where drug absorption occurs
- Onset of action: time from administration until therapeutic effect begins
- Peak concentration level: maximum blood concentration level achieved through absorption
- Duration of action: time a drug produces a therapeutic effect
- Bioavailability: percentage of drug absorbed into systemic circulation for activity
- Half-life: time required for a drug's plasma concentration to decrease by 50%

● **Distribution**
- Refers to movement of a drug from the systemic circulation into the tissues
- May be affected by several physiologic factors, including blood-brain barrier, cardiac output, body composition (amount of adipose tissue), blood supply to target tissues, degree of vessel constriction or dilation, and degree to which the drug binds to plasma proteins such as albumin
  - Blood–brain barrier refers to limited distribution of drugs into the central nervous system; only highly lipid-soluble drugs can pass through tightly packed glial cells
  - As the drug comes in contact with proteins such as albumin, part of the drug will bind to the protein. The portion bound to the protein is inactive and can't exert a therapeutic effect. A drug that's more than 80% bound to a protein is considered highly protein bound

● **Metabolism**
- Refers to alteration of a drug from its dosage form to a more water-soluble form that can be excreted
- Usually occurs in the liver; may occur in plasma, kidneys, or intestinal membranes
- May be affected by genetics, patient's age and physical condition, or the drug itself (for example, the suitability of the metabolites for drug activity or the drug's lipid solubility)
- First pass effect
  - Can influence the effectiveness of orally administered drugs, which pass through the liver and are partially metabolized before entering the systemic circulation
  - Usually requires higher doses; some drugs have almost complete first-pass metabolism and are ineffective when given orally

● **Excretion**
- Refers to elimination of a drug from the circulation
- Major excretion routes: kidneys via urine; liver via bile, then in feces; lungs via exhaled air; breast milk
- Minor excretion routes: saliva, tears, sweat

● **Factors that determine proper dosing schedules**
- Route of administration—area of the body where drug absorption will take place; bioavailability may change when route of administration is changed
- Onset of action—time interval from when the drug is administered until its therapeutic effects begin
- Peak concentration level—maximum blood concentration level achieved through absorption; at this level, most of the drug reaches the site of action and provides the therapeutic response
- Duration of action—length of time a drug produces its therapeutic effect
- Bioavailability—percentage of a drug absorbed into systemic circulation for activity; drugs injected I.V. have 100% bioavailability

- Drug's half-life—time required for a drug's plasma concentration to decrease by 50%

PHARMACOTHERAPEUTICS

● **General information**
  - Refers to the use of drugs to treat a specific disease or produce a desired effect
  - Includes acute, empiric, supportive, palliative, maintenance, supplemental, and replacement drug therapies
  - Involves several therapeutic steps, including:
    - Assessing the nature and extent of the patient's health problem
    - Assessing therapy options
    - Selecting type of therapy
    - Implementing therapy
    - Monitoring effectiveness of therapy and reassessing the problem
  - Affected by various factors
    - Patient's disease or disorder
    - Route of administration
    - Patient's body size, weight, sex, and past or current medical conditions
    - Psychological and emotional issues
    - Drug tolerance and dependence
  - Loading dose
    - Refers to administration of one or more doses at the onset of therapy to quickly reach the therapeutic blood level and hasten a therapeutic effect
    - Commonly larger than the maintenance dose
  - Drug efficacy
    - Refers to a drug's maximal effectiveness
    - May be measured by the patient's vital signs, body weight, and easing of symptoms that the drug is expected to relieve; the nurse can document efficacy using these parameters
  - Therapeutic drug levels
    - Refer to drug levels that provide adequate action but minimal adverse effects
    - May be monitored to individualize drug dosage, evaluate toxicity, and monitor compliance

ADVERSE REACTIONS

● **Definition**
  - Refers to unwanted or potentially harmful drug effects (all drugs have one or more adverse reactions in addition to producing a desired effect)

Types of drug therapy

- Acute
- Empiric
- Supportive
- Palliative
- Maintenance
- Supplemental
- Replacement

Factors affecting pharmacotherapeutics

- Patient's disease or disorder
- Administration route
- Patient's size, weight, sex, or medical condition
- Psychological and emotional issues
- Drug tolerance and dependance

Key facts about adverse reactions

- Range from mild responses to debilitating, chronic or life-threatening problems
- Can be dose-related or sensitivity-related

Types of adverse reactions

- Dose-related reactions: reactions to the drug's primary or secondary effect
- Sensitivity-related: reaction due to hypersensitivity or allergy
- Iatrogenic: mimics a pathologic condition
- Toxicity: reaction when drug levels exceed therapeutic range
- Idiosyncrasy: reaction that's unexpected or peculiar
- Miscellaneous: includes blood dyscrasias, nephrotoxicity, hepatic toxicity, carcinogenicity, teratogenicity, photosensitivity, and disease-related effects

Key facts about interactions

- Can produce additive effects, potentiation, antagonistic effects, altered metabolism, and altered excretion
- Include contraindications and precautions that warn against drug use or advise caution in patients with specific medical conditions, patients in a specific age-group, or patients who are taking another, potentially incompatible or interacting drug

● **Types of adverse reactions**
- May range from mild responses that resolve spontaneously or disappear upon discontinuing the drug to debilitating, potentially chronic or life-threatening problems
- Reactions associated with starting a new drug—occur shortly after starting a drug but lessen with time
- Reactions inseparable from drug's intended effect, such as when a patient taking an anticoagulant develops bruising and excessive bleeding
- Dose-related reactions
  - Include reactions related to a drug's primary effect (such as bleeding from anticoagulants) or secondary effect (such as drowsiness after taking antihistamines), and overdose
  - Can be prevented in most cases with careful prescribing and administration
- Sensitivity-related reaction—hypersensitivity or an allergic response to a drug or one of its components (can be dose-related)
  - In hypersensitivity or allergic reactions, sensitized patient is exposed to a drug that elicits an antigen-antibody reaction
  - Reactions may be immediate (resulting in anaphylaxis or urticaria) or delayed (as in serum sickness)
- Iatrogenic effect—reaction that mimics a pathologic condition, such as when aspirin or nonsteroidal anti-inflammatory drugs cause GI irritation and bleeding
- Toxicity—reaction that occurs when drug levels exceed the therapeutic range, possibly causing additional adverse effects
  - May develop because of overdosage resulting from failure to consider hepatic impairment, renal function, or the patient's age
  - May result from the patient misunderstanding dosage or administration instructions
  - May require dosage modification
  - Can commonly be prevented by closely following and monitoring established therapeutic blood levels
- Idiosyncrasy—an unexpected or peculiar response to a drug; for example, diphenhydramine (Benadryl) may cause hyperexcitability in children
- Miscellaneous reactions—include blood dyscrasias, nephrotoxicity, hepatic toxicity, carcinogenicity, teratogenicity, photosensitivity, and disease-related effects

INTERACTIONS

● **General information**
- Refer to alterations of the pharmacokinetic, pharmacodynamic, or pharmacotherapeutic characteristics of drugs, which affect overall therapeutic effects
- Can produce additive effects, potentiation, antagonistic effects, increased or decreased metabolism, and increased or decreased excretion

- May be the result of other drugs, foods, herbs, or the environment; for example, taking monoamine oxidase inhibitors with tyramine-containing foods (aged cheese, beer) may lead to hypertensive crisis
- Include contraindications or precautions, which warn against the drug's use or advise cautious use in certain circumstances such as specific medical conditions or age-groups, or when used in combination with other, potentially incompatible or interacting drugs
- May be desired in some cases for their therapeutic benefits; for example, one drug may block the elimination of another drug, thus keeping the drug in systemic circulation longer
- May affect and alter laboratory test values
- Categorized as incompatibilities, pharmacokinetic interactions, and pharmacodynamic interactions

Incompatibilities
- Result from chemical or physical reactions between two or more drugs
- May occur when preparing I.V. admixtures, administering medications in an I.V. bolus or piggyback, or mixing medications in a syringe
- Usually seen as a crystallization of a solution or a change in solution color

Pharmacokinetic interactions
- Altered drug absorption—may result from changes in stomach pH, presence or absence of food in the GI tract, or the presence of other drugs or herbs in the stomach
- Toxicity—can occur when protein-bound drugs compete for protein binding sites, causing the drugs to displace one another and circulate
- Induction or inhibition of hepatic metabolism—may occur with increases or decreases of some hepatically metabolized drugs
- Altered drug excretion—may be planned or coordinated to enhance or inhibit excretion of certain drugs; for example, probenecid may be administered with penicillin to delay renal excretion and prolong the antibiotic's effect

Pharmacodynamic interactions
- Additive effect—combining two or more drugs to cause an effect equal to the sum of their separate effects; for example, aspirin and codeine may be combined to increase pain relief
- Synergism—combining two or more drugs to cause an effect greater than the sum of their separate effects; for example, administration of promethazine (Phenergan) and meperidine (Demerol) provides greater pain relief than meperidine alone
- Potentiation—type of synergism in which one of two or more combined drugs exerts an action greater than if it were given alone; for example, vitamin D helps with the absorption and the action of calcium in the body
- Antagonistic effect—combining two or more drugs to produce an effect less than the sum of their separate effects; for example, a drug antidote

Types of interactions
- Incompatibilities
- Pharmacokinetic interactions
- Pharmacodynamic interactions

Incompatibilities
- Chemical or physical reactions between two or more drugs

Pharmacokinetic interactions
- Altered drug absorption
- Toxicity
- Induction or inhibition of hepatic metabolism
- Altered drug excretion

Pharmacodynamic interactions
- Additive effect
- Synergism
- Potentiation
- Antagonistic effect

FDA regulations

- All drugs need testing for harmful effects in four stages of clinical trials
- Drug labels need to be complete and accurate
- Durham-Humphrey Amendment: distinguishes between prescription and OTC drugs
- Controlled Substances Act groups controlled substances and limits the number of refills
- Drug Price Competition and Patent Time Restoration Act allows generic version equivalents without duplicating trials

DRUG LEGISLATION IN THE UNITED STATES

● **Federal Food, Drug, and Cosmetic Act of 1906**
- Empowers federal government to enforce standards set by the United States Pharmacopeia and the National Formulary
- Requires that drugs meet standards of strength and purity
- Requires that the type and amount of opioid be listed on the label of opiate mixtures
- Was amended in 1912 (Sherley Amendment) to prohibit drug companies from using fraudulent therapeutic claims

● **Food, Drug, and Cosmetic Act—Amendment of 1938**
- Requires that all drugs and drug products be tested for harmful effects in four stages of clinical trials involving animal and human subjects before Food and Drug Administration (FDA) approval of a new drug for sale
- Mandates that all drug labels and literature be complete and accurate and include:
  - Drug dose
  - Manufacturer's name and address
  - Names and amounts of potentially harmful ingredients
  - Warning if the drug might be habit-forming
  - Directions for use
  - Contraindications

● **Food, Drug, and Cosmetic Act—Durham-Humphrey Amendment of 1952**
- Distinguishes between prescription and over-the-counter (OTC) medications
- States that a prescription for opioids, hypnotics, habit-forming drugs, and potentially harmful drugs can be refilled only with a new prescription; requires that the label state this fact

● **Food, Drug, and Cosmetic Act—Kefauver-Harris Amendment of 1962**
- Increases FDA's control over drug safety
- Allows FDA to evaluate the testing methods of drug manufacturers
- Requires manufacturers to prove that a drug is effective, not just nontoxic

● **Controlled Substances Act or Comprehensive Drug Abuse Prevention Act of 1970**
- Groups controlled substances (drugs with the potential for abuse or physical and psychological dependence such as opioids, sedatives, barbiturates, and amphetamines) into five categories (schedules) (see *Schedules of controlled substances*)
- Limits the number of prescription refills for controlled substances and requires specific guidelines and procedures; for example, practitioners must use specially designated prescription pads

Schedules of controlled substances

Controlled substances are grouped into five categories (schedules) based on a drug's medical effectiveness and potential for abuse or physical and psychological dependence. These drugs must be handled properly; any violations by a nurse may result in suspension or loss of nursing license.

SCHEDULE I
Schedule I drugs carry the highest risk of abuse. These drugs, which include cannabinols, such as marijuana, and hallucinogens, such as LSD, heroin, and mescaline, aren't acceptable for prescription use; they may be available for investigational use.

SCHEDULE II
Schedule II drugs carry high potential for abuse and may lead to physical and psychological dependence. This group includes certain barbiturates, opioids, and stimulants.

SCHEDULE III
Schedule III drugs carry a lesser abuse potential than schedules I and II. This group includes barbiturates such as butabarbital, opioids used in combination with other drugs, stimulants, androgens, anabolic steroids, and paregoric.

SCHEDULE IV
Schedule IV drugs carry a low abuse potential, with psychological dependence more common than physical dependence. This group includes benzodiazepines, propoxyphene (Darvon), and chlordiazepoxide (Librium).

SCHEDULE V
Schedule V drugs carry the least abuse potential. Most drugs in this class have a small amount of an opioid combined with an antitussive or antidiarrheal.

● **Drug Price Competition and Patent Time Restoration Act of 1984**
  - Allows for the marketing of generic versions of bioequivalent drugs without duplicating clinical trials

NURSING PROCESS IN DRUG ADMINISTRATION

● **Assessment**
  - Determine whether the patient has food or drug allergies; document clearly on the patient's chart all food and drug allergies
  - Find out:
    - Which prescription and nonprescription medications the patient currently takes
    - The frequency of administration
    - The purpose of each medication for the patient
    - Whether the patient has experienced adverse effects
  - Obtain a history of the patient's medical conditions, socioeconomic status, and psychosocial support
  - Perform a physical examination; pay particular attention to body systems that may be affected by current or newly prescribed medications or to areas where the patient has complaints or concerns

Nursing diagnosis and planning

- Begin by addressing immediate threat to patient's health.
- Include deficient knowledge, injury risk, ineffective mangement of therapeutic regimen, noncompliance.
- Develop manageable outcomes using the nursing diagnosis.

● **Nursing diagnosis**
- Develop a nursing diagnosis consisting of the patient's disease and its etiology
- Begin by addressing problems that pose immediate threats to the patient's health
- Commonly listed nursing diagnoses related to drug administration include:
  – Deficient knowledge
  – Risk for injury
  – Ineffective therapeutic regimen management
  – Noncompliance

● **Planning**
- Develop outcomes using the nursing diagnosis; if possible, obtain input from the patient and his family
- Use these goals as outcome criteria for evaluation

● **Implementation**
- Put the care plan into action
- Include all relevant nursing interventions, including drug therapy, to meet the patient's health care needs
- A multidisciplinary team approach is usually needed

● **Evaluation**
- Evaluate whether interventions enabled the patient to achieve the desired outcomes
- Include appropriate evaluation statements, such as:
  – The patient experiences expected effects of the prescribed medication
  – The patient avoids adverse effects or interactions with other drugs, foods, or alcohol
  – The patient demonstrates an understanding of information taught
  – The patient complies with the therapeutic regimen (if the patient doesn't comply, determine the reasons for noncompliance)
  – Therapeutic drug levels are maintained
- Based on patient evaluation, modify outcomes and interventions, as needed

AVOIDING MEDICATION ERRORS

Six rights of drug administration

- Right drug
- Right route
- Right dose
- Right time
- Right patient
- Right documentation

● **Follow the six rights of drug administration**
- Verify the medication order for the RIGHT DRUG
  – Ensure that the medication order is properly composed and includes:
    · Patient's full name
    · Drug name
    · Dosage form
    · Dose amount
    · Administration route
    · Time schedule

Sample dosage calculations

Proper dosage calculations can help ensure that the right dose of a drug is administered. For example, if you have an order to administer meperidine (Demerol) 75 mg I.M. taken from a 1 ml prefilled syringe containing 100 mg of Demerol, you can calculate the ordered dose in one of two ways.

RATIO AND PROPORTION METHOD

The ratio for this calculation would be 75 mg is to X ml as 100 mg is to 1 ml; the equation would read as follows:

$$75 \text{ mg} : X :: 100 \text{ mg} : 1 \text{ ml}$$
$$75 \text{ mg} \times 1 \text{ ml} = 100 \text{ mg} \times X$$

Solve for X:
$$X = 75/100 \text{ or } X = 0.75 \text{ ml}$$

DOSE DESIRED VERSUS DOSE ON HAND METHOD

Alternatively, you may use the dose desired/dose on hand $\times$ ml method. The equation using this method would be:

$$75/100 \times 1 \text{ ml} = 0.75 \text{ ml}$$

- Practitioner's signature
- Date and time of order
  - Check the medication order against the drug label three times
  - Know why the patient is receiving this specific drug at this time
- Check the order and medication supplied to ensure the RIGHT ROUTE
  - Drugs can be administered orally (by mouth or through a gastric tube), parenterally (by intradermal, subcutaneous [subQ], I.M., or I.V. injection), topically, otically, ophthalmically, or via the mucous membranes (by sublingual, buccal, vaginal, rectal, intranasal, transdermal, or inhaled methods)
  - Be aware of the routes available for the specified drug ordered; if the patient can't swallow the pill form of a drug, suggest to the practitioner an alternative route, such as I.M. or I.V.
  - Be aware that drug forms or types aren't always interchangeable
- Perform a dosage calculation to ensure the RIGHT DOSE (see *Sample dosage calculations*)
- Verify the frequency of dosage with the medication order to ensure the RIGHT TIME
- Confirm the patient's identity by checking his identification bracelet before administering each drug to ensure the RIGHT PATIENT
- Make sure the practitioner's order is clear and complete to ensure the RIGHT DOCUMENTATION
  - Compare the original order with the medication label to ensure accuracy
  - Record the medication in the patient's chart immediately after administering it
  - If the patient doesn't take the medication, document that the drug wasn't given and why; notify the practitioner if appropriate

Topics for patient discussion

- Drug name and purpose
- How to monitor the drug's effectiveness
- Drugs that could interact with the prescribed drug
- Possible adverse effects

Key medication guidelines

- Never give a drug poured or prepared by someone else.
- Never allow the medication cart or tray out of your sight once you have prepared a dose.
- Never leave a drug at a patient's bedside; rather, watch the patient swallow the drug.
- Never return unwrapped or prepared drugs to the stock supply; instead, dispose of the medication and notify the pharmacist.
- Keep the medication cart locked at all times.
- Take care to avoid medication errors that can easily be caused by similar sounding drug names, unclear orders, wrong route of administration, and miscalculation of dosages.

When to question a medication order

- When handwriting is difficult to read
- When the drug's use in the patient's condition is questionable
- When dosages are unclear
- When drug incompatibilities or interactions may occur

 TIME-OUT FOR TEACHING

Teaching about drug therapy

Be sure to include these topics in your teaching plan for the patient receiving drug therapy:
- drug's name
- drug's purpose
- how and when to take the drug as well as what to do about missed doses
- how to monitor the drug's effectiveness (for example, monitoring blood glucose level when taking a hypoglycemic)
- drugs that may interact with the prescribed drug (including over-the-counter and herbal drugs)
- required dietary changes, including use of alcohol
- possible adverse effects and what to do if these occur
- signs and symptoms to bring to the practitioner's attention
- required follow-up procedures
- storing and handling drug.

Medication administration guidelines

- Administer the medication as prescribed and according to the manufacturer's instructions
- If there's any concern or question regarding the look, consistency, dosage, or proper administration technique for a drug, consult the pharmacist and document the consultation
- Follow these safety procedures:
  - Never give a drug poured or prepared by someone else
  - Never allow the medication cart or tray out of your sight after you've prepared a dose
  - Never leave a drug at a patient's bedside; rather, watch the patient swallow the drug
  - Never return unwrapped or prepared drugs to the stock supply; instead, dispose of the medication and notify the pharmacist
  - Keep the medication supply secure at all times
  - Follow standard precautions as appropriate
- Monitor the patient for therapeutic effects; regularly evaluate the serum drug level and the results of relevant laboratory tests
- Evaluate the patient for adverse reactions; notify the practitioner if adverse reactions occur and intervene, as necessary
- Provide patient teaching essential to proper medication administration; include family members in patient teaching (see *Teaching about drug therapy*)
- Consider legal aspects associated with drug therapy
  - Make sure the medication order is present and complete
  - Question an order when:
    - Handwriting is difficult to read
    - Drug's use in the patient's condition is questionable
    - Dosages are unclear
    - Drug incompatibilities or interactions may occur

- Consider ethical principles when dealing with medication errors, medications during pregnancy, and investigational protocols
- Remember that medication errors can easily be caused by similar sounding drug names, unclear orders, wrong routes of administration, and miscalculation of dosages; take extra care to avoid these errors

DRUG ADMINISTRATION ROUTES

● Oral administration

- Most commonly prescribed route because it's safe, convenient, and least expensive
- May be necessary to administer oral drugs at higher doses than their parenteral equivalents because of first-pass metabolism or poor bioavailability
- Includes formulations such as tablets, enteric-coated tablets, capsules, syrups, elixirs, oils, liquids, suspensions, powders, and granules
- May require special preparation before administration, such as mixing with juice to improve palatability
- Can sometimes be mixed with juice or foods if the patient has difficulty taking medications; check whether the drug can be crushed or mixed with foods because some drugs are sustained-release formulations
- May be administered via the nasogastric (NG) route; for example in patients with NG tubes in place who can't swallow or take drugs orally
  - Requires consideration of which tablets shouldn't be crushed and which capsules shouldn't be opened; consult the pharmacist if needed
  - May interact with tube feedings, causing decreased drug absorption; tube feeding should be held for at least 1 hour before and 2 hours after drug administration
  - Requires adjustments if the NG tube is hooked to suction (suction should be held for 20 to 30 minutes after drug administration)
- Buccal and sublingual administration
  - Involves placing medication between the cheek and teeth (buccal) or placing medication under the tongue (sublingual)
  - Drugs are immediately absorbed into systemic circulation because they bypass the digestive tract
  - Requires either concentrated liquid formulations or specially formulated disintegrating tablets
  - Can't be swallowed because involving the digestive tract in absorption eliminates immediate absorption

● Parenteral administration

- May be used when medications can't be delivered orally
- Involves administering drugs via injection directly into the vein (I.V.), into the muscle (I.M.), into the subcutaneous tissue (subQ), or intradermally
  - I.V. administration

Oral administration

- Most medications delivered orally; safe, convenient, and least expensive
- Oral forms include tablets, enteric-coated tablets, capsules, syrups, elixirs, oils, liquids, suspensions, powders, and granules
- Remember that many drugs can be mixed with juice or foods
- Make sure that the drug is able to be crushed or mixed with foods because some drugs are sustained-release formulations

Buccal and sublingual administration

- Buccally administered medications are placed between the cheek and the teeth
- Sublingually administered medications are placed under the tongue
- These drugs bypass the digestive tract and are immediately absorbed into systemic circulation

Four methods of parenteral administration

1. Intravenous: deposits drug directly into the systemic circulation
2. Intramuscular: deposits drug into the muscle
3. Subcutaneous: deposits drug directly into fatty tissue
4. Intradermal: deposits drug into corium

Topical administration

- Lotions, creams, ointments, drops, and transdermal patches applied directly to the skin
- When applying, never place a heating pad over the application site; never place a defibrillator paddle over a transdermal patch

Ophthalmic administration

- Ointments or drops used for local effects within the eye
- Absorbed into mucus membrane
- When administering, never instill the drug directly onto the eyeball; never touch the eye or lid with applicator tip

Otic administration

- Drugs administered to the ear to treat local infection and inflammation, soften cerumen, and provide local anesthesia
- When administering, straighten the patient's ear canal; in adults, gently pull the auricle up and back; in infants or children younger than age 3, gently pull the auricle down and back

Inhalation administration

- Topical medications delivered into the respiratory tract by inhaler or nebulizer
- Lung's mucosal lining absorbs the drug almost immediately

- Provides direct delivery of drugs into the systemic circulation and 100% bioavailability of drug
- May be administered by bolus infusion or continuous infusion
- Produces immediate effects
- Bypasses absorption process and enters directly in the systemic circulation
- I.M. administration
  - Deposits the drug into the muscle at varying tissue depths
  - Requires avoiding areas that look inflamed, edematous, or irritated and areas that contain moles, birthmarks, scars, or other lesions
  - Commonly uses dorsogluteal and ventrogluteal muscle groups (see *Locating I.M. injection sites*); vastus lateralis in children
- SubQ administration
  - Involves injection into fatty tissue
  - Allows for a slower, more sustained administration than I.M. injection; more rapid absorption than oral administration
- Intradermal administration
  - Involves injection into the corium, a skin layer consisting of dense vascular tissue
  - Usually used for diagnostic testing

● **Topical administration**
- Involves applying medication directly to the skin
- Includes use of lotions, creams, ointments, and transdermal patches
  - Effects may be local, as with lotions, creams, and ointments
  - Effects may be systemic, as with transdermal delivery systems (includes some ointments and patches), which are designed to deliver drug into systemic circulation after absorption through the skin
- Requires applying drug only to areas of skin that are intact, clean, and dry (unless the drug is prescribed to treat a skin lesion); application of the drug to callused or scarred areas may result in impaired absorption

● **Ophthalmic administration**
- Is used for local effects within the eye
- Is absorbed into the mucous membrane
- Is available as ointments or drops (see *Administering eyedrops or eye ointment,* page 16)

● **Otic administration**
- Involves instilling drugs into the ear to treat local infection and inflammation, to soften cerumen, or to provide local anesthesia (see *Administering eardrops,* page 16)

● **Inhalation administration**
- Involves administering topical medications via the respiratory tract for local and systemic effects; the lung's mucosal lining absorbs the drug almost immediately
- Commonly given by inhaler or nebulizer

Locating I.M. injection sites

Use these illustrations to help you locate the most common I.M. injection sites used in adults.

DELTOID

Find the lower edge of the acromial process and the point on the lateral arm in line with the axilla. Insert the needle 1″ to 2″ (2.5 to 5 cm) below the acromial process, usually two or three fingerwidths, at a 90-degree angle or angled slightly toward the process. Typical injection: 0.5 ml (range: 0.5 to 2 ml).

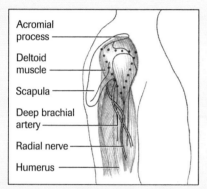

Acromial process
Deltoid muscle
Scapula
Deep brachial artery
Radial nerve
Humerus

DORSOGLUTEAL

Inject above and outside a line drawn from the posterior superior iliac spine to the greater trochanter of the femur. Alternatively, divide the buttock into quadrants, and inject in the upper outer quadrant, about 2″ to 3″ (5 to 7.5 cm) below the iliac crest. Insert the needle at a 90-degree angle. Typical injection: 1 to 4 ml (range: 1 to 5 ml).

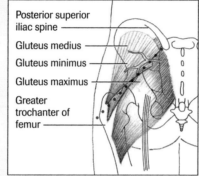

Posterior superior iliac spine
Gluteus medius
Gluteus minimus
Gluteus maximus
Greater trochanter of femur

I.M. injection sites

- Deltoid
- Dorsogluteal
- Ventrolgluteal
- Vastus lateralis

VENTROGLUTEAL

Locate the greater trochanter of the femur with the heel of your hand. Then spread your index and middle fingers from the anterior superior iliac spine to as far along the iliac crest as you can reach. Insert the needle between the two fingers at a 90-degree angle to the muscle. (Remove your fingers before inserting the needle.) Typical injection: 1 to 4 ml (range: 1 to 5 ml).

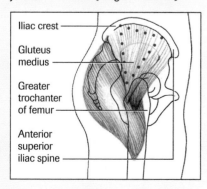

Iliac crest
Gluteus medius
Greater trochanter of femur
Anterior superior iliac spine

VASTUS LATERALIS

Use the lateral muscle of the quadriceps group, from a handbreadth below the greater trochanter to a handbreadth above the knee. Insert the needle into the middle third of the muscle parallel to the surface on which the patient is lying. You may have to bunch the muscle before insertion. Typical injection: 1 to 4 ml (range: 1 to 5 ml; 1 to 3 ml for infants)

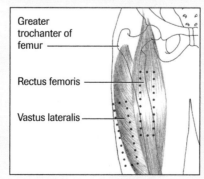

Greater trochanter of femur
Rectus femoris
Vastus lateralis

Administering eyedrops or eye ointment

Follow these steps to administer eyedrops or ointment:
- Place the patient in a supine position, and tilt his head back and toward the affected eye (this will direct flow of the drug away from the tear duct and minimize the risk of systemic absorption through the nasal mucosa).

- Gently pull down the lower lid of the affected eye, and instill the drops or ointment into the conjunctival sac.
- Never instill the drug directly onto the eyeball.
- Never touch the eye or lid with the applicator tip.

Administering eardrops

Follow these steps to administer eardrops:
- Have the patient lie on the side opposite the affected ear; straighten the patient's ear canal (for adults, gently pull the auricle up and back; for an infant or child younger than age 3, gently pull the auricle down and back).

- Gently massage the anterior area of the ear, and instruct the patient to remain on his side for an additional 5 minutes.
- If ordered, insert a cotton ball into the external ear and observe for reactions.

Vaginal administration
- Topical treatments used to treat vaginal infections and inflammation
- Includes suppositories or creams

Rectal administration
- Drugs administered rectally to treat constipation, nausea and vomiting, hemorrhoids, colitis, and pain
- Used when other routes aren't available
- Absorbed into the large intestine

● Vaginal administration
- Involves administering topical treatments for vaginal infections and inflammation
- Includes use of suppositories and creams

● Rectal administration
- Is used when other routes of administration aren't available
- Is used to administer drugs to treat constipation, nausea and vomiting, hemorrhoids, colitis, and pain
- Involves drug absorption into the large intestine; degree of absorption depends on the patient's ability to retain the suppository or enema
- Requires the patient to be in Sims' position; urge him to remain in this position for 30 minutes, if possible

● Specialized (site-specific) infusions
- Epidural—infuses drug into the epidural space
- Intrapleural—infuses drug into the pleural cavity
- Intraperitoneal—infuses drug into peritoneal cavity
- Intraosseous—administers drug into the vascular network of a long bone
- Intra-articular—administers drug directly into a joint

Pregnancy risk categories

Category A: Controlled studies failed to demonstrate a risk to the fetus.

Category B: Animal studies showed no risk to the fetus or there were no studies performed on pregnant women.

Category C: Either animal studies showed adverse effects to the fetus or no studies in women or animals are available.

Category D: Fetal risk exists.

Category X: Fetal risk has been shown in animals and in women. Drug is contraindicated in women who are or who may become pregnant.

Category NR: No rating is available.

ADMINISTERING DRUGS TO SPECIAL POPULATIONS

● Pregnant or breast-feeding women
- The FDA has established six pregnancy risk categories for pregnant patients or patients considering pregnancy (see *Pregnancy risk categories*)
- Teratogenic effects may occur in the fetus secondary to drug exposure, including topically administered drugs
- Caution the pregnant patient to avoid all drugs except those that are approved by her practitioner; instruct her to check with her practitioner before taking any drugs, including herbal and over-the-counter drugs
- Drugs may appear in breast milk, producing a pharmacologic effect in the infant; may warrant discontinuing the drug or avoiding breast-feeding
- Weigh the potential fetal and neonatal risks and potential benefits to the mother when administering medications

● Children
- Usually, pediatric dosing is based on milligram of drug per kilogram of body weight (mg/kg) or body surface area expressed as milligrams per square meter (mg/m^2)
- Pharmacokinetics in children
  - Absorption—may vary between neonates and infants; thin epidermis in children causes increased absorption of topical drugs
  - Distribution—may be altered in neonates because they have a larger percentage of body water, lower protein levels, and less fat than adults, which may result in reduced plasma levels of water-soluble drugs and less storage
  - Metabolism—immaturity of the liver may delay metabolism in infants; some drugs may be metabolized more rapidly in children than in adults
  - Excretion—immaturity of the kidneys may delay excretion in infants

Drug considerations in pregnant and breast-feeding women

- Six pregnancy risk categories guide drug administartion for pregnant women.
- Teratogenic effects may occur in the fetus secondary to drug exposure.
- Drugs may appear in breast milk, producing a pharmacologic effect in the infant; this may warrant discontinuing the drug or avoiding breast-feeding.

Drug considerations in children

- Pediatric dosing is based on mg of drug/kg of body weight or mg/m^2.
- Immaturity of liver may delay metabolism; some drugs may be metabolized more rapidly in children than adults.
- Immaturity of the kidneys may delay excretion in infants.

Drug considerations in elderly patients

- Drug absorption, distribution, and elimination are less efficient.
- Decreased dosage is usually required.
- Multiple disorders are more likely.
- Adverse reactions and toxicities may occur.

TOP 6

Items to study for your next test on fundamentals of nursing pharmacology

1. Pharmacodynamic and pharmacokinetic phases of drug action
2. Patients at risk for drug toxicities
3. Use of the nursing process with patients and families when administering medications
4. Measures to avoid or reduce the risk of medication errors
5. Techniques for administering I.M., subQ, and intradermal medications
6. Special drug considerations in pregnant women, children, and elderly patients

● Elderly patients

- Elderly patients tend to absorb, distribute, and eliminate drugs less efficiently; therefore, they usually require decreased drug dosages
- They're at higher risk for having multiple disorders (such as cardiac disease, renal disease, hepatic disturbances, and diabetes), which may alter drug action and excretion; this places them at increased risk for adverse reactions and drug toxicities
- Drugs requiring careful monitoring for adverse reactions and toxicities in the elderly include:
  - Antiarrhythmics
  - Diuretics
  - Antihypertensives
  - Corticosteroids
  - Anticoagulants
  - Benzodiazepines
  - Opioids
- Factors affecting poor compliance with drug regimen include lack of family support, fixed income and decreased access to transportation or resources
- Patient teaching is sometimes difficult because of sensory deficits (hearing impairment, poor eyesight) and cognitive deficits (poor memory)

NCLEX CHECKS

It's never too soon to begin your NCLEX® examination preparation. Now that you've reviewed this chapter, carefully read each of the following questions and choose the best answer. Then compare your responses with the correct answers.

1. A client carefully follows a diabetic diet and exercise program prescribed by his physician. Because his blood glucose level remains elevated, his physician orders glipizide (Glucotrol) daily. The nurse wants to learn more about this drug's absorption, distribution, metabolism, and excretion. Which branch of pharmacology provides this information?
- ☐ 1. Pharmacognosy
- ☑ 2. Pharmacokinetics
- ☐ 3. Pharmacodynamics
- ☐ 4. Pharmacotherapeutics

2. A nurse is preparing to give a client his scheduled 9 a.m. drugs. The nurse realizes the client is in the bathroom. Through the door, the client tells the nurse to leave the pills by his bed and he'll take them when he comes out. Which action is most appropriate for the nurse to take?
- ☑ 1. Take the drugs away, but return in 10 minutes to give them.
- ☐ 2. Return the drugs to the client's drug drawer, and chart "drugs refused."
- ☐ 3. Go into the bathroom and give the pills to the client to take while standing there.
- ☐ 4. Leave the drugs at the bedside with a note for the client to take them as soon as possible.

3. In 1938, Congress passed an amendment to the Federal Food, Drug, and Cosmetic Act. As a result of this amendment, drug labels must consist of:

- ☐ **1.** only the name of the distributor.
- ☐ **2.** a warning if the drug comes from a foreign source.
- ☐ **3.** the name of the scientist who discovered the drug.
- ☑ **4.** a statement describing the contents of the package.

4. A nurse is reviewing a new drug order written for a client. After reviewing the order, the nurse thinks that the dosage is unusually high. How should the nurse proceed?

- ☐ **1.** Ignore the drug order.
- ☐ **2.** Give the drug exactly as prescribed.
- ☐ **3.** Question the physician about the dosage.
- ☑ **4.** Have another nurse double-check the order.

5. A nurse is preparing to give cortisone to a client. Which item must always be checked before giving a drug?

- ☐ **1.** Family history
- ☑ **2.** Blood pressure
- ☐ **3.** Respiratory rate
- ☐ **4.** Identification bracelet

6. A nurse is teaching a client about a newly prescribed drug. What could cause an elderly client to have difficulty learning about prescribed medications?

- ☐ **1.** Decreased drug excretion
- ☑ **2.** Sensory deficits
- ☐ **3.** Lack of family support
- ☐ **4.** Fixed income

7. During an acute infection, a client with diabetes develops severe hyperglycemia and requires insulin therapy. Which administration route provides an immediate systemic response?

- ☐ **1.** I.M.
- ☐ **2.** Intradermal
- ☑ **3.** I.V.
- ☐ **4.** SubQ

8. A cardiologist prescribes digoxin (Lanoxin) 125 mcg orally every morning for a client diagnosed with heart failure. The pharmacy dispenses tablets that contain 0.25 mg each. How many tablets should the nurse administer in each dose? Record your answer using one decimal place.

_____ tablet(s)

9. A nurse is administering an I.M. injection to a 2-year-old child. The best place for the nurse to give the injection is:
- ☐ **1.** 1″ to 2″ (2.5 to 5 cm) below the acromial process, with the needle angled toward the process.
- ☐ **2.** in the middle third of the lateral muscle of the quadriceps group, from a handbreadth below the greater trochanter to a handbreadth above the knee.
- ☒ **3.** in the upper outer quadrant of the buttock, below the iliac crest.
- ☐ **4.** within 1″ (2.5 cm) of the umbilicus, with the needle at a 45-degree angle.

10. A client taking ibuprofen (Motrin) for joint pain is admitted for GI bleeding. The nurse would document this as what type of adverse reaction?
- ☐ **1.** Dose-related
- ☐ **2.** Sensitivity-related
- ☐ **3.** Iatrogenic
- ☒ **4.** Toxicity

ANSWERS AND RATIONALES

1. CORRECT ANSWER: 2
Pharmacokinetics refers to the absorption, distribution, metabolism, and excretion of the drug in a living organism. Pharmacognosy deals with natural drug resources. Pharmacodynamics is the study of the biochemical and physical effects of drugs and the mechanism of drug actions in living organisms. Pharmacotherapeutics, also known as *clinical pharmacology,* is a general term covering the use of drugs to prevent and treat diseases.

2. CORRECT ANSWER: 1
Legally, a nurse must witness the client taking the drugs. Thus, coming back with the drugs in 10 minutes would be the best action to make sure the client takes his drugs. The client didn't refuse to take the drugs, so it wouldn't be appropriate to chart this information. Going into the bathroom wouldn't be the best option because the nurse wouldn't be respecting the client's privacy. Drugs should never be left at the bedside.

3. CORRECT ANSWER: 4
Drug labels must be clear and list the contents of the package. The manufacturer, packager, and distributor also must be listed. The other information isn't required to be listed on the drug label.

4. CORRECT ANSWER: 3
The nurse is obliged to act as the client's advocate and legally is required to question an order that doesn't seem safe or correct. To ignore the drug order or give an unusually high dose can harm the client. Because the physician ordered the dosage, the nurse should question him, not another nurse.

5. CORRECT ANSWER: 4

Remember the six "rights" of drug administration—right drug, right dose, right client, right time, right route, and right documentation. The nurse should always check the client's identification bracelet before giving a drug. Checking the client's history (not the family history) is also important before giving a drug. Checking blood pressure and respiratory rate is needed only when the drug to be given affects these factors. Cortisone doesn't affect blood pressure or respiratory rate.

6. CORRECT ANSWER: 2

Sensory deficits could cause an elderly client to have difficulty retaining knowledge about prescribed medications. Decreased drug excretion doesn't alter the client's knowledge about a drug. A lack of family support or limited finances may affect compliance, but not knowledge retention.

7. CORRECT ANSWER: 3

The I.V. route bypasses the body's absorption barriers and provides an immediate systemic response. Drugs given intradermally, I.M., or subQ require absorption.

8. CORRECT ANSWER: 0.5

The nurse should begin by converting 125 mcg to milligrams:
$$125 \text{ mcg}/1,000 = 0.125 \text{ mg}$$
Then the nurse should use this formula to calculate the drug dosage:
$$\text{Dose on hand}/\text{Quantity on hand} = \text{Dose desired}/X$$
$$0.25 \text{ mg}/1 = 0.125 \text{ mg}/X \text{ tablet}$$
$$0.25X = 0.125$$
$$X = 0.5 \text{ tablet}$$

9. CORRECT ANSWER: 2

The most common I.M. injection site for a child is the vastus lateralis. The acromial process is the landmark used to give a deltoid muscle injection. The upper outer quadrant of the buttocks is used for a dorsogluteal injection. Although this quadrant is sometimes used in children, it usually isn't used in children younger than age 3 because the muscle isn't well developed. The area around the umbilicus is typically used for subQ injections.

10. CORRECT ANSWER: 3

An iatrogenic adverse reaction mimics a pathologic condition. A dose-related reaction is related to the drug's primary or secondary effect. A sensitivity-related reaction occurs when the client is allergic to the drug or one of its components. Toxicity occurs when the drug levels exceed the therapeutic range and cause additional adverse effects.

2

Drugs and the autonomic nervous system

1. Cholinergic agonists stimulate which receptors?

☐ 1. Adrenergic

☐ 2. Alpha$_1$

☐ 3. Beta$_2$

☐ 4. Cholinergic

CORRECT ANSWER: 4

2. Edrophonium is used to treat:

☐ 1. myasthenia gravis.

☐ 2. inner ear infection.

☐ 3. paralytic ileus.

☐ 4. bradycardia.

CORRECT ANSWER: 1

3. Terbutaline (Brethine) is commonly used for:

☐ 1. treating glaucoma.

☐ 2. stopping preterm labor.

☐ 3. treating hyperthyroidism.

☐ 4. controlling seizures.

CORRECT ANSWER: 2

4. A nurse should monitor a client taking ergotamine (Ergomar) for:

- ☐ 1. ringing in the ears.
- ☐ 2. blurred vision.
- ☐ 3. tingling in the fingers and toes.
- ☐ 4. bradycardia.

CORRECT ANSWER: 3

5. Which drug is most appropriate to give an intubated client who's fighting the use of a mechanical ventilator?

- ☐ 1. Metoprolol (Lopressor)
- ☐ 2. Dobutamine (Dobutrex)
- ☐ 3. Cisatracurium (Nimbex)
- ☐ 4. Dicyclomine (Antispas)

CORRECT ANSWER: 3

LEARNING OBJECTIVES

After studying this chapter, you should be able to:

- Correlate the mechanisms of action of certain drugs to the receptor that's stimulated or blocked.
- Identify indications for the various types of drugs.
- Describe nursing responsibilities related to cholinergics, adrenergic agonists, adrenergic blockers, and neuromuscular blockers.

CHAPTER OVERVIEW

Cholinergics include parasympathomimetics, which mimic the effects of the parasympathetic nervous system, and parasympatholytics, which oppose or block the effects of the parasympathetic system. Parasympathomimetics include cholinergic agonists, acetylcholinesterase inhibitors, and Alzheimer's treatment drugs. Parasympatholytics include anticholinergics.

Sympathomimetics mimic the effects of the sympathetic system. This drug type includes the adrenergic agonists catecholamines and noncatecholamines. Sympatholytics (also known as *adrenergic* blockers) antagonize or inhibit the adrenergic activity. Types of sympatholytics are alpha-adrenergic blockers and beta-adrenergic blockers. Neuromuscular blockers include nondepolarizing drugs and depolarizing drugs.

A&P highlights

- The ANS consists of the sympathetic nervous system, the parasympathetic nervous system, and the enteric nervous system.
- ANS pathways consist of two neurons, which transmit information to the effector organs: preganglionic neuron and postganglionic neuron.
- The ANS controls involuntary body functions, glands, and organs.
- The sympathetic system helps the body cope with external stimuli and functions during stress (triggers "fight or flight" response).
- The parasympathetic system works to save energy, aids in digestion, and supports restorative, resting body functions.

ANATOMY AND PHYSIOLOGY

- **Anatomy of the autonomic nervous system (ANS)**
  - Composed of three systems
    - Sympathetic nervous system (adrenergic system)
    - Parasympathetic nervous system (cholinergic system)
    - Enteric nervous system (usually not discussed)
  - Includes pathways that consist of two types of neurons, which transmit information to the effector organs
    - Preganglionic neuron—extends from the central nervous system (CNS) to a ganglion
    - Postganglionic neuron—extends from the ganglion to the effector organ or gland

- **Function of ANS**
  - Controls involuntary (automatic) body functions, glands, and organs, such as cardiac muscle activity and the smooth muscle of blood vessels, eyes, stomach, and intestines
  - Sympathetic system
    - Helps the body cope with external stimuli and functions during stress
    - Triggers fight-or-flight response (vasoconstriction, increased heart and respiratory rate; cold, sweaty palms; and pupil dilation)
  - Parasympathetic system
    - Works to save energy
    - Activates the GI system (aids in digestion)
    - Supports restorative, resting body functions (decreased heart rate, increased GI tract tone and peristalsis, urinary sphincter relaxation, and vasodilation)

- **ANS neurotransmitters**
  - Acetylcholine
    - Helps neurons transmit impulses in the CNS
    - Released from the axons of preganglionic neurons in response to a stressful event

Adrenergic receptor uses and effects

RECEPTOR ACTIVATED	THERAPEUTIC USES	ADVERSE EFFECTS
Alpha$_1$	• Control topical superficial bleeding • Treat nasal decongestion • Elevate blood pressure • Delay absorption of local anesthetics • Decrease intraocular pressure	• Hypertension • Necrosis with extravasation • Bradycardia
Alpha$_2$	• Treat glaucoma	• Burning sensation • Ptosis • Redness and swelling of eyelid
Beta$_1$	• Treat heart failure, cardiac arrest, and shock	• Tachycardia • Arrhythmias • Angina
Beta$_2$	• Produce bronchodilation • Delay preterm labor	• Hyperglycemia • Tremors
Dopamine	• Increase renal blood flow • Increase cardiac output • Elevate blood pressure	• Ectopy • Nausea and vomiting • Tachycardia • Palpitations

  – Stimulates postganglionic neurons, causing the release of epinephrine and norepinephrine
  – Activates effector organs by combining with cholinergic receptors on effector organs
  – Inactivated by cholinesterase
 • Norepinephrine
  – Helps neurons transmit impulses in the CNS
  – Released from postganglionic neurons
  – Causes sympathetic stimulation by triggering the release of epinephrine and more norepinephrine
  – Produces its effects by combining with adrenergic receptors found on effector organs
   • Adrenergic receptors are divided into alpha and beta receptors; most effector organs contain both alpha and beta receptors (see *Adrenergic receptor uses and effects*)
   • Alpha receptors include two subgroups: alpha$_1$ and alpha$_2$
    - Stimulation of alpha$_1$ receptors produces contractions (vasoconstriction) of smooth-muscle walls of blood vessels
    - Stimulation of alpha$_2$ receptors produces the opposite effect by inhibiting norepinephrine release from sympathetic nerve endings
   • Beta receptors include two subgroups: beta$_1$ and beta$_2$
    - Stimulation of beta$_1$ receptors (found mostly in the heart) causes the heart to beat faster and more forcefully

Key facts about ANS neurotransmitters

• Acetylcholine
 – Is released in response to a stressful event
 – Helps neurons transmit impulses in the CNS
 – Stimulates postganglionic neurons, causing epinephrine and norepinephrine release
 – Activates effector organs by combining with cholinergic receptors
 – Is inactivated by cholinesterase
• Norepinephrine
 – Causes sympathetic stimulation by triggering release of epinephrine and more norepinephrine
 – Combines with adrenergic receptors on effector organs

- Stimulation of beta$_2$ receptors (found mostly in smooth muscles of the bronchial walls and blood vessels) dilates bronchi and relaxes blood vessels
– Inactivated by reuptake (some norepinephrine is taken back into the synaptic vesicles in the axon terminals) or by the enzymes catechol O-methyl-transferase or monoamine oxidase

CHOLINERGICS (PARASYMPATHOMIMETICS)

CHOLINERGIC AGONISTS

● **Mechanism of action**
  - Directly stimulate cholinergic receptors, mimicking the action of acetylcholine

● **Pharmacokinetics**
  - Absorption: Varies widely
    – Usually given orally or subcutaneously (subQ)
    – Rarely administered I.M. or I.V. because drug would be subject to immediate breakdown by cholinesterases
  - Distribution: Widely distributed
  - Metabolism: Metabolized by cholinesterases in plasma and liver
  - Excretion: Excreted in urine

● **Drug examples**
  - Bethanechol (Duvoid, Myotonachol), pilocarpine (Isopto Carpine, Pilocar)

● **Indications**
  - Treat atonic bladder conditions and postoperative and postpartum urine retention
  - Treat GI disorders (such as postoperative abdominal distention and GI atony)
  - Decrease eye pressure in patients with glaucoma and during eye surgery
  - Treat salivary gland hypofunction caused by radiation therapy or Sjögren's syndrome

● **Contraindications and precautions**
  - Contraindicated in patients with prostate enlargement, possible urinary or GI obstruction, hyperthyroidism, bradycardia or atrioventricular (AV) conduction defects, asthma, and coronary artery disease
  - Used cautiously in pregnant or breast-feeding patients

● **Adverse reactions**
  - Hypotension, headache, sweating, increased salivation, abdominal cramps, nausea, vomiting, diarrhea, blurred vision, urinary frequency, decreased heart rate, and shortness of breath

● **Interactions**
  - Use with anticholinergic drugs decreases drug's effect
  - Use with anticholinesterase drugs produces additive effects and increases risk of toxicity
  - Use with quinidine decreases effect of cholinergic agonists

---

Key facts about cholinergic agonists

- Directly stimulate cholinergic receptors
- Mimic action of acetylcholine
- Metabolized by cholinesterases in plasma and liver
- Excreted in urine

When to use cholinergic agonists

- Glaucoma
- Atonic bladder
- Postoperative and postpartum urine retention
- Abdominal distention and GI atony
- Salivary gland hypofunction

When NOT to use cholinergic agonists

- Prostate enlargement
- Possible urinary or GI obstruction
- Hyperthyroidism
- Bradycardia or AV conduction defects
- Asthma
- Coronary artery disease

Adverse reactions

- Hypotension, headache, sweating, increased salivation, abdominal cramps, nausea, vomiting, diarrhea, blurred vision, urinary frequency, decreased heart rate, shortness of breath

● **Nursing responsibilities**
  – Assess the patient's urinary status
  – Assess bowel sounds and abdomen for possible paralytic ileus
  – Never give bethanechol I.V. or I.M. (only give by mouth or subQ)
  – Observe the patient for 20 to 60 minutes after subQ administration
  – Monitor the patient for signs and symptoms of drug toxicity (urinary urgency, excessive secretions, respiratory depression or spasm, bradycardia, abdominal cramping, and involuntary defecation)
  – Administer atropine as the antidote for toxicity, as prescribed

ACETYLCHOLINESTERASE INHIBITORS (PARASYMPATHOMIMETICS)

● **Mechanism of action**
  • Inhibit acetylcholinesterase, the enzyme that inactivates acetylcholine; as acetylcholine builds up, cholinergic receptors are stimulated

● **Pharmacokinetics**
  • Absorption: Absorbed readily in the GI tract, subcutaneous tissues, and mucous membranes, except for neostigmine, which is absorbed poorly if given orally
  • Distribution: Widely distributed
  • Metabolism: Metabolized in plasma
  • Excretion: Excreted in urine

● **Drug examples**
  • Ambenonium (Mytelase), edrophonium (Enlon, Reversol, Tensilon), neostigmine (Prostigmin), physostigmine (Antilirium), pyridostigmine (Mestinon, Regonol)

● **Indications**
  • Treat myasthenia gravis and glaucoma
  • Diagnose myasthenia gravis (edrophonium and neostigmine)
  • Prevent or treat postoperative paralytic ileus
  • Promote muscle contraction
  • Increase bladder tone
  • Used as an antidote to anticholinergic drugs, tricyclic antidepressants, belladonna alkaloids, and opioids

● **Contraindications and precautions**
  • Contraindicated in patients with possible urinary or GI obstruction
  • Used cautiously in patients with asthma, peptic ulcer disease, bradycardia, arrhythmias, hyperthyroidism, and seizure disorders
  • Contraindicated in patients with allergy to sulfites (edrophonium)

● **Adverse reactions**
  • Nausea, vomiting, diarrhea, dyspnea, arrhythmias, headaches, anorexia, seizures, insomnia, pruritis, urinary frequency, and nocturia

Key nursing actions

- Assess urinary status.
- Assess bowel sounds and abdomen.
- Administer by mouth or subQ; never give I.V. or I.M.
- Observe patient for 20 to 60 minutes after subQ administration.
- Monitor for toxicity; administer atropine as an antidote as prescribed.

Key facts about acetylcholinesterase inhibitors

- Inhibit acetylcholinesterase, the enzyme that inactivates acetylcholine; as acetylcholine builds up it stimulates the cholinergic receptors
- Metabolized in plasma
- Excreted in urine

When to use acetylcholinesterase inhibitors

- Myasthenia gravis
- Glaucoma
- Anticholinergic poisoning
- Paralytic ileus

When NOT to use acetylcholinesterase inhibitors

- Possible urinary or GI obstruction

Adverse reactions

- Nausea, vomiting, diarrhea, dyspnea, arrhythmias, headaches, anorexia, seizures, insomnia, pruritis, urinary frequency, and nocturia

Key nursing actions

- Assess the patient's neuromuscular status before and during drug therapy.
- Monitor for drug toxicity; administer atropine as an antidote, as prescribed.
- Monitor vital signs and breath sounds every 4 hours.
- Take seizure precautions.

Key facts about Alzheimer's treatment drugs

- Inhibit cholinesterase, leading to elevated acetylcholine levels in the cortex
- Metabolized in the liver
- Excreted in feces and urine

When to use Alzheimer's treatment drugs

- Mild to moderate Alzheimer's-type dementia
- Moderate to severe Alzheimer's-type dementia (memantine)

● **Interactions**

- Pyridostigmine administered with depolarizing muscle relaxants (such as succinylcholine) prolongs and increases neuromuscular blockade
- Use with cholinergic agonists (such as pilocarpine, bethanechol, or carbachol) increases risk of toxic effects
- Use with anticholinergics (such as atropine or scopolamine) aminoglycoside antibiotics, magnesium, corticosteroids, or antiarrhythmics decreases anticholinesterase effect and could mask signs of cholinergic crisis

● **Nursing responsibilities**

- Assess the patient's neuromuscular status (gait, muscle strength, reflexes, and heart rate) before and during drug therapy
- Assess the patient for urine retention and bladder distention
- Assess the patient's bowel sounds and abdomen for signs of paralytic ileus
- Administer with meals to minimize GI upset
- Monitor the patient for signs and symptoms of toxicity (generalized weakness, dysphagia, and respiratory weakness); administer atropine as the antidote for toxicity, as prescribed
- Monitor the patient's vital signs and auscultate for breath sounds at least once every 4 hours
- Take seizure precautions

ALZHEIMER'S TREATMENT DRUGS

● **Mechanism of action**

- Centrally act to inhibit cholinesterase, leading to elevated acetylcholine levels in the cortex, thereby slowing the neuronal degradation that occurs in Alzheimer's disease

● **Pharmacokinetics**

- Absorption: Absorbed orally
- Distribution: Widely distributed
- Metabolism: Metabolized in liver
- Excretion: Excreted in urine

● **Drug examples**

- Donepezil (Aricept, Aricept ODT), galantamine (Razadyne), memantine (Namenda), rivastigmine (Exelon)

● **Indications**

- Treat mild to moderate dementia of the Alzheimer's type
- Treat moderate to severe dementia of the Alzheimer's type (memantine)

● **Contraindications and precautions**

- Used cautiously in patients with sick sinus syndrome, GI bleeding, seizures, and asthma
- Used cautiously in patients with severe hepatic and renal impairment (galantamine)

Adverse reactions

- Insomnia, fatigue, dizziness, confusion, ataxia, depression, syncope, bradycardia, nausea, vomiting, diarrhea, anorexia, and abdominal pain
- Hepatotoxicity (donepezil)
- Hypertension (memantine)

Interactions

- Use with theophylline increases drug levels and risk of toxicity
- Use with anticholinergics decreases drug effects
- Use with nonsteroidal anti-inflammatory drugs increases risk of GI bleeding
- Increased effects and risk of galantamine toxicity if administered with cimetidine, ketoconazole, paroxetine, erythromycin, succinylcholine, or bethanechol; dosages may need to be adjusted

Nursing responsibilities

- Establish a functional baseline to evaluate drug effectiveness
- Administer with food to decrease GI upset
- If GI upset continues, instruct the patient to eat small, frequent meals
- Before surgery, notify the surgeon about the patient's use of Alzheimer's drugs because of the risk of exaggerated muscle relaxation
- Inform the patient that these drugs don't cure Alzheimer's; they merely slow degeneration associated with the disease
- Administer donepezil daily at bedtime, as ordered

ANTICHOLINERGICS (PARASYMPATHOLYTICS)

Mechanism of action

- Interrupt parasympathetic nerve impulses in the CNS and ANS and prevents acetylcholine from stimulating cholinergic receptors
- Are also referred to as *cholinergic blockers*

Pharmacokinetics

- Absorption: Absorbed in the GI tract
- Distribution: Most are widely distributed
- Metabolism: Metabolized in liver
- Excretion: Excreted in the feces and the urine

Drug examples

- Belladonna alkaloids: atropine, belladonna, hyoscyamine (Anaspaz, Levsin, Levsin/SL), scopolamine (Transderm-Scop)
- Quaternary ammoniums: glycopyrrolate (Robinul), methscopolamine (Pamine), propantheline (Pro-Banthine)
- Tertiary amines: benztropine (Cogentin), dicyclomine (Antispas, Bentyl), oxybutynin (Ditropan, Oxytrol), trihexyphenidyl (Artane)

Indications

- Reduce oral, gastric, and respiratory secretions, especially preoperatively
- Reverse heart block
- Paralyze ciliary muscles of the eye and induce mydriasis

Adverse reactions to anticholinergics

Common dose-related adverse reactions to anticholinergics are listed below. Use this illustration as a head-to-toe guide when assessing a patient.

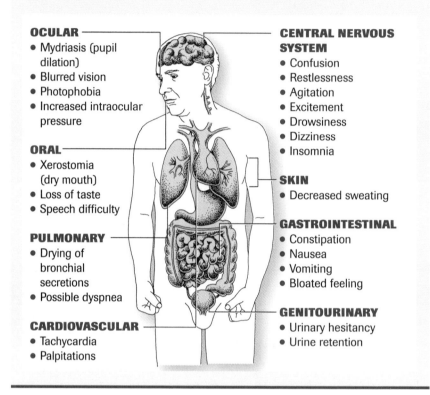

OCULAR
- Mydriasis (pupil dilation)
- Blurred vision
- Photophobia
- Increased intraocular pressure

ORAL
- Xerostomia (dry mouth)
- Loss of taste
- Speech difficulty

PULMONARY
- Drying of bronchial secretions
- Possible dyspnea

CARDIOVASCULAR
- Tachycardia
- Palpitations

CENTRAL NERVOUS SYSTEM
- Confusion
- Restlessness
- Agitation
- Excitement
- Drowsiness
- Dizziness
- Insomnia

SKIN
- Decreased sweating

GASTROINTESTINAL
- Constipation
- Nausea
- Vomiting
- Bloated feeling

GENITOURINARY
- Urinary hesitancy
- Urine retention

- Treat Parkinson's disease, GI spasms, motion sickness, and enuresis
- Treat symptomatic bradycardia (atropine drug of choice)
- Prevent bradycardia caused by vagal nerve stimulation during general anesthesia
- Treat biliary colic (belladonna alkaloids together with morphine)
- Antidote to cholinergic and anticholinergic drugs (atropine and hyoscyamine)
- Prevent nausea and vomiting resulting from motion sickness (scopolamine)

● **Contraindications and precautions**
- Contraindicated in patients with angle-closure glaucoma, uncontrolled tachycardia, urinary or GI tract obstruction, hypersensitivity, bladder neck obstruction, chronic obstructive pulmonary disease (COPD), severe ulcerative colitis, myasthenia gravis, tachycardia caused by cardiac insufficiency or thyrotoxicosis, acute or severe hemorrhage, and unstable cardiovascular status
- Contraindicated in breast-feeding women

When NOT to use anticholinergics

- Angle-closure glaucoma, uncontrolled tachycardia, urinary or GI tract obstruction, bladder neck obstruction, COPD, severe ulcerative colitis, myasthenia gravis, acute or severe hemorrhage, and unstable cardiovascular status
- Breast-feeding women

- Used cautiously in patients with fever, diarrhea, hyperthyroidism, heart failure, hypertension, or renal disease

● **Adverse reactions**
- Commonly dose-related (see *Adverse reactions to anticholinergics*)

● **Interactions**
- Use with tricyclic antidepressants, disopyramide, antidyskinetics, antiemetics, antipsychotics, cyclobenzaprine, or orphenadrine may increase anticholinergic adverse effects
- Use with cholinergic agonists or anticholinesterase drugs decreases drug effects
- Use with digoxin increases risk of digoxin toxicity
- Absorption of sublingual nitroglycerin decreased when given with anticholinergics

● **Nursing responsibilities**
- Assess the patient for relief of symptoms
- Monitor the patient for adverse reactions
- Teach the patient to reduce dry mouth by using ice chips, hard candy, or gum and to reduce constipation by exercising and increasing fiber and fluid intake
- Instruct the patient to consult the practitioner before taking nonprescription drugs to prevent adverse drug interactions
- Administer anticholinergics 30 minutes before meals and at bedtime when used to reduce GI motility
- Monitor the patient's intake and output, and watch for signs and symptoms of urine retention (urinary frequency, voiding of minimal amounts)

ADRENERGIC AGONISTS

CATECHOLAMINES (SYMPATHOMIMETICS)

● **Mechanism of action**
- Stimulate nervous system by combining with either alpha-adrenergic or beta-adrenergic receptors

● **Pharmacokinetics**
- Absorption: Rapidly absorbed if given sublingually, subQ, or I.V.
- Distribution: Widely distributed
- Metabolism: Metabolized primarily in liver
- Excretion: Excreted in urine

● **Drug examples**
- Dobutamine (Dobutrex), dopamine (Intropin), epinephrine (Adrenalin), isoproterenol (Isuprel), norepinephrine (Levophed)

● **Indications**
- Treat bradycardia, heart blocks, and decreased cardiac output
- Treat bronchodilation in acute and chronic bronchial asthma
- Treat acute drug-induced allergic reaction

Adverse reactions
- Commonly dose-related

Key nursing actions
- Administer before meals.
- Monitor for adverse reactions.
- Teach the patient to consult the practitioner before taking nonprescription drugs.
- Advise the patient on how to reduce dry mouth and constipation.
- Monitor intake and output.

Key facts about catecholamines
- Stimulate nervous system by combining with either alpha-adrenergic or beta-adrenergic receptors
- Metabolized primarily in the liver
- Excreted in urine

When to use catecholamines
- Bradycardia, heart blocks, and decreased cardiac output
- Acute hypotension and shock
- Acute drug-induced allergic reaction

When NOT to use catecholamines

- Acute MI or tachyarrhythmias
- During pregnancy
- With caution in patients with diabetes, atherosclerosis, Raynaud's disease, and cardiac insufficiency

Adverse reactions

- Arrhythmias, tachycardia, angina
- Restlessness, anxiety, dizziness
- Headache, hypertension, stroke
- Increased blood glucose levels

Key nursing actions

- Monitor ECG, hemodynamic parameters, vital signs and urine output.
- Correct hypovolemia.
- Administer through a large vein to prevent extravasation. Always administer with an infusion pump.
- Monitor for a sudden drop in blood pressure after stopping the drug.

Key facts about noncatecholamines

- Stimulate sympathetic nervous system by directing stimulating alpha or beta$_2$ receptors or indirectly affecting adrenergic receptors
- Metabolized in the liver
- Excreted in urine

- Treat mild renal failure caused by decreased cardiac output (dopamine, which dilates renal arteries in low doses)
- Stimulate the heart in cardiac arrest
- Increase blood pressure through vasoconstriction in acute hypotension and shock
- Increase myocardial force and cardiac output in patients with acute heart failure and those undergoing cardiopulmonary bypass

● **Contraindications and precautions**
- Contraindicated in patients with acute myocardial infarction (MI) or tachyarrhythmias and during pregnancy
- Used cautiously in patients with diabetes, atherosclerosis, Raynaud's disease, and cardiac insufficiency

● **Adverse reactions**
- Arrhythmias, tachycardia, angina, restlessness, anxiety, dizziness, headache, hypertension, stroke, and increased blood glucose levels

● **Interactions**
- Use with alpha-adrenergic blockers may cause hypotension
- Diabetic patients receiving epinephrine may need an increased dose of insulin or oral antidiabetic medication
- Use with other adrenergic drugs may cause additive effects (such as hypertension and arrhythmias)
- Use with tricyclic antidepressants may cause hypertension

● **Nursing responsibilities**
- Monitor electrocardiogram, hemodynamic parameters, vital signs, and urine output while the patient is receiving the drug
- Correct hypovolemia before infusing dopamine or norepinephrine to ensure the drug's effectiveness
- Administer drugs through a large vein to prevent extravasation
  - If extravasation occurs during infusion of dopamine or norepinephrine, infiltrate the skin with phentolamine (Regitine) and normal saline solution, as ordered
  - Always administer catecholamines with an infusion pump
- Base patient evaluation on improved vital signs, urine output, and hemodynamics or on relief of bronchospasms without serious adverse effects
- After stopping the drug, monitor the patient for a sudden drop in blood pressure

NONCATECHOLAMINES

● **Mechanism of action**
- Stimulate sympathetic nervous system by directing stimulating alpha or beta$_2$ receptors or indirectly affecting adrenergic receptors

● **Pharmacokinetics**
- Absorption: Varies by drug
- Distribution: Varies by drug

- Metabolism: Metabolized in liver
- Excretion: Excreted in urine

● **Drug examples**
- Albuterol (Proventil, Ventolin), ephedrine, isoetharine, mephentermine, metaproterenol (Alupent), phenylephrine (Neo-Synephrine), terbutaline (Brethine)

● **Indications**
- Treat hypotension and severe shock
- Stop preterm labor (terbutaline)
- Treat bronchodilation (albuterol and metaproterenol)
- Treat nasal congestion (ephedrine and phenylephrine)

● **Contraindications and precautions**
- Contraindicated in patients with tachyarrhythmias, hypertension, coronary artery disease, history of stroke, angle-closure glaucoma, and thyrotoxicosis
- Used cautiously in elderly patients and those with diabetes, hyperthyroidism, angina, prostatic hypertrophy, or a history of seizures
- Mephentermine contraindicated in patients taking monoamine oxidase (MAO) inhibitors

● **Adverse reactions**
- Headache, restlessness, anxiety, irritability, trembling, drowsiness, seizures, hypertension, palpitations, tachycardia, irregular heart rhythm, angina, and tingling or coldness in the arms or legs

● **Interactions**
- General anesthetics, cyclopropane, and halogenated hydrocarbons may cause arrhythmias in patients receiving noncatecholamines
- MAO inhibitors may cause severe hypertension and death when taken with noncatecholamines
- Use with tricyclic antidepressants may cause hypertension and arrhythmias

● **Nursing responsibilities**
- If giving the drug via inhalation, administer the bronchodilator inhaler first, then wait 2 minutes and administer the corticosteroid inhaler
- Monitor the patient's respiratory status before, during, and after treatment
- Administer terbutaline I.M. in the lateral deltoid area

ADRENERGIC BLOCKERS (SYMPATHOLYTICS)

ALPHA-ADRENERGIC BLOCKERS

● **Mechanism of action**
- Interrupt the action of epinephrine and norepinephrine at alpha receptors

---

When to use noncatecholamines

- Hypotension and severe shock
- Preterm labor
- Bronchodilation treatment
- Nasal congestion

When NOT to use noncatecholamines

- Tachyarrhythmias, hypertension, coronary artery disease, history of stroke, angle-closure glaucoma, and thyrotoxicosis
- With caution in elderly patients and those with diabetes, hyperthyroidism, angina, or a history of seizures

Key nursing actions

- If given via inhalation, administer the bronchodilator inhaler, wait 2 minutes and administer the corticosteroid inhaler.
- Monitor respiratory status.

Key facts about alpha-adrenergic blockers

- Interrupt the action of epinephrine and norepinephrine at the alpha-receptors
- Metabolized by the liver
- Excreted in feces

When to use alpha-adrenergic blockers

- Peripheral vascular disorders
- Raynaud's disease
- Vascular headaches
- Adrenergic excess

When NOT to use alpha-adrenergic blockers

- MI
- Coronary insufficiency
- Evidence of coronary artery disease
- Pregnancy

Adverse reactions

- Orthostatic hypotension, tachycardia, dizziness, arrhythmias, ergotism (characterized by numbness, tingling of fingers and toes, weakness, and blindness)

Key nursing actions

- Monitor blood pressure for signs of orthostatic hypotension, as appropriate.
- Instruct patient to change positions slowly to minimize orthostatic hypotension.
- Administer drug with milk or food.
- If patient experiences a shock-like state, place in the Trendelenburg position, notify practitioner, and begin emergency resuscitation, as appropriate.

● **Pharmacokinetics**
- Absorption: Absorption erratic when administered orally; more rapid and complete when administered sublingually
- Distribution: Unknown
- Metabolism: Metabolized by liver
- Excretion: Excreted in feces

● **Drug examples**
- Doxazosin (Cardura), ergotamine (Cafergot, Ergomar), phenoxybenzamine (Dibenzyline), phentolamine (Regitine), prazosin (Minipress), terazosin (Hytrin)

● **Indications**
- Treat peripheral vascular disorders, Raynaud's disease, hypertension, and adrenergic excess (for example, pheochromocytoma)
- Treat vascular headache (ergotamine)

● **Contraindications and precautions**
- Used cautiously in patients who have had an MI, coronary insufficiency, or other evidence of coronary artery disease; pregnant patients; and those with impaired liver or renal function
- Contraindicated in patients with peripheral vascular disease, hypertension, and coronary artery disease (ergotamine)

● **Adverse reactions**
- Orthostatic hypotension, tachycardia, dizziness, arrhythmias, severe hypertension, edema, shortness of breath, flushing, and angina
- Ergotism (chronic poisoning from excessive ergot use), characterized by numbness, tingling of fingers and toes, weakness, and blindness (ergotamine)

● **Interactions**
- Use of antihypertensives with terazosin potentiates hypotensive effects
- Use of adrenergic agonists with other adrenergics causes additive effects
- Use of adrenergic blockers with other sympatholytics increases effects
- Use of prazosin with diuretics, propranolol, or beta-adrenergic blockers increases frequency of syncopal episodes
- Doxazosin and terazosin decrease effectiveness of clonidine
- Use of ergotamine and caffeine suppository with potent CYP3A4 inhibitors (such as macrolides and protease inhibitors) can cause ergot toxicity (vasospasms, ischemic extremities, and cerebral ischemia)

● **Nursing responsibilities**
- During administration, monitor blood pressure for signs of orthostatic hypotension; instruct the patient to change positions slowly to minimize orthostatic hypotension
- If a phentolamine test (for pheochromocytoma) is scheduled, withhold all antihypertensives, as ordered, and explain the test to the patient
- Instruct the patient with vascular headache to take ergotamine at onset of headache and then lie down in a dark, quiet room

- Monitor the patient receiving ergotamine for signs and symptoms of vascular insufficiency caused by ergotism (numbness, tingling, or weakness in extremities)
- Administer with milk or food to minimize gastric irritation; administer at bedtime to minimize dizziness and light-headedness
- If the patient experiences a shocklike state, place him in the Trendelenburg position, notify the practitioner, and begin emergency resuscitation, as appropriate

BETA-ADRENERGIC BLOCKERS

● Mechanism of action
- Prevent stimulation of the sympathetic nervous system by inhibiting the action of catecholamines at the beta-adrenergic receptors
- Selective beta-adrenergic blockers block $beta_1$ receptors (found predominantly in the heart)
- Nonselective beta-adrenergic blockers block $beta_1$ and $beta_2$ receptors (found mainly in the lungs)

● Pharmacokinetics
- Absorption: Absorbed rapidly and well from the GI tract
- Distribution: Widely distributed
- Metabolism: Metabolized in liver
- Excretion: Excreted in feces and urine

● Drug examples
- Selective: acebutolol (Sectral), atenolol (Tenormin), betaxolol (Betoptic, Kerlone), carteolol (Cartrol), esmolol (Brevibloc), metoprolol (Lopressor, Toprol)
- Nonselective: carvedilol (Coreg), labetalol (Normodyne, Trandate), levobunolol (Betagan), nadolol (Corgard), penbutolol (Levatol), pindolol (Visken), propranolol (Inderal), sotalol (Betapace), timolol (Blocadren)

● Indications
- Treat hypertension, angina, tachyarrhythmias, open-angle glaucoma, pheochromocytoma, and hypertrophic cardiomyopathy (beta-adrenergic blockers)
- Treat mild to severe heart failure and left ventricular dysfunction after MI (carvedilol)
- Prevent migraine headaches, MI, and acute anxiety reactions

● Contraindications and precautions
- Contraindicated in patients with bradyarrhythmias, heart block, COPD, and asthma
- Used cautiously in patients with diabetes, hepatic or renal impairment, and those receiving general anesthesia

● Adverse reactions
- Bradycardia, bronchospasm, nausea, vomiting, diarrhea, decreased blood pressure, peripheral vascular insufficiency, atrioventricular heart block, heart failure, abdominal discomfort, and rash

Key facts about beta-adrenergic blockers

- Prevent stimulation of sympathetic nervous system
- Usually metabolized in the liver
- Excreted in feces and urine

When to use beta-adrenergic blockers

- Hypertension
- Angina
- Tachyarrhythmias
- Migraines
- MI
- Glaucoma
- Acute anxiety reaction
- Mild to severe heart failure
- Left ventricular dysfunction after MI

When NOT to use beta-adrenergic blockers

- Bradyarrhythmias
- COPD
- Heart block
- Asthma

Adverse reactions

- Bradycardia, bronchospasm, nausea, vomiting, diarrhea, hypotension

Topics for patient discussion

- Medication regimen, including proper administration
- Methods to assess pulse and blood pressure
- Signs and symptoms of adverse reactions
- Avoidance of over-the-counter drugs
- Importance of carrying identification about disease and drug regimen
- Follow-up care

Key nursing actions

- Assess pulse rate; withhold drug and notify practitioner if rate is below 50 beats/minute (or according to hospital policy).
- Advise patient receiving long-term therapy not to discontinue the drug suddenly because of the risk of MI or arrhythmia.

 TIME-OUT FOR TEACHING

Teaching about beta-adrenergic blockers

Be sure to include these topics in your teaching plan for the patient receiving a beta-adrenergic blocker:
- medication prescribed, including name, dose, frequency, action, and adverse effects
- proper technique for administration
- methods to assess pulse and blood pressure
- signs and symptoms of adverse reactions
- avoidance of over-the-counter products
- follow-up care.

Interactions
- Increased effect and risk of toxicity if taken with digoxin, calcium channel blockers, or cimetidine
- Decreased effect if taken with antacids, calcium salts, barbiturates, anti-inflammatories, or rifampin
- May alter the requirement for insulin and oral antidiabetic agents
- Nonselective beta-adrenergic blockers may decrease the ability of theophylline to produce bronchodilation
- Nonselective beta-adrenergic blockers used with sympathomimetics may cause hypertension and reflex bradycardia

Nursing responsibilities
- Assess the patient's pulse rate; withhold the drug and notify the practitioner if the rate is less than 50 beats/minute (or according to facility policy)
- After administering eyedrops, apply pressure to the inner canthus of the eye for 1 minute to minimize systemic absorption
- Teach the patient to monitor pulse and blood pressure for adverse changes (see *Teaching about beta-adrenergic blockers*)
- If appropriate, encourage the patient to comply with other recommended antihypertensive interventions (such as weight reduction, smoking cessation, dietary sodium restriction, moderation of alcohol consumption, regular exercise, and stress management)
- Instruct the patient to carry identification describing the disease and drug regimen
- Advise the patient receiving long-term therapy not to discontinue the drug suddenly because doing so may precipitate an MI or arrhythmias
- Observe the patient with diabetes for sweating, hunger, and fatigue; signs of hypoglycemic shock may be masked
- Administer drug with meals to increase absorption

NEUROMUSCULAR BLOCKERS

NONDEPOLARIZING DRUGS

● **Mechanism of action**
- Compete with acetylcholine at the cholinergic receptor sites of the skeletal muscle membrane, thereby blocking acetylcholine transmitter action and preventing muscle membranes from depolarizing
- Are also referred to as *competitive* or *stabilizing* drugs

● **Pharmacokinetics**
- Absorption: Given parenterally because of poor absorption after oral administration; I.V. is the preferred route of administration
- Distribution: Distributed rapidly throughout the body
- Metabolism: Partially metabolized in liver
- Excretion: Most drugs excreted unchanged in urine

● **Drug examples**
- Cisatracurium (Nimbex), pancuronium, vecuronium (Norcuron)

● **Indications**
- Reduce intensity of muscle spasms in drug-induced or electrically induced seizures
- Provide skeletal muscle relaxation during surgery
- Manage patients who are fighting the use of a ventilator to help with breathing

● **Contraindications and precautions**
- Contraindicated in patients hypersensitive to the drug and in neonates because these drugs contain benzyl alcohol
- Used cautiously in pregnant and breast-feeding patients

● **Adverse reactions**
- Apnea, hypotension, skin reactions, bronchospasms, excessive bronchial or salivary excretions
- Pancuronium may cause tachycardia, arrhythmias, and hypertension

● **Interactions**
- Aminoglycoside antibiotics and anesthetics potentiate or exaggerate neuromuscular blockers
- Drugs that alter the serum levels of potassium, magnesium, or calcium may also alter the effects of nondepolarizing drugs
- Use with clindamycin, polymyxin, verapamil, quinine, ketamine, lithium, nitrates, thiazide diuretics, tetracycline, or magnesium salts may increase the intensity and duration of paralysis
- Carbamazepine, hydantoin, ranitidine, and theophylline may decrease the effects of nondepolarizing drugs
- Use with corticosteroids may cause prolonged muscle weakness
- Anticholinesterases (neostigmine, pyridostigmine, and edrophonium) are antagonistic and used as antidotes to nondepolarizing blockers

Key facts about nondepolarizing drugs

- Compete with acetylcholine at cholinergic receptor sites of skeletal muscle membrane, thereby blocking acetylcholine transmitter action and preventing muscle membranes from depolarizing
- Partially metabolized in the liver
- Excreted in urine

When to use nondepolarizing drugs

- Prolonged or intermediate muscle relaxation for surgery or ET intubation

When NOT to use nondepolarizing drugs

- Hypersensitivity
- Neonates
- Pregnancy
- Breast-feeding

Adverse effects

- Apnea, hypotension, skin reactions, bronchospasms, excessive bronchial or salivary excretions

Key nursing actions

- Monitor for adverse reactions.
- Have oxygen and ET and suction equipment available.
- Monitor respirations frequently until the patient is fully recovered.
- Suction the patient as needed.
- Frequently check the mechanical ventilator settings and functions to ensure proper functioning.
- Always administer with sedation or general anesthesia.

Key facts about depolarizing drugs

- Cause persistent depolarization followed by muscle fasciculations and paralysis or flaccidity
- Metabolized in the liver and plasma
- Excreted in urine

When to use depolarizing drugs

- Skeletal muscle relaxation for surgery or mechanical ventilation

● Nursing responsibilities

- Monitor the patient for adverse reactions, especially apnea or bronchospasm, during drug therapy
- Have oxygen and endotracheal (ET) and suction equipment available at all times in case respiratory support is needed
- Monitor respirations frequently until the patient is fully recovered from the neuromuscular blockade, as evidenced by increased muscle strength (peripheral nerve stimulation, hand grip, head lift, and ability to cough)
- Keep drugs refrigerated to maintain their potency
- Suction the patient as needed because the drug will suppress the cough reflex and increase respiratory secretions
- Frequently check the mechanical ventilator's settings and function to ensure it's working properly; never turn off the ventilator alarm
- Monitor serum electrolyte levels while the patient is receiving the drug
- Assess skin for pressure areas and breakdown, and provide skin care per facility policy
- Neuromuscular blockers don't decrease consciousness or alter the pain threshold; always administer sedation or general anesthesia concurrently
- Have atropine, edrophonium, or neostigmine readily available as an antidote

DEPOLARIZING DRUGS

● Mechanism of action

- Mimic the action of acetylcholine but aren't inactivated by cholinesterase, causing persistent depolarization and muscle fasciculation, paralysis, and flaccidity

● Pharmacokinetics

- Absorption: I.V. administration is preferred; absorbed poorly in the GI tract
- Distribution: Unknown
- Metabolism: Metabolized in the liver and plasma by pseudocholinesterase
- Excretion: Excreted in urine

● Drug examples

- Succinylcholine (Anectine, Quelicin)

● Indications

- Short-term muscle relaxation
- Induce skeletal muscle relaxation during surgery or mechanical ventilation

● Contraindications and precautions

- Contraindicated in patients with a known hypersensitivity to the drug or its components, a genetic disorder of plasma pseudocholinesterase, personal or family history of malignant hyperthermia, myopathies associated

with elevated creatine phosphokinase levels, acute angle-closure glaucoma, or penetrating eye injuries
- Used cautiously in pregnant or breast-feeding patients, children, and those with cardiovascular, hepatic, pulmonary, metabolic, or renal disorders

● Adverse reactions
- Prolonged apnea and cardiovascular effects, hypotension, and possible muscle pain and increased intraocular pressure

● Interactions
- Anticholinesterases increase succinylcholine blockade
- Many antibiotics and anesthetics increase action of succinylcholine

● Nursing responsibilities
- Maintain airway patency at all times
- Check the patient's respiratory rate and pattern every 5 minutes during drug infusion
- Monitor the patient closely until recovery from neuromuscular blockade is complete; signs of recovery include renewed ability to cough and return of previous levels of muscle strength on hand-grip and head-lift tests
- Have oxygen and suction equipment available at all times in case respiratory support is needed
- Keep the drug refrigerated to maintain potency
- Assess skin for pressure areas and breakdown, and provide skin care per facility policy
- Neuromuscular blockers don't decrease consciousness or alter the pain threshold; always administer sedation or general anesthesia concurrently
- Don't use a reversing agent because it may worsen the effect of the neuromuscular block

NCLEX CHECKS

It's never too soon to begin your NCLEX® examination preparation. Now that you've reviewed this chapter, carefully read each of the following questions and choose the best answer. Then compare your responses with the correct answers.

1. A client with Parkinson's disease asks the nurse why he's taking trihexyphenidyl. The nurse should respond by explaining that the drug:
- ☐ **1.** helps clients relax so they can sleep.
- ☐ **2.** counteracts the adverse reactions of levodopa.
- ☐ **3.** prevents clients from developing depression.
- ☐ **4.** controls the symptoms of drooling and muscle rigidity.

When NOT to use depolarizing drugs

- Hypersensitivity
- Genetic disorder of plasma pseudocholinesterase
- History of malignant hyperthermia
- Myopathies associated with elevated creatine phosphokinase levels
- Acute angle-closure glaucoma
- Penetrating eye injuries

Adverse effects

- Prolonged apnea and cardiovascular effects, hypotension, muscle pain, increased intraocular pressure

Key nursing actions

- Maintain airway patency.
- Monitor closely; check respiratory rate and pattern every 5 minutes.
- Keep oxygen and suction equipment available.
- Always administer with sedation or general anesthesia.

TOP 4

Items to study for your next test on drugs and the autonomic nervous system

1. Mechanisms of action of cholinergics and adrenergics
2. Indications for various autonomic nervous system drugs
3. Nursing responsibilities related to each class of cholinergic and adrenergic
4. Indications and mechanisms of action for neuromuscular blockades

2. A client is scheduled for a cholecystectomy. The physician orders preoperative sedation with meperidine (Demerol), 75 mg I.M., and the cholinergic blocker atropine, 0.4 mg I.M. Which statement describes the purpose of atropine as a preanesthetic agent?

☐ **1.** Atropine reduces hyperreflexia during surgery.
☐ **2.** Atropine minimizes the risk of postoperative ileus.
☐ **3.** Atropine prevents respiratory depression during surgery.
☐ **4.** Atropine reduces excess salivation and gastric secretions.

3. A client with an ET tube receiving mechanical ventilation becomes more conscious and begins to fight both the ET tube and the ventilator. Pancuronium, 0.1 mg/kg of body weight, is ordered. This drug exerts its therapeutic effect by:

☐ **1.** stimulating muscarinic receptors at effector organs.
☐ **2.** inhibiting the action of cholinesterase at the motor end plate.
☐ **3.** enhancing the muscle's ability to respond to the neurotransmitter acetylcholine.
☐ **4.** competing with acetylcholine at cholinergic receptor sites in the skeletal muscle.

4. A client with a history of asthma occasionally has bronchospasm attacks. The nurse reviews the client's drug history, questioning the use of which drug?

☐ **1.** Ergotamine (Ergomar)
☐ **2.** Metoprolol (Lopressor)
☐ **3.** Phenoxybenzamine (Dibenzyline)
☐ **4.** Phentolamine (Regitine)

5. Essential hypertension, Raynaud's disease, and pheochromocytoma respond effectively to which class of drugs?

☐ **1.** Alpha-adrenergic blockers
☐ **2.** Beta-adrenergic blockers
☐ **3.** CNS stimulants
☐ **4.** Cholinergic blockers

6. A client taking an anticholinergic for 1 month arrives at an outpatient clinic with complaints of constipation, dry mouth, and decreased sweating. The nurse realizes that these complaints are:

☐ **1.** rare.
☐ **2.** normal.
☐ **3.** dose-related adverse reactions.
☐ **4.** symptoms of an anaphylactic reaction.

7. A nurse is caring for a client with a T5 complete spinal cord injury. On assessment, the nurse notes flushed skin, diaphoresis above T5, and a blood pressure of 162/96 mm Hg. The client reports a severe, pounding headache. Which nursing intervention would be appropriate for this client? Select all that apply.

- ☐ **1.** Elevate the head of the bed 90 degrees.
- ☐ **2.** Loosen constrictive clothing.
- ☐ **3.** Use a fan to reduce diaphoresis.
- ☐ **4.** Assess for bladder distention and bowel impaction.
- ☐ **5.** Administer antihypertensive medication.
- ☐ **6.** Place the client in the supine position with legs elevated.

8. The wife of a client taking donepezil (Aricept) asks the nurse when her husband's Alzheimer's disease will be cured. The nurse's best response is:

- ☐ **1.** "This medication takes about 6 weeks to cure Alzheimer's."
- ☐ **2.** "Your husband will be cured in 2 weeks."
- ☐ **3.** "This medication slows the degeneration of the disease. It doesn't cure it."
- ☐ **4.** "This medication alone doesn't cure Alzheimer's; you have to take two other medications to cure the disease."

9. A nurse is caring for a client taking ergotamine (Ergomar) for vascular headaches. Which complaint by the client requires immediate further investigation?

- ☐ **1.** "My fingers and toes are tingling."
- ☐ **2.** "I'm having hot flashes every day."
- ☐ **3.** "I feel my heart racing every now and then."
- ☐ **4.** "My ankles are puffy after I sit up for a couple of hours."

10. A nurse is caring for a client on a mechanical ventilator who complains of pain. The physician orders succinylcholine (Anectine). What should the nurse do next?

- ☐ **1.** Administer the drug as ordered.
- ☐ **2.** Withhold the drug, call the physician, and ask for pain medication or sedation.
- ☐ **3.** Position the client for an I.M. injection.
- ☐ **4.** Insert a nasogastric tube to administer the medication.

ANSWERS AND RATIONALES

1. CORRECT ANSWER: 4

Anticholinergics antagonize functions controlled by the parasympathetic nervous system. Trihexyphenidyl, an anticholinergic, is used to control the symptoms of drooling and muscle rigidity associated with Parkinson's disease. It isn't used to help with sleep, adverse reactions of levodopa, or depression.

2. CORRECT ANSWER: 4

The ultimate goal of giving atropine is to prevent the client from aspirating. Atropine will reduce the amount of excess salivation and gastric secretions preoperatively by preventing stimulation of the receptors that cause these effects. This effect aims to prevent nausea, vomiting, and possible aspiration intraoperatively and postoperatively. Atropine isn't used to reduce hyperreflexia, minimize postoperative ileus, or prevent respiratory depression during surgery.

3. CORRECT ANSWER: 4

Pancuronium is a neuromuscular blocking agent. It disrupts nerve impulse transmission at the motor end plate by competing with acetylcholine at receptor sites. This drug doesn't stimulate muscarinic receptors at effector organs, inhibit cholinesterase, or enhance muscle response to acetylcholine.

4. CORRECT ANSWER: 2

Metoprolol is a beta-adrenergic blocker. The most common respiratory adverse reaction is bronchospasm. Beta-adrenergic blockers must be used cautiously in clients with bronchial asthma, bronchitis, or emphysema. Ergotamine, phenoxybenzamine, and phentolamine are alpha-adrenergic blockers, which cause smooth-muscle relaxation and vasodilation, not bronchospasm.

5. CORRECT ANSWER: 1

Alpha-adrenergic blockers increase blood flow by relaxing smooth muscles and causing vasodilation. This mechanism makes them useful in treating essential hypertension, Raynaud's disease, and pheochromocytoma. Beta-adrenergic blockers, cholinergic blockers, and CNS stimulants don't produce this action.

6. CORRECT ANSWER: 3

Constipation, dry mouth, and decreased sweating are dose-related adverse reactions to anticholinergics. These effects usually decrease as treatment continues. These symptoms aren't normal or rare, and some physicians will try to reduce the dose to decrease them. Anticholinergics don't cause anaphylactic reactions, but client sensitivity reactions (including urticaria and allergic rashes that may lead to exfoliation) may occur.

7. CORRECT ANSWER: 1, 2, 4, 5

The client is exhibiting signs and symptoms of autonomic dysreflexia. The condition is a potentially life-threatening emergency caused by an uninhibited response from the sympathetic nervous system resulting from a lack of control over the autonomic nervous system. The nurse should immediately elevate the head of the bed to 90 degrees and place the client's extremities in a dependent position to decrease venous return to the heart and increase venous return from the brain. Because tactile stimuli can trigger autonomic dysreflexia, any constrictive clothing should be loosened. The nurse should also assess for bladder distension and bowel impaction—which may trigger autonomic dysreflexia—and correct any problems. Elevated blood pressure is the most life-threatening complication of autonomic dysreflexia because it can cause stroke, myocardial infarction, or seizure activity. If removing the triggering event doesn't reduce the client's blood pressure, I.V. antihypertensives should be administered. A fan shouldn't be used because cold drafts may trigger autonomic dysreflexia.

8. CORRECT ANSWER: 3
Telling the client's wife that the medication slows the degeneration of the disease is appropriate because currently Alzheimer's disease has no cure. Although the client may take the other medications in addition to donepezil, the combination of drugs won't cure the disease.

9. CORRECT ANSWER: 1
Tingling fingers and toes is a sign of ergotism, or chronic poisoning from ergot use. Other signs of ergotism include numbness, weakness, and blindness. Flushing, tachycardia, and edema are common adverse reactions; although they should be investigated, they aren't immediate priorities.

10. CORRECT ANSWER: 2
Succinylcholine is a depolarizing drug that causes paralysis and flaccidity but doesn't alter level of consciousness or the pain threshold. The nurse shouldn't administer the medication; she should call the physician and obtain an order for pain medication or sedation. Depolarizing drugs are never administered I.M. or by mouth; they're administered I.V.

3

Drugs and the central nervous system

PRETEST

1. A common adverse effect of central nervous system (CNS) stimulants such as dextroamphetamine (Adderall) is:

☐ 1. weight loss.
☐ 2. blurred vision.
☐ 3. nausea.
☐ 4. diarrhea.

CORRECT ANSWER: 1

2. What's an important teaching topic for a client taking phenytoin (Dilantin)?

☐ 1. Restrict fluid intake.
☐ 2. Take the medication at night.
☐ 3. Use good oral hygiene.
☐ 4. Take the medication on an empty stomach.

CORRECT ANSWER: 3

3. Dopaminergic agonists work by:

☐ 1. suppressing acetylcholine activity.
☐ 2. increasing the amount of dopamine available in the CNS.
☐ 3. raising the seizure threshold.
☐ 4. blocking acetylcholine breakdown at the neuromuscular junction.

CORRECT ANSWER: 2

4. When administering I.V. phenobarbital, a nurse should have:

☐ 1. emergency resuscitation equipment readily available.

☐ 2. an indwelling urinary catheter or straight catheter on hand.

☐ 3. the practitioner at the client's bedside.

☐ 4. a signed consent form for the drug.

CORRECT ANSWER: 1

5. A client should take antimyasthenics according to schedule because:

☐ 1. doing so helps the client remember to take them on time.

☐ 2. he must make an appointment at the clinic to obtain the medication.

☐ 3. it's necessary to take these drugs 2 hours before eating.

☐ 4. taking them on time helps prevent weakness.

CORRECT ANSWER: 4

LEARNING OBJECTIVES

After studying this chapter, you should be able to:

- Explain the general mechanism of action of central nervous system (CNS) stimulants, anticonvulsants, antiparkinsonians, antimigraine drugs, and antimyasthenics.

- Name the most common adverse effects of the various CNS stimulants, anticonvulsants, antiparkinsonians, antimigraine drugs, and antimyasthenics.

- Identify nursing responsibilities for administering CNS stimulants, anticonvulsants, antiparkinsonians, antimigraine drugs, and antimyasthenics.

- Discuss appropriate teaching for the patient who's receiving a CNS stimulant, anticonvulsant, antiparkinsonian, antimigraine drug, or antimyasthenic.

CHAPTER OVERVIEW

Central nervous system (CNS) drugs include CNS stimulants, anticonvulsants, antiparkinsonians, antimigraine drugs, and antimyasthenics. CNS stimulants increase neurotransmitter levels in the CNS, causing CNS and respiratory stimulation, pupil dilation, increased motor activity, heightened mental alertness, brighter spirits, and a diminished sense of fatigue.

Anticonvulsants reduce or eliminate seizures. The current trend in anticonvulsant therapy is maintenance with one drug (monotherapy) to avoid drug interactions.

Antiparkinsonians treat Parkinson's disease, an imbalance of neurotransmitters, particularly excess acetylcholine and insufficient dopamine, in the CNS. Drug therapy reduces cholinergic activity and enhances dopamine activity. Antiparkinsonians include dopaminergic agonists, anticholinergics, and catechol-O-methyltransferase (COMT) inhibitors.

Antimigraine drugs, also known as *5-hydroxytryptamine (HT) agonists,* treat acute to moderate severe migraines and cluster headaches. Antimyasthenics (cholinergics) are used to treat myasthenia gravis, an autoimmune disease caused by a deficiency of acetylcholine that causes muscle weakness exacerbated by physical or emotional stress or infection.

Nursing responsibilities for all these drugs focus on monitoring the drug's therapeutic effectiveness, as evidenced by improvement in the condition and avoidance of overdosage, and patient education about all aspects of the drug therapy, complications, and possible adverse effects.

ANATOMY AND PHYSIOLOGY

Anatomy of the CNS
- Spinal cord
  - Carries messages from the body to the brain
  - Protected by vertebrae and cerebrospinal fluid
- Brain
  - Receives message, analyzes and interprets it, and sends a response message through the spinal cord to the rest of the body
  - Protected by skull and membranous meninges
- Neurons—the basic functional unit of the CNS

Function of the CNS
- Relays messages
- Processes, compares, and analyzes information
- Uses neurons to conduct impulses across a synapse to and from muscles, glands, and organs and the CNS

CNS neurotransmitters
- Help neurons transmit impulses in the CNS
- Include acetylcholine, norepinephrine, serotonin, dopamine, and gamma-aminobutyric acid (GABA)
- Inactivated by reuptake or enzymatic action

A&P highlights

- The CNS consists of the spinal cord and the brain.
- The spinal cord carries messages from the body to the brain.
- The brain analyzes and interprets messages and sends response messages, through the spinal cord, to the rest of the body.
- Neurons are the basic functional unit of the nervous system.
- Neurons conduct impulses across a synapse to and from muscles, glands, and organs and the CNS.

Five CNS neurotransmitters

1. Acetylcholine
2. Norepinephrine
3. Serotonin
4. Dopamine
5. GABA

- CNS neurotransmitter types
  - Acetylcholine—inactivated by the enzyme cholinesterase
  - Norepinephrine—inactivated by reuptake (when some of it is taken back into the synaptic vesicles in the axon terminals) or by the enzymes COMT or monoamine oxidase (MAO)
  - Serotonin—inactivated by reuptake and by enzymatic (MAO) breakdown
  - Dopamine—inactivated by reuptake or by COMT or MAO
  - GABA—inactivated by enzymatic breakdown

CNS STIMULANTS

● **Mechanism of action**
- Increase neurotransmitter levels in the CNS, either by increasing neuronal discharge or by blocking an inhibitory neurotransmitter

● **Pharmacokinetics**
- Absorption: Absorbed in GI tract after oral administration
- Distribution: Widely distributed
- Metabolism: Metabolized by liver
- Excretion: Excreted in urine

● **Drug examples**
- Amphetamine-dextroamphetamine (Adderall), dexmethylphenidate (Focalin), dextroamphetamine (Dexedrine), doxapram (Dopram), methylphenidate (Concerta, Metadate, Ritalin), modafinil (Provigil), pemoline (PemADD)

● **Indications**
- Increase mental alertness and respiratory rate
- Treat attention deficit hyperactivity disorder (ADHD)
- Treat narcolepsy (dextroamphetamine, methylphenidate, modafinil, and pemoline)
- Treat respiratory stimulation after anesthesia (doxapram)

● **Contraindications and precautions**
- Contraindicated in patients with glaucoma and severe cardiovascular (CV) disease
- Used with caution in patients with psychosis and in pregnant and breast-feeding patients

● **Adverse reactions**
- Acute adverse effects (toxicity), including restlessness, tremor, irritability, insomnia, hypotension, arrhythmias, angina, and CV collapse
- Chronic adverse effects, including marked weight loss, fatigue, irritability, depression, and growth suppression (in children)

● **Interactions**
- Use with similar-acting drugs causes additive sympathomimetic effects
- Altered urine pH may alter drug effectiveness
  - Urine acidification enhances renal excretion of the drug

Key facts about CNS stimulants

- Increase neurotransmitter levels in the CNS
- Metabolized by the liver
- Excreted in urine

When to use CNS stimulants

- ADHD
- Narcolepsy
- Respiratory stimulation after anesthesia

When NOT to use CNS stimulants

- Glaucoma
- Severe CV disease

Adverse reactions

- Restlessness, tremor, irritability, insomnia, hypotension, arrhythmias, angina, CV collapse, weight loss, fatigue, depression, growth suppression

Key nursing actions

- Assess patient behavior to determine drug effectiveness.
- Monitor growth in a child receiving long-term therapy.
- Instruct patient to take last daily dose 6 hours before bedtime to prevent insomnia.
- Instruct patient to avoid caffeine.

Key facts about anticonvulsants

- Inhibit seizure activity
- Metabolized in the liver
- Excreted in urine

When to use anticonvulsants

- Tonic-clonic seizures
- Status epilepticus
- Complex partial seizures
- Arrhythmias
- Painful conditions, such as trigeminal neuralgia

– Urine alkalinization enhances renal absorption of the drug
- Risk of increased pressor effects when given with MAO inhibitors

● **Nursing responsibilities**

- Assess the patient's behavior to determine drug effectiveness
- Monitor growth in a child receiving long-term therapy
- When administering doxapram, assess the patient's respiratory status (including breath sounds and rate and depth of respirations) and arterial blood gas (ABG) measurements for changes
- Keep in mind that most CNS stimulants are controlled substances and that amphetamines may cause dependence and abuse
- Instruct the patient to take the last daily dose at least 6 hours before bedtime to prevent insomnia
- Instruct the patient to avoid beverages containing caffeine to prevent added stimulation
- Base patient evaluation on the reason for using the drug
    – For patient with narcolepsy: increased activity and alertness, diminished fatigue, and brighter spirits
    – For patient with ADHD: increased calmness, decreased hyperactivity, and prolonged attention span (effects usually appear in 3 to 4 weeks)
    – For patient receiving doxapram to treat respiratory depression after anesthesia: improved respiratory status and ABG measurements

ANTICONVULSANTS

HYDANTOINS

● **Mechanism of action**

- Inhibit seizure activity by promoting sodium outflow from the neurons, thereby depressing abnormal neuronal stimulation and discharge

● **Pharmacokinetics**

- Absorption: Varies by drug
- Distribution: Protein-bound
- Metabolism: Metabolized in liver
- Excretion: Excreted in urine

● **Drug examples**

- Ethotoin (Peganone), fosphenytoin (Cerebyx), phenytoin (Dilantin, Phenytek)

● **Indications**

- Treat tonic-clonic (grand mal) seizures and complex partial seizures
- Treat arrhythmias and such painful conditions as trigeminal neuralgia (phenytoin)
- Short-term control of general convulsive status epilepticus (fosphenytoin given I.V.)

Contraindications and precautions

- Contraindicated in patients hypersensitive to drug or its components; pregnant or breast-feeding patients; and those with sinus bradycardia, sinoatrial block, second- or third-degree heart block, Adams-Stokes syndrome, hematologic disorders, or hepatic abnormalities
- Used cautiously in patients with acute intermittent porphyria, severe myocardial insufficiency, and diabetes

Adverse reactions

- Gingival hyperplasia, rare blood dyscrasias, diplopia, nystagmus, ataxia, drowsiness, headache, dizziness, vertigo, anorexia, depressed atrial and ventricular conduction, irritability, and restlessness
- May cause ventricular fibrillation in toxic states
- I.V. administration may cause bradycardia, hypotension, and cardiac arrest

Interactions

- Amiodarone, allopurinol, chloramphenicol, cimetidine, disulfiram, isoniazid, oral anticoagulants, sulfamethizole, and valproate may increase phenytoin activity, leading to phenytoin toxicity
- Oral tube feedings may interfere with absorption of oral phenytoin, diminishing the drug's effectiveness; feedings should be scheduled at least 1 hour before or 2 hours after phenytoin dose
- Phenytoin incompatible with dextrose and any dextrose-containing solutions
- Phenobarbital, diazoxide, theophylline, carbamazepine, rifampin, antacids, and sucralfate may decrease the drug's effectiveness
- Hydantoins decrease the effects of oral anticoagulants, carbamazepine, levodopa, amiodarone, corticosteroids, doxycycline, methadone, metyrapone, valproic acid, cyclosporine, quinidine, theophylline, thyroid hormones, and hormonal contraceptives

Nursing responsibilities

- Monitor the patient for signs and symptoms of toxicity (ataxia, nystagmus, and dysarthria), hypotension, coma, or unresponsive pupils; treatment for toxicity is nonspecific
- Monitor therapeutic hydantoin, complete blood count, and liver enzyme levels to avoid or detect toxicity
- When administering phenytoin I.V., dilute in normal saline solution (dextrose solutions cause a precipitate); infuse no faster than 50 mg/ minute
- Monitor vital signs, blood pressure, and electrocardiogram (ECG) during I.V. administration
- Teach the patient about the importance of good oral hygiene and regular dental examinations to prevent gingival hyperplasia
- If GI upset occurs, give drug with food
- Instruct the patient to consult the practitioner or pharmacist before changing drug brands because bioavailability may differ among brands (see *Teaching about oral hydantoin anticonvulsant therapy*, page 50)

When NOT to use anticonvulsants

- Hypersensitivity
- Sinus bradycardia
- Sinoatrial block
- Second- and third-degree heart block
- Adam-Stokes syndrome

Adverse reactions

- Gingival hyperplasia, rare blood dyscrasias, diplopia, nystagmus, ataxia, drowsiness
- Ventricular fibrillation in toxic states

Key nursing actions

- Monitor for signs and symptoms of toxicity.
- Monitor therapeutic hydantoin, complete blood count, and liver enzyme levels.
- If GI upset occurs, administer drug with food.
- Monitor vital signs, blood pressure, and ECG during I.V. administration.

Signs of anticonvulsant toxicity

- Ataxia
- Nystagmus
- Dysarthria

Topics for patient discussion

- Medication regimen
- Signs and symptoms to discuss with the practitioner
- Oral hygiene measures to minimize gingival hyperplasia
- Urine discoloration
- Activity allowances and restriction
- Avoidance of alcohol and over-the-counter drug use
- Compliance with therapy
- Follow-up care
- Care during and after a seizure
- Community resources for support and information

Key facts about barbiturates

- Depress sensory cortex and motor activity and alter cerebellar function, causing drowsiness, sedation, and hypnosis
- May induce anesthesia
- Metabolized by the liver
- Excreted in urine

When to use barbiturates

- Tonic-clonic seizures
- Partial seizures
- Acute convulsive episodes

When NOT to use barbiturates

- Hypersensitivity
- Pregnancy
- Breast-feeding
- Hepatic impairment
- Severe respiratory disease
- Previous addiction to sedative or hypnotic

 TIME-OUT FOR TEACHING

Teaching about oral hydantoin anticonvulsant therapy

Be sure to include these topics in your teaching plan for the patient receiving an oral hydantoin anticonvulsant:

- medication prescribed, including name, dose, frequency, action, and possible adverse effects
- signs and symptoms to discuss with practitioner, including adverse effects
- oral hygiene measures to minimize gingival hyperplasia
- possible (though harmless) urine discoloration
- activity allowances and restrictions, such as avoiding driving and other hazardous activities until drug's effect is known
- avoidance of alcohol and self-medication with over-the-counter products
- compliance with therapy, including adherence to regimen, avoidance of abrupt discontinuation, and consistent use of same drug preparation
- importance of follow-up care, including laboratory tests and primary care visits
- care during and after a seizure
- community resources for support and information.

BARBITURATES

Mechanism of action
- Depress the sensory cortex and motor activity and alter cerebellar function, causing drowsiness, sedation, and hypnosis; in high doses, may induce anesthesia

Pharmacokinetics
- Absorption: Absorbed slowly in GI tract
- Distribution: Protein-bound and well distributed in body tissues
- Metabolism: Metabolized by liver
- Excretion: Excreted in urine

Drug examples
- Mephobarbital (Mebaral), pentobarbital (Nembutal), phenobarbital (Luminal), primidone (Mysoline)

Indications
- Treat tonic-clonic seizures, partial seizures, and febrile seizures
- Adjunct to anesthesia; may be used as an emergency control for acute convulsive episodes
- Treatment of choice for chronic epilepsy (primidone)

Contraindications and precautions
- Contraindicated in patients who are sensitive to barbiturates; pregnant or breast-feeding patients; patients with hepatic impairment, severe respiratory distress or disease, or porphyria; and those who have had a previous addiction to a sedative or hypnotic

- Used cautiously in patients with acute or chronic pain, fever, hyperthyroidism, diabetes, and anemia

● **Adverse reactions**
- Dizziness, drowsiness, lethargy, nystagmus, confusion, ataxia, lupus-like syndrome
- Acute psychosis, hair loss, impotence, and osteomalacia (primidone)
- Laryngospasm, respiratory depression, and hypotension (I.V. administration)

● **Interactions**
- Increased risk of toxicity with CNS depressants, valproic acid, chloramphenicol, felbamate, cimetidine, and phenytoin
- Increased metabolism and decreased effects of corticosteroids, cimetidine, and phenytoin if taken with phenobarbital
- Barbiturates reduce the effectiveness of hormonal contraceptives, beta-adrenergic blockers, corticosteroids, digoxin, estrogens, doxycycline, oral anticoagulants, quinidine, phenothiazines, metronidazole, tricyclic antidepressants, theophylline, cyclosporine, carbamazepine, felodipine, and verapamil

● **Nursing responsibilities**
- Assess the patient's respiratory status before and during drug therapy
- Discourage alcohol use during drug therapy
- Monitor blood levels closely to maintain therapeutic drug levels
- Administer with food to minimize GI upset
- Administer I.V. phenobarbital in emergency situations only, and have emergency resuscitation equipment available
- Know that barbiturates may be habit forming; tolerance and psychological and physical dependence may occur, especially following prolonged use at high doses
- Monitor the patient for withdrawal symptoms
  - Minor symptoms (anxiety, muscle twitching, hand and finger tremors, weakness, dizziness, and nausea and vomiting) may appear 8 to 12 hours after last dose
  - Severe symptoms (seizures and delirium) may occur within 16 hours of last dose after abrupt cessation of drug; may last up to 5 days
  - Notify practitioner immediately if the patient develops fever, sore throat, mouth sores, bruising, bleeding, or tiny broken blood vessels under the skin during drug therapy

BENZODIAZEPINES

● **Mechanism of action**
- Depress the CNS at the limbic and subcortical levels, suppressing seizure activity; action is poorly understood

● **Pharmacokinetics**
- Absorption: Absorbed rapidly and completely in GI tract

When to use benzodiazepines

- Absence seizures
- Lennox-Gastaut syndrome
- Akinetic and myoclonic seizures
- Long-term treatment of epilepsy (clonazepam only)
- Partial seizures
- Acute alcohol withdrawal
- Acute status epilepticus
- Anxiety
- Skeletal muscle spasms

When NOT to use benzodiazepines

- Hypersensitivity
- Acute angle-closure glaucoma
- Acute alcohol intoxication

Adverse reactions

- Ataxia, drug dependence, drowsiness, dizziness, tremors, confusion

Key nursing actions

- Caution patient not to stop drug abruptly (could produce status epilepticus or worsen disorder).
- Administer I.V. diazepam no faster than 5 mg/minute in adults and over at least 3 minutes in children.
- Don't mix I.V. diazepam with other drugs in same syringe.

- Distribution: Highly protein-bound
- Metabolism: Metabolized by liver
- Excretion: Excreted in urine

● Drug examples
- Clonazepam (Klonopin), clorazepate (Tranxene), diazepam (Valium), lorazepam (Ativan)

● Indications
- Treat absence seizures, Lennox-Gastaut syndrome (petit mal variant), and akinetic and myoclonic seizures (clonazepam)
- Long-term treatment of epilepsy (clonazepam only)
- Adjunctive treatment of partial seizures and treatment of acute alcohol withdrawal (clorazepate)
- Treat acute status epilepticus, anxiety, and skeletal muscle spasms (diazepam)
- Treat acute status epilepticus (I.V. lorazepam is drug of choice)

● Contraindications and precautions
- Contraindicated in patients with hypersensitivity, acute angle-closure glaucoma, psychoses, and acute alcohol intoxication
- Used cautiously in patients with impaired liver or kidney function

● Adverse reactions
- Ataxia, drug dependence, drowsiness, dizziness, tremors, confusion, weakness, nystagmus, vertigo, fainting, and headache
- I.V. diazepam may cause respiratory depression with decreased heart rate

● Interactions
- Increased CNS depression if given with CNS depressants, alcohol, hormonal contraceptives, or cimetidine
- Increased digoxin levels and digoxin toxicity if given concurrently
- If given with phenobarbital, increased effects of both drugs

● Nursing responsibilities
- Caution the patient not to stop the drug abruptly; doing so could produce status epilepticus or worsen the seizure disorder
- Be aware that psychological dependence may develop with use of clonazepam or diazepam
- When administering I.V. diazepam:
  - Administer no faster than 5 mg/minute in adults; over at least 3 minutes in children
  - Avoid giving in small veins
  - Don't mix with other drugs in same syringe
  - Give by direct I.V. push only; don't give as an infusion
  - Keep emergency equipment and oxygen at the bedside

SUCCINIMIDES

- **Mechanism of action**
  - Raise seizure threshold by depressing neural transmission in the motor cortex and basal ganglia

- **Pharmacokinetics**
  - Absorption: Readily absorbed in GI tract
  - Distribution: Widely distributed
  - Metabolism: Metabolized by liver
  - Excretion: Excreted in urine

- **Drug examples**
  - Ethosuximide (Zarontin), methsuximide (Celontin)

- **Indications**
  - To control absence seizures

- **Contraindications and precautions**
  - Contraindicated in patients who are hypersensitive to drug or its components
  - Used cautiously in patients with hepatic or renal impairment or blood dyscrasias

- **Adverse reactions**
  - Anorexia, nausea, vomiting, drowsiness, fatigue, hiccups, and headache
  - Rarely, blood dyscrasias, rashes, and psychotic behavior

- **Interactions**
  - Carbamazepine increases the metabolism of succinimides
  - Valproic acid may increase or decrease succinimide levels
  - Use with phenytoin may elevate serum phenytoin levels

- **Nursing responsibilities**
  - Don't withdraw the drug abruptly because it may precipitate absence seizures
  - If GI upset occurs, give the drug with food or milk
  - Monitor the patient for adverse reactions
  - Notify the practitioner if the patient develops rashes, joint pain, unexplained fever, sore throat, unusual bleeding or bruising, drowsiness, dizziness, or blurred vision; these may be symptoms of overdose
  - Notify the practitioner if the patient becomes pregnant
  - Instruct the patient to avoid alcohol during therapy

SULFONAMIDES

- **Mechanism of action**
  - Unknown, but raises the threshold for generalized seizures (in rats) and increases dopaminergic and serotonergic neurotransmission
  - Also blocks sodium channels, stabilizes neuronal membranes, and suppresses neuronal hypersynchronization

Key facts about succinimides

- Raise seizure threshold by depressing neural transmission in the motor cortex and basal ganglia
- Metabolized in the liver
- Excreted in urine

When to use succinimides

- Absence seizures

When NOT to use succinimides

- Hypersensitivity

Adverse reactions

- Anorexia, nausea, vomiting

Key nursing actions

- Don't withdraw the drug abruptly.
- If GI upset occurs, give drug with food or milk.
- Monitor for adverse reactions.
- Notify practitioner if rashes, joint pain, unexplained fever, sore throat, unusual bleeding or bruising, drowsiness, dizziness, or blurred vision develops.
- Tell patient to avoid alcohol during therapy.

Key facts about sulfonamides

- Action unknown; raise the threshold for generalized seizures in rats
- Increase dopaminergic and serotonergic neurotransmission
- Block sodium channels
- Stabilize neuronal membranes
- Suppress neuronal hypersynchronization

When to use sulfonamides

- Partial seizures related to epilepsy

When NOT to use sulfonamides

- Hypersensitivity

Adverse reactions

- Somnolence, ataxia, dizziness, headache, anorexia, Stevens-Johnson syndrome, toxic epidermal necrolysis

Key nursing actions

- Monitor for adverse reactions.
- If rash or seizures worsen, contact practitioner immediately.
- Also notify the practitioner if the patient develops fever, easy bruising, sore throat, or oral ulcers.

Key facts about other anticonvulsants

- Action largely unknown; may reduce polysynaptic responses and block posttetanic potentiation by blocking voltage-sensitive sodium channels
- Metabolized in the liver
- Excreted in urine

● **Pharmacokinetics**
- Absorption: Orally absorbed
- Distribution: Extensively binds to erythrocytes, so plasma levels are higher in red blood cells than in plasma
- Metabolism: Metabolized in liver
- Excretion: Excreted in urine

● **Drug examples**
- Zonisamide (Zonegran)

● **Indications**
- Adjunctive therapy in treatment of partial seizures in adults with epilepsy

● **Contraindications and precautions**
- Contraindicated in patients who are hypersensitive to drug or its components
- Used cautiously in patients with impaired hepatic, renal, or cardiac function

● **Adverse reactions**
- Somnolence, ataxia, dizziness, headache, anorexia, nausea, diarrhea, rash, confusion, Stevens-Johnson syndrome, toxic epidermal necrolysis, and psychosis

● **Interactions**
- Drugs that induce liver enzymes (CYP-450) increase the metabolism and clearance of zonisamide and decrease its half-life

● **Nursing responsibilities**
- Monitor the patient for adverse reactions; if rash occurs or seizures worsen, contact the practitioner immediately
- Monitor serum drug levels
- Don't suddenly discontinue the drug; taper gradually
- Risk of renal calculi is increased with zonisamide, so encourage the patient to drink plenty of fluids to reduce risk of calculus formation; notify the practitioner if the patient complains of sudden back pain, abdominal pain, or hematuria
- Notify the practitioner if the patient develops a fever, easy bruising, sore throat, or oral ulcers

MISCELLANEOUS ANTICONVULSANTS

● **Mechanism of action**
- Largely unknown; thought to reduce polysynaptic responses and block posttetanic potentiation by blocking the voltage-sensitive sodium channels

● **Pharmacokinetics**
- Absorption: Rate varies with each drug
- Distribution: Varies with each drug
- Metabolism: Metabolized in liver
- Excretion: Excreted in urine

Drug examples

- Carbamazepine (Tegretol), divalproex (Depakote), felbamate (Felbatol), gabapentin (Neurontin), lamotrigine (Lamictal), levetiracetam (Keppra), oxcarbazepine (Trileptal), pregabalin (Lyrica), tiagabine (Gabitril), topiramate (Topamax), valproic acid (Depakene)

Indications

- Treat tonic-clonic seizures, simple and complex partial seizures, trigeminal neuralgia, and neurogenic pain (carbamazepine, lamotrigine, and topiramate)
- Treat simple and absence seizures (divalproex and valproic acid)
- Adjunctive therapy in the treatment of partial seizures with or without secondary generalization (felbamate, gabapentin, levetiracetam, oxcarbazepine, and tiagabine)
- Treat postherpetic neuralgia (gabapentin and pregabalin)

Contraindications and precautions

- Contraindicated in patients hypersensitive to drug or its components, in pregnant or breast-feeding patients, and in those with bone marrow suppression
- Contraindicated within 14 days of MAO inhibitor therapy

Adverse reactions

- Sedation, photophobia, drowsiness, ataxia, headache, nausea, vomiting, and diarrhea
- Serious rashes, including Stevens-Johnson syndrome (lamotrigine)
- Hepatic failure and pancreatitis (valproic acid)
- Leukopenia, weight gain, and diplopia (gabapentin)
- Psychomotor slowing, impaired concentration, memory impairment, liver failure, and hypohidrosis (topiramate)

Interactions

- Lithium and carbamazepine given concurrently increase the risk of toxic neurogenic effects
- Valproic acid decreases the effectiveness of lamotrigine, phenobarbital, primidone, benzodiazepines, CNS depressants, warfarin, and zidovudine
- Cimetidine, danazol, diltiazem, erythromycin, isoniazid, selective serotonin reuptake inhibitors, propoxyphene, ketoconazole, valproic acid, and verapamil increase the metabolism of carbamazepine and increase the risk of toxicity
- Use with aspirin, erythromycin, or felbamate increases drug effectiveness
- Additive effect when lamotrigine is given with folate inhibitors
- Decreased effectiveness when lamotrigine is given with carbamazepine, phenytoin, phenobarbital, primidone, or acetaminophen
- Decreased effectiveness when topiramate is given with carbamazepine, phenytoin, or valproic acid
- Topiramate decreases effectiveness of hormonal contraceptives and valproic acid

● **Nursing responsibilities**
- Assess seizure characteristics, including location and duration
- Implement seizure precautions as indicated
- Watch for signs and symptoms of anticonvulsant toxicity, including CNS depression, ataxia, nausea and vomiting, drowsiness, dizziness, vision disturbances, and restlessness
- Monitor serum drug levels
- Consider giving anticonvulsants with food to decrease GI irritation
- Instruct the patient not to discontinue the drug without consulting the practitioner because this may precipitate tonic-clonic seizures
- Warn the patient not to consume alcohol during anticonvulsant therapy to prevent potentiation of CNS depressant effects
- Urge the patient to use caution when driving or performing other activities requiring alertness until response to drug is known (typically, the practitioner gives permission to drive based on adequacy of seizure control)
- Instruct the patient to carry identification describing the disorder and drug regimen
- Encourage the patient on long-term anticonvulsant therapy to comply with periodic blood studies (these determine serum drug levels and detect serious hematologic toxicity)
- Notify the practitioner if the patient develops fever, sore throat, oral ulcers, easy bruising or bleeding, or fatigue because these may indicate aplastic anemia, which may be fatal

ANTIPARKINSONIANS

DOPAMINERGIC AGONISTS

● **Mechanism of action**
- Restore the natural balance of the neurotransmitters acetylcholine and dopamine in the CNS or enhance the amount and neurotransmission of dopamine in the CNS, thereby decreasing the signs and symptoms of Parkinson's disease
- Levodopa and levodopa-carbidopa: Restore dopamine levels (levodopa is converted to dopamine by enzymes in the brain); carbidopa is used with levodopa because it makes more levodopa available for transport to the brain, thereby allowing a lower levodopa dosage and reduced adverse effects
- Amantadine: Increases amount of dopamine in the brain by increasing dopamine's release from intact neurons
- Bromocriptine, pramipexole, and ropinirole: Activate dopamine receptor sites, producing effects similar to those of dopamine
- Selegiline: Possibly inhibits MAO activity, thereby increasing dopaminergic activity

● **Pharmacokinetics**
  - Absorption: Rapidly absorbed
  - Distribution: Extensively distributed throughout body
  - Metabolism: Metabolized in brain, periphery, and liver
  - Excretion: Primarily excreted in urine

● **Drug examples**
  - Amantadine (Symmetrel), bromocriptine (Parlodel), levodopa (Dopar), levodopa-carbidopa (Sinemet), pergolide (Permax), pramipexole (Mirapex), ropinirole (Requip), selegiline (Eldepryl)

● **Indications**
  - Treat Parkinson's disease and drug-induced extrapyramidal reactions (amantadine, bromocriptine, levodopa, levodopa-carbidopa, ropinirole, and pramipexole)
  - Treat Parkinson's disease (concurrent use of pergolide, selegiline, or bromocriptine with levodopa-carbidopa)
  - Antiviral to prevent and treat influenza A (amantadine)
  - Treat hyperprolactinemia and acromegaly (bromocriptine)
  - Treat restless leg syndrome (ropinirole)

● **Contraindications and precautions**
  - Contraindicated in breast-feeding patients and patients with psychoses or severe ischemic heart disease
  - Used cautiously in patients with residual arrhythmias after myocardial infarction (MI); patients with a history of peptic ulcer disease or seizure disorders; pregnant patients; and those experiencing hallucinations, confusion, or dyskinesia
  - Contraindicated in patients with glaucoma or a history of melanoma; used cautiously in those with severe cardiovascular, pulmonary, renal, hepatic, or endocrine disease (levodopa)

● **Adverse reactions**
  - Vary by drug
  - Dizziness, insomnia, orthostatic hypotension, and constipation (amantadine)
  - Persistent orthostatic hypotension, ventricular tachycardia, angina, nausea, and vomiting (bromocriptine)
  - Nausea, vomiting, orthostatic hypotension, anorexia, neuroleptic malignant syndrome, arrhythmias, irritability, and confusion (levodopa and levodopa-carbidopa)
  - Nausea (selegiline)
  - Peripheral edema, confusion, dyskinesia, hallucinations, nausea, and vomiting (pergolide)
  - Orthostatic hypotension, dizziness, confusion, and insomnia (pramipexole and ropinirole)

● **Interactions**
  - Use with MAO inhibitors increases risk of hypertensive crisis

When to use dopaminergic agonists

- Parkinson's disease
- Influenza A (amantadine)
- Hyperprolactinemia

When NOT to use dopaminergic agonists

- Glaucoma
- Breast-feeding
- Ischemic heart disease
- Psychoses

Adverse reactions

- Dizziness, confusion, mood changes, involuntary body movements, orthostatic hypotension, nausea, vomiting, dry mouth, altered tastes, tremors, insomnia, agitation, hallucinations

Topics for patient discussion

- Medication regimen
- Signs and symptoms to discuss with practitioner
- Time required for drug to reach maximum effectiveness
- Safety measures
- Avoidance of alcohol and over-the-counter drug use
- Follow-up care

TIME-OUT FOR TEACHING

Teaching about dopaminergic agonists

Be sure to include these topics in your teaching plan for the patient receiving a dopaminergic agonist:

- medication prescribed, including name, dose, frequency, duration, and possible adverse effects
- signs and symptoms to discuss with practitioner, including adverse effects
- time required for drug to reach maximum effectiveness
- safety measures, including possible need for assistive devices
- avoidance of alcohol and self-medication with over-the-counter products
- compliance with therapy, including adherence to regimen and prescribed dosage; avoidance of discontinuation of therapy if longterm
- importance of follow-up care.

- Use of levodopa with pyridoxine (vitamin B_6), phenytoin, benzodiazepines, reserpine, or papaverine may increase peripheral metabolism of levodopa, decreasing the amount of drug available to the brain
- Antipsychotics may decrease effectiveness of levodopa and pergolide
- Amantadine potentiates the anticholinergic adverse effects of anticholinergic drugs and decreases absorption of levodopa
- Meperidine administered with high-dose selegiline may cause a fatal reaction
- Erythromycin increases bromocriptine serum levels, increasing its pharmacologic effects and toxicity
- Pramipexole levels increase when drug is administered with other drugs that are eliminated via the kidneys
- Ropinirole administered with alcohol increases CNS depression

● **Nursing responsibilities**

- Assess for signs and symptoms of parkinsonism (rigidity, tremors, akinesia, and bradykinesia)
- Base patient evaluation on improvement in signs and symptoms of parkinsonism without severe adverse effects
- Monitor the patient for adverse effects
- Administer drug with food to decrease GI upset
- Don't suddenly stop medication; taper dose slowly to prevent serious adverse reactions
- When administering levodopa, instruct the patient to avoid excessive vitamin B_6 intake to prevent adverse drug interactions (see *Teaching about dopaminergic agonists*)
- When administering levodopa, bromocriptine, or pergolide, instruct the patient to change position slowly to minimize orthostatic hypotension

Key nursing actions

- Assess for signs and symptoms of parkinsonism.
- Base patient evaluation on improvement in signs and symptoms of parkinsonism without severe adverse effects.
- Taper medication slowly to prevent serious adverse reactions.

ANTICHOLINERGICS (CHOLINERGIC BLOCKERS)

- **Mechanism of action**
  - Block acetylcholine receptors in the CNS and autonomic nervous system, thereby suppressing acetylcholine activity

- **Pharmacokinetics**
  - Absorption: Well absorbed from GI tract
  - Distribution: Unknown
  - Metabolism: Metabolized in liver
  - Excretion: Excreted in urine

- **Drug examples**
  - Benztropine (Cogentin), biperiden (Akineton), trihexyphenidyl (Trihexy-2, Trihexy-5)

- **Indications**
  - Treat Parkinson's disease, postencephalitic parkinsonism, acute dystonic reactions, and drug-induced extrapyramidal reactions

- **Contraindications and precautions**
  - Contraindicated in patients with angle-closure glaucoma, stenosing peptic ulcers, achalasia, prostatic hypertrophy, bladder neck obstructions, and myasthenia gravis
  - Used cautiously in patients with tachycardia, arrhythmias, hypertension, and hepatic or renal dysfunction

- **Adverse reactions**
  - Blurred vision, dry mouth, constipation, urine retention, confusion, restlessness, increased intraocular pressure, tachycardia, palpitations, nausea, and vomiting

- **Interactions**
  - Use of drug with alcohol increases CNS depression
  - Use with antipsychotics decreases antipsychotic effectiveness and increases anticholinergic adverse effects
  - Use with amantadine increases anticholinergic adverse effects
  - Anticholinergics decrease absorption of levodopa

- **Nursing responsibilities**
  - Assess the patient's bowel and urinary function for evidence of adverse effects
  - Monitor for development of adverse effects
  - Monitor vital signs during initiation of therapy and with dosage changes
  - Instruct the patient to consult the practitioner or pharmacist before taking any nonprescription drugs to prevent adverse drug interactions
  - Teach the patient to minimize dry mouth by increasing fluid intake and by using ice chips, hard candy, or gum
  - Instruct the patient to take the drug with food if GI upset occurs
  - Teach the patient to reduce constipation by increasing fluid and fiber intake

Key facts about cholinergic blockers

- Block acetylcholine receptors in the CNS and ANS, thereby suppressing acetylcholine activity

When to use cholinergic blockers

- Parkinson's disease
- Postencephalitic parkinsonism
- Acute dystonic reactions
- Drug-induced extrapyramidal reactions

When NOT to use cholinergic blockers

- Angle-closure glaucoma
- Myasthenia gravis
- Stenosing peptic ulcers
- Achalasia
- Prostatic hypertrophy
- Bladder neck obstructions

Adverse reactions

- Blurred vision, constipation, dry mouth, urine retention

Key nursing actions

- Assess bowel and urinary function for evidence of adverse effects.
- Instruct patient to consult practitioner or pharmacist before taking nonprescription drugs.
- If GI upset occurs, administer drug with food.

Key facts about COMT inhibitors

- Inhibit transmission of COMT leading to sustained dopaminergic stimulation of the brain
- Metabolized by the liver
- Excreted in urine

When to use COMT inhibitors

- Parkinson's disease; adjunctive treatment with levodopa and carbiodopa

When NOT to use COMT inhibitors

- Liver disease

Adverse reactions

- Disorientation, hallucinations, dizziness, nausea, muscular weakness, diarrhea

Key nursing actions

- Administer with levodopa-carbiodopa; COMT inhibitors aren't single-therapy agents.
- Monitor for hallucinations and orthostatic hypotension.
- Discontinue drug slowly.

- Advise patients (especially elderly, chronically ill, alcoholic, or those with CNS diseases) to use the drug cautiously in hot weather; may cause severe anhidrosis and fatal hyperthermia

COMT INHIBITORS

● **Mechanism of action**
- Inhibit transmission of COMT—the major metabolizing enzyme for levodopa in the presence of a decarboxylase inhibitor such as carbidopa—leading to sustained plasma levels of levodopa, thus sustained dopaminergic stimulation of the brain

● **Pharmacokinetics**
- Absorption: Rapidly absorbed from GI tract
- Distribution: Highly bound to albumin with limited distribution to tissues
- Metabolism: Metabolized in liver
- Excretion: Excreted in urine

● **Drug examples**
- Entacapone (Comtan), tolcapone (Tasmar)

● **Indications**
- Adjunctive treatment with levodopa and carbidopa for signs and symptoms of Parkinson's disease

● **Contraindications and precautions**
- Used cautiously in breast-feeding patients and those with hypertension, hypotension, and hepatic or renal dysfunction (entacapone)
- Contraindicated in patients with liver disease (tolcapone)

● **Adverse reactions**
- Disorientation, confusion, hallucinations, light-headedness, dizziness, drowsiness, nausea, vomiting, muscular weakness, and diarrhea
- Tolcapone has been shown to cause liver failure
- Entacapone can cause dyskinesias and hyperkinesias, brown-orange urine discoloration, and hypotension

● **Interactions**
- Use with MAO inhibitors can cause increased toxicity and serum levels
- Probenecid, cholestyramine, erythromycin, rifampin, ampicillin, and chloramphenicol can cause decreased excretion of entacapone
- Use with norepinephrine, dopamine, dobutamine, methyldopa, isoetharine, bitolterol, isoproterenol, or epinephrine can cause increased heart rate, arrhythmias, and excessive blood pressure changes
- Concurrent use of CNS depressants may cause additive CNS effects
- Iron absorption may be decreased when taken with entacapone
- Use with dopaminergic drugs may increase orthostatic effects

● **Nursing responsibilities**
- Administer drug only if the patient is taking levodopa-carbidopa; this isn't a single-therapy agent

- Administer the drug at the same time as the levodopa-carbidopa dose
- If the patient is taking tolcapone, monitor liver function tests
- Monitor the patient for hallucinations
- Discontinue the drug slowly because abrupt withdrawal may lead to hyperpyrexia and confusion
- Monitor the patient for orthostatic hypotension
- Observe the patient for urine discoloration
- Administer without regard to food

ANTIMIGRAINE DRUGS (5-HT AGONISTS)

● **Mechanism of action**
- Cause 5-HT to bind to serotonin receptors, causing cranial vessel constriction, thereby inhibiting and reducing the inflammatory process along the trigeminal nerve pathway

● **Pharmacokinetics**
- Absorption: Varies by drug
- Distribution: Widely distributed
- Metabolism: Metabolized by liver
- Excretion: Varies by drug

● **Drug examples**
- Almotriptan (Axert), eletriptan (Relpax), frovatriptan (Frova), naratriptan (Amerge), rizatriptan (Maxalt, Maxalt-MLT), sumatriptan (Imitrex), zolmitriptan (Zomig, Zomig-ZMT)

● **Indications**
- Treat acute moderate to severe migraines with or without aura
- Treat cluster headaches (sumatriptan injection)

● **Contraindications and precautions**
- Contraindicated in patients with any type of triptan allergy; in patients with coronary artery disease, ischemic heart disease, any significant underlying cardiovascular condition, or uncontrolled hypertension; in patients with basilar or hemiplegic migraines or a history of strokes, temporary ischemic attacks, or any type of peripheral vascular disease
- Avoid use in pregnant patients because of risk of serious birth defects

● **Adverse reactions**
- Dizziness, vertigo, weakness, myalgia, blood pressure alterations, chest pressure or tightness, tingling sensations, feeling hot or flushed, numbness, nausea, palpitations, and injection site discomfort (with sumatriptan)
- Rarely, MI, cerebrovascular events, and ventricular arrhythmias (frovatriptan)

● **Interactions**
- Concurrent use with MAO inhibitors, ergot-containing drugs, and other triptans may cause prolonged vasoactive reactions; the patient should be off MAO inhibitors for 2 weeks before taking triptans

Key facts about antimigraine drugs

- Cause 5-HT to bind to serotonin receptors, reducing inflammatory process along the trigeminal nerve pathway
- Metabolized by the liver
- Excretion varies by drug

When to use antimigraine drugs

- Moderate to severe migraines
- Cluster headaches

When NOT to use antimigraine drugs

- Triptan allergy; coronary artery disease, ischemic heart disease, uncontrolled hypertension; basilar or hemiplegic migraines; history of stroke, temporary ischemic attacks, peripheral vascular disease; pregnancy

Adverse reactions

- Dizziness, vertigo, blood pressure alterations, chest tightness, weakness, tingling, nausea, palpitations

- Bioavailability increases with concurrent use of hormonal contraceptives
- Increased risk of severe reaction if used with St. John's wort
- Almotriptan has increased effects and possible toxicity when taken with antifungals, macrolide antibiotics, or antivirals

Nursing responsibilities

- Administer the drug as soon as migraine or aura begins; drug shouldn't be used as a prophylactic measure
- Provide appropriate concurrent pain relief measures if needed
- Monitor injection sites for redness or irritation
- Provide additional therapeutic treatments (dim lights, cool cloth, and quiet environment) as needed
- Teach the patient to use an auto-injector for certain triptans
- Don't administer more than two doses within 24 hours
- Instruct the patient to contact the practitioner immediately if severe, persistent chest pain or pressure occurs
- Instruct the patient about possible adverse effects and to avoid driving or using heavy machinery while taking these drugs
- Administer naratriptan with food to help prevent GI upset
- Administer sumatriptan with fluids

ANTIMYASTHENICS (CHOLINERGICS)

Mechanism of action

- Relieve muscle weakness associated with myasthenia gravis by blocking acetylcholine breakdown at the neuromuscular junction

Pharmacokinetics

- Absorption: Usually poorly absorbed in GI tract; duration of action varies in patients with myasthenia gravis, depending on physical and emotional stress suffered and severity of disease
- Distribution: 15% to 25% protein-bound; may cross placental barrier in large doses
- Metabolism: Either undergo hydrolysis by cholinesterases or are metabolized by liver
- Excretion: Excreted in urine

Drug examples

- Ambenonium (Mytelase), edrophonium (Tensilon), neostigmine (Prostigmin), pyridostigmine (Mestinon)

Indications

- Treat or diagnose myasthenia gravis
- Control myasthenic symptoms (neostigmine, ambenonium, and pyridostigmine)
- Diagnose myasthenia gravis and distinguish cholinergic crisis from myasthenic crisis (edrophonium)

● Contraindications and precautions
- Contraindicated in patients with hypersensitivity to the drug
- Edrophonium, neostigmine, and pyridostigmine contraindicated in patients with bromide allergy

● Adverse reactions
- Abdominal pain, nausea, vomiting, diarrhea, sweating, miosis, increased salivation, increased bronchial secretions, and difficulty breathing resulting from cholinergic overstimulation

● Interactions
- Use with similar-acting drugs causes additive cholinergic effects
- Use with guanethidine and other ganglionic blockers may increase myasthenic symptoms and hypertension

● Nursing responsibilities
- Assess the patient's neuromuscular status, including reflexes, muscle strength, and gait
- Have emergency resuscitation equipment (suction equipment, oxygen, and mechanical ventilator) on hand if edrophonium is used
- Monitor the patient for signs and symptoms of drug overdose (cholinergic crisis) and underdose (possible myasthenic crisis)
  - Cholinergic crisis usually develops within 1 hour of drug administration; signs and symptoms include muscle weakness, dyspnea, dysphagia, increased respiratory secretions and saliva, nausea, vomiting, cramping, diarrhea, and diaphoresis
  - Myasthenic crisis usually doesn't occur for 3 or more hours after drug administration; signs and symptoms include extreme muscle weakness, dyspnea, and dysphagia
- Know that atropine is the antidote for cholinergic overdose and increasing the anticholinesterase dosage is the treatment for myasthenic crisis
- Explain to the patient that antimyasthenic therapy is long-term
- Teach the patient the importance of taking doses according to schedule
  - Timely administration prevents weakness
  - Profound weakness can impair ability to breathe and swallow
- Urge the patient to carry identification describing the disease and drug regimen
- Base patient evaluation on improvement of neuromuscular symptoms or strength without cholinergic signs or symptoms
- Know that parenteral doses of neostigmine and pyridostigmine should be much smaller than oral doses because absorption increases with the parenteral route

---

When NOT to use antimyasthenics
- Hypersensitivity
- Bromide allergy

Adverse reactions
- Abdominal pain, nausea, vomiting, diarrhea, sweating, miosis, increased salivation, increased bronchial secretions, difficulty breathing

Key nursing actions
- Assess neuromuscular status.
- Monitor patient for signs and symptoms of drug overdose or underdose.
- Urge patient to carry identification describing the disease and drug regimen.
- Base patient evaluation on improvement of neuromuscular symptoms or strength without cholinergic signs or symptoms.
- Know that atropine is the antidote for cholinergic overdose and increasing anticholinesterase dosage is the treatment for myasthenic crisis.

TOP 6

Items to study for your next test on drugs and the CNS

1. Mechanism of action of CNS stimulants, anticonvulsants, antiparkinsonians, and antimyasthenics

2. Common adverse effects of the various CNS stimulants, anticonvulsants, antiparkinsonians, and antimyasthenics

3. Nursing responsibilities when administering CNS stimulants, anticonvulsants, antiparkinsonians, and antimyasthenics

4. Teaching for the patient who is receiving a CNS stimulant, an anticonvulsant, an antiparkinsonian, or an antimyasthenic

5. Differences between dopaminergic and cholinergic blocking drugs

6. Importance of patient compliance with antimyasthenic therapy

NCLEX CHECKS

It's never too soon to begin your NCLEX® examination preparation. Now that you've reviewed this chapter, carefully read each of the following questions and choose the best answer. Then compare your responses with the correct answers.

1. A client with Parkinson's disease is being treated with levodopa (Dopar). The nurse would become most concerned if the client develops:

☐ **1.** edema.
☐ **2.** tachycardia.
☐ **3.** irritability.
☐ **4.** nausea and vomiting.

2. A physician suspects that a client has myasthenia gravis. Which anticholinesterase can be used to diagnose this disorder?

☐ **1.** Ambenonium (Mytelase)
☐ **2.** Edrophonium (Tensilon)
☐ **3.** Physostigmine (Antilirium)
☐ **4.** Pyridostigmine (Mestinon)

3. A client being treated with diazepam (Valium), a benzodiazepine, is most likely to experience which adverse reaction?

☐ **1.** Hypertension
☐ **2.** Rash
☐ **3.** Sedation
☐ **4.** Tachycardia

4. A nurse is preparing a female client with tonic-clonic seizure disorder for discharge. Which instructions should the nurse include about phenytoin (Dilantin)? Select all that apply.

☐ **1.** Monitor for skin rash.
☐ **2.** Maintain adequate amounts of fluid and fiber in the diet.
☐ **3.** Perform good oral hygiene, including daily brushing and flossing.
☐ **4.** Follow up with necessary, periodic blood work.
☐ **5.** Report to the physician any problems with walking, coordination, slurred speech, or nausea.
☐ **6.** Feel safe about taking this drug, even during pregnancy.

5. A nurse would expect a client taking entacapone (Comtan) to also be taking:

☐ **1.** famotidine (Pepcid).
☐ **2.** levodopa-carbidopa (Dopar).
☐ **3.** tolcapone (Tasmar).
☐ **4.** furosemide (Lasix).

6. A 12-year-old child who's taking methylphenidate (Concerta) is in with his mother for a check-up. Which statement by the mother warrants further investigation?

☐ **1.** "He hasn't grown in over 1 year."
☐ **2.** "I noticed he's starting to get acne."
☐ **3.** "He still takes his medication at noon every day."
☐ **4.** "He likes to drink soy milk."

7. A nurse should question the use of sumatriptan (Imitrex) in which client?

☐ **1.** An 18-year-old who's taking a hormonal contraceptive
☐ **2.** A 21-year-old with frequent cluster headaches
☐ **3.** A 34-year-old who's 15 weeks pregnant
☐ **4.** A 65-year-old with diabetes

8. A nurse warns a client taking mephobarbital (Mebaral) about which possible adverse effect?

☐ **1.** Diarrhea
☐ **2.** Seizures
☐ **3.** Restlessness
☐ **4.** Lethargy

9. Gabapentin (Neurontin) may be ordered for a client with which disorder?

☐ **1.** Postherpetic neuralgia
☐ **2.** Tonic-clonic seizures
☐ **3.** Parkinson's disease
☐ **4.** A history of pancreatitis

10. A nurse suspects a client receiving neostigmine (Prostigmin) is having a myasthenic crisis. Which finding is the nurse likely to assess?

☐ **1.** The client begins vomiting 30 minutes after administration of the medication.
☐ **2.** The client experiences extreme muscle weakness 4 hours after the medication is given.
☐ **3.** The client has diaphoresis 45 minutes after the medication is given.
☐ **4.** Increased respiratory secretions are seen 90 minutes after the medication is given.

ANSWERS AND RATIONALES

1. CORRECT ANSWER: 2

Levodopa is a dopamine agonist. Cardiac symptoms such as tachycardia are considered levodopa's most serious adverse reactions because they may lead to ventricular tachycardia and death. Edema isn't a common adverse reaction to this drug. Although nausea, vomiting, and irritability are common adverse reactions, they aren't as serious as cardiovascular effects.

2. CORRECT ANSWER: 2

Edrophonium or neostigmine may be used to diagnose myasthenia gravis. Ambenonium and pyridostigmine are used to treat myasthenia gravis, not diagnose it. Physostigmine is used to reverse the effects of tricyclic antidepressant and anticholinergic poisoning.

3. CORRECT ANSWER: 3

Sedation is the most common adverse reaction of diazepam, affecting 4% to 12% of all patients taking diazepam. Rash is a less likely effect. Tachycardia and hypertension aren't adverse reactions to this drug.

4. CORRECT ANSWER: 1, 3, 4, 5

A rash may occur 10 to 14 days after starting phenytoin. If a rash appears, the client should notify the physician and discontinue the medication. Because phenytoin may cause gingival hyperplasia, the client must practice good oral hygiene and see a dentist regularly. Periodic blood work is necessary to monitor complete blood counts, platelet levels, hepatic function, and drug levels. Signs and symptoms of phenytoin toxicity include problems with walking, coordination, slurred speech, nausea, lethargy, diplopia, nystagmus, and disturbances in balance. These symptoms must be reported to the physician immediately. Although adequate amounts of fluid and fiber are part of a healthy diet, they aren't required for a client taking phenytoin. Phenytoin must be used cautiously during pregnancy because of the increased incidence of birth defects; phenobarbital is a safer drug to take during pregnancy.

5. CORRECT ANSWER: 2

Entacapone is a COMT inhibitor, which helps sustain plasma levels of levodopa, resulting in sustained dopaminergic stimulation of the brain. The drug must be administered with levodopa-carbidopa. Although a client may be taking famotidine or furosemide while taking entacapone, these drugs aren't needed to achieve the therapeutic benefits of entacapone. Tolcapone is another COMT inhibitor.

6. CORRECT ANSWER: 1

Methylphenidate is a CNS stimulant, commonly used to treat attention deficit hyperactivity disorder in children. One adverse effect of CNS stimulants in children is growth suppression. The fact that the child hasn't grown in 1 year warrants further investigation. Acne, another adverse effect of CNS stimulants in children, usually doesn't require follow-up action. Taking methylphenidate at noon is an appropriate action; it should be taken 6 hours before bedtime to prevent insomnia. Drinking soy milk while taking CNS stimulants isn't a problem; however, caffeine should be limited to avoid added stimulation.

7. CORRECT ANSWER: 3

Pregnant clients shouldn't take 5-HT agonists such as sumatriptan because of the risk of serious birth defects. Sumatriptan is indicated for the treatment of cluster headaches. Diabetes isn't a contraindication to taking sumatriptan. Hormonal contraceptives may increase the bioavailability of sumatriptan, but there's no reason the client shouldn't take the drug.

8. CORRECT ANSWER: 4

Lethargy is an adverse reaction to mephobarbital. Mephobarbital is used to treat seizures; it doesn't cause them. Diarrhea and restlessness aren't adverse reactions to this medication.

9. CORRECT ANSWER: 1

Gabapentin is used to treat postherpetic neuralgia. It's also used as an adjunctive therapy to treat partial seizures, not tonic-clonic seizures. It isn't used to treat Parkinson's disease or pancreatitis.

10. CORRECT ANSWER: 2

A myasthenic crisis is usually caused by underdosing of an antimyasthenic. The signs and symptoms of a myasthenic crisis are usually seen 3 hours or more after administration of the drug and include extreme muscle weakness, dyspnea, and dysphagia. Vomiting, diaphoresis, and increased respiratory secretions are signs of a cholinergic crisis, which occurs with overdose of an antimyasthenic.

Drugs and pain

---

1. One way that a nonopioid analgesic acts is by:
- [ ] 1. inhibiting stimulation of pain receptors.
- [ ] 2. binding to opiate receptors to alter perception of pain.
- [ ] 3. blocking the effects of opioids.
- [ ] 4. locking nerve impulse transmission across nerve cell membranes.

CORRECT ANSWER: 1

2. Before administering a dose of pain medication, a nurse should always:
- [ ] 1. give the client something to eat.
- [ ] 2. assess the client's pain level.
- [ ] 3. reposition the client.
- [ ] 4. have emergency resuscitation equipment available.

CORRECT ANSWER: 2

3. Which statement is appropriate for a nurse to make to a client who's about to have surgery using an inhalation anesthetic?
- [ ] 1. "I'll monitor the area for a rash after surgery."
- [ ] 2. "Your sense of touch will decrease, and then you'll lose motor function."
- [ ] 3. "It's normal for you to shiver after surgery."
- [ ] 4. "You may not have feeling in the surgical area when you wake up."

CORRECT ANSWER: 3

4. When caring for a client who's about to receive an injectable anesthetic, a nurse should have:

☐ 1. atropine (Sal-Tropine) ready for injection.

☐ 2. food for the client to prevent GI upset.

☐ 3. naloxone (Narcan) in case of overdose.

☐ 4. equipment for endotracheal intubation readily available.

CORRECT ANSWER: 4

5. Which measure may enhance a client's therapeutic response to an analgesic?

☐ 1. Having a loud television playing

☐ 2. Providing soft, quiet music

☐ 3. Allowing the patient to walk around the unit

☐ 4. Waiting as long as possible to administer medication

CORRECT ANSWER: 2

LEARNING OBJECTIVES

After studying this chapter, you should be able to:

● Describe the mechanisms of action of nonopioid analgesics, opioid agonists and mixed opioid agonist-antagonists, opioid antagonists, and general, local, and topical anesthetics.

● Describe nursing responsibilities when administering analgesics.

● Compare the effects of general anesthesia with those of local anesthesia for the patient undergoing surgery.

● Identify nursing responsibilities that may enhance the therapeutic response to analgesics.

● Identify nursing responsibilities when caring for a patient receiving a general or local anesthetic.

● Discuss appropriate teaching for the patient who's receiving an analgesic and for the patient who's receiving an anesthetic.

CHAPTER OVERVIEW

Effective pain management requires knowledge of analgesic pharmacology and careful evaluation of the patient's response. Drugs used for pain include nonopioid analgesics, opioid agonists and mixed opioid agonists-antagonists, opioid antagonists, and general, local, and topical anesthetics.

Nonopioid analgesics are used for relief of mild to moderate pain, inflammation, and fever and as prophylaxis for thromboembolic disorders. Opioid agonists and mixed opioid agonists-antagonists treat pain that's unresponsive to nonopioid analgesics. Opioid antagonists are used to reverse effects of the opioid analgesic when respiratory or central nervous system (CNS) depression has occurred.

Nursing responsibilities related to analgesics include monitoring vital signs and the patient's satisfaction, preventing constipation, and evaluating pain relief. Additionally, except during palliative care or in oncology patients, a nurse must balance concerns about addiction to opioids with the goal of relieving pain and knowledge of drug tolerance, dependence, and abuse.

General anesthetics cause analgesia, muscle relaxation, and a decreased level of consciousness (LOC). Local anesthetics block sensation on the skin, in body tissues when infiltrated, and in epidural or spinal blocks. Topical anesthetics are used to relieve or prevent pain and anesthetize injection or catheter insertion sites. Nursing responsibilities related to anesthetics include maintaining airway patency, having resuscitation equipment on hand, and observing the patient for arrhythmias.

A&P highlights

- Nociceptors are where pain begins
- Myelinated A-delta fibers are fast-conducting fibers that signal sharp, well-localized pain
- Unmyelinated C fibers are more numerous, smaller, and slower than the A-delta fibers and signal dull, poorly localized pain
- Dorsal horn of the spinal cord is where nociceptors terminate
- Pain acts as a protective mechanism that indicates an underlying physiologic or psychological problem
- Pain is subjective and varies widely from person to person, based upon a person's perception, emotional state, and ethnic, cultural, or religious influences
- Analgesics may block the effect of these neurotransmitters

ANATOMY AND PHYSIOLOGY

- ### Anatomy of pain
  - Nociceptors
    - Are free nerve endings located primarily in the skin, periosteum, joint surfaces, and arterial walls
    - Are part of the afferent neurons
    - Are the origin of pain sensation
    - Include two types
      - Myelinated A-delta fibers—fast-conducting fibers that signal sharp, well-localized pain
      - Unmyelinated C fibers—more numerous, smaller, and slower than A-delta fibers; signal dull, poorly localized pain
  - Chemical mediators
    - Stimulate nociceptors
    - Are released or synthesized in response to tissue damage
    - Include prostaglandins, histamine, bradykinin, and serotonin
  - Dorsal horn of spinal cord
    - Receives pain impulse after activation of nociceptors, which have afferent neuron neurotransmitters (somatostatin, cholecystokinin, substance P)
    - Is where nociceptors end

– Is the control center for:
  · Incoming information from afferent neurons
  · Pain impulse regulation
  · Descending influences from higher centers in the CNS

● **Function of pain**
- Acts as protective mechanism indicating an underlying physiologic or psychological problem
- Is subjective and varies widely from person to person, based upon a person's perception, emotional state, and ethnic, cultural, or religious influences

● **Pain theory (Gate-control theory)**
- Most widely accepted pain theory
- States that the dorsal horn is the regulator between the peripheral fibers and the CNS; it acts as gatekeeper of pain and nonpain signals before sending an impulse to the CNS
- States that pain perception may be inhibited by simultaneously activating nonpain signals to the CNS

NONOPIOID ANALGESICS

● **Mechanism of action**
- Act peripherally to prevent prostaglandin formation in inflamed tissues with two actions
  – Inhibit stimulation of pain receptors
  – Inhibit prostaglandin synthesis in the CNS and stimulate peripheral vasodilation to reduce fever (antipyretic action)

● **Pharmacokinetics**
- Absorption
  – Salicylates: Absorbed mainly in upper part of small intestine through passive diffusion and partly in stomach
  – Acetaminophen (para-aminophenol derivatives): Absorbed rapidly and completely in GI tract and absorbed well from rectal mucosa
  – Nonsteroidal anti-inflammatory drugs (NSAIDs): Absorbed in GI tract
  – Cyclooxygenase-2 (COX-2) drugs: Absorbed in GI tract
- Distribution
  – Salicylates: Distributed widely throughout body
  – Acetaminophen: Distributed widely in body fluids; crosses placental barrier
  – NSAIDs: Distributed widely
  – COX-2 drugs: Distributed widely
- Metabolism
  – Salicylates: Metabolized by liver
  – Acetaminophen: Metabolized by liver
  – NSAIDs: Metabolized by liver
  – COX-2 drugs: Metabolized by liver

Key facts about nonopioid analgesics

- Act peripherally to prevent prostaglandin formation in inflamed tissues by two actions:
  - inhibit stimulation of pain receptors
  - inhibit prostaglandin synthesis in the CNS and stimulate peripheral vasodilation to reduce fever
- Metabolized in liver
- Excreted in urine, breast milk, and feces

- Excretion
  - Salicylates: Excreted in urine
  - Acetaminophen: Excreted in urine and breast milk
  - NSAIDs: Primarily excreted in urine
  - COX-2 drugs: Excreted in urine and feces

● **Drug examples**
- Salicylate analgesics: aspirin (ASA), choline and magnesium salicylates (Trilisate), choline salicylate (Arthropan), diflunisal (Dolobid), salsalate (Disalcid)
- Para-aminophenol derivative nonopioid analgesics: acetaminophen (Tempra, Tylenol)
- NSAIDs: diclofenac (Cataflam, Voltaren), fenoprofen calcium (Nalfon), flurbiprofen (Ansaid), ibuprofen (Advil, Motrin, Nuprin, ketoprofen, ketorolac tromethamine (Toradol), mefenamic acid (Ponstel), naproxen (Naprosyn), naproxen sodium (Anaprox), piroxicam (Feldene), sulindac (Clinoril), tolmetin (Tolectin)
- COX-2 drugs: celecoxib (Celebrex)

● **Indications**
- Treat mild to moderate pain (acetaminophen, aspirin, choline salicylate, diflunisal, fenoprofen, ibuprofen, naproxen, ketoprofen, ketorolac, magnesium salicylate, mefenamic acid, and salsalate)
- Treat arthritis and osteoarthritis (all drugs except mefenamic acid)
- Reduce fever (acetaminophen, aspirin, and ibuprofen)
- Reduce inflammation (aspirin, naproxen, and sulindac)
- Prevent transient ischemic attacks and myocardial infarction (MI) by smoothing platelets (aspirin)
- Treat dysmenorrhea (celecoxib, ibuprofen, ketoprofen, mefenamic acid, naproxen, and naproxen sodium)

● **Contraindications and precautions**
- Used cautiously in patients with asthma or nasal polyps
- All drugs except acetaminophen: Contraindicated in pregnant patients and those with aspirin hypersensitivity
- Aspirin
  - Contraindicated in patients with bleeding disorders or GI ulcers; shouldn't be given to children (unless under practitioner's supervision) because of increased risk of Reye's syndrome
  - Used cautiously in patients with impaired hepatic function and those scheduled for surgery within 1 week
- Celecoxib contraindicated in patients with a history of heart disease or sulfa allergies

● **Adverse reactions**
- GI pain and upset, nausea, vomiting, diarrhea, heartburn, dizziness, headache, and tinnitus

- Rarely, rash, hypoglycemia, and neutropenia; high doses (more than 4 grams daily) can cause serious liver toxicity (acetaminophen)
- Hemostatic defects; signs of acute aspirin toxicity include respiratory alkalosis, hyperpnea, hemorrhage, confusion, pulmonary edema, and lethargy (aspirin)
- Severe thromboembolic events, such as MI and stroke (celecoxib)
- Ulcers, bladder infection, hematuria, kidney necrosis, hypertension, and heart failure (NSAIDs)

● Interactions

- Use with opioid analgesics enhances pain relief
- Use of NSAIDs with oral anticoagulants prolongs bleeding time and increases anticoagulant effects
- Use of aspirin with other NSAIDs or corticosteroids may exacerbate the GI adverse effects of aspirin and reduce aspirin effectiveness
- Long-term use of acetaminophen with NSAIDs increases the risk of renal toxicity or failure
- NSAIDs and celecoxib exacerbate GI adverse effects of alcohol
- Aspirin used with anticoagulants increases the risk of bleeding
- Angiotensin-converting enzyme (ACE) inhibitors and beta-adrenergic blockers have decreased antihypertensive properties when given with aspirin
- Celecoxib decreases the clearance of lithium, increasing the risk of lithium toxicity
- Celecoxib decreases the antihypertensive effects of ACE inhibitors and diuretics; increases prothrombin time (PT) when given with warfarin

● Nursing responsibilities

- For a more rapid effect, administer the drug before meals; to reduce GI irritation, administer with meals
- Instruct the patient to inform the practitioner or dentist of the prescribed drug regimen before undergoing medical or dental treatment or surgery
- Assess the patient's pain level before and after administering the drug
- Monitor complete blood count, platelet, PT, and hepatic and renal function tests
- Don't crush enteric-coated aspirin
- Closely monitor the patient taking a COX-2 drug for thromboembolic events
- Don't administer more than the recommended dosage because of increased risk of toxicity
- Advise the patient that the Centers for Disease Control and Prevention (CDC) warns against giving salicylates (including aspirin) to children or adolescents with influenza, varicella (chickenpox), or viral illness because these drugs may be linked to Reye's syndrome

Key nursing actions

- Administer the drug before meals for a rapid effect and with meals for GI irritation reduction.
- Advise the patient that the CDC warns against giving salicylates to children or adolescents with influenza, varicella, or viral illness.
- Closely monitor the patient taking a COX-2 drug for thromboembolic events.

Key facts about opioid agonists and mixed agonists-antagonists

- Bind to opiate receptors in the CNS to alter the perception of and emotional response to pain
- Metabolized in liver
- Excreted in urine

When to use opioid agonists and mixed agonists-antagonists

- Adjuncts to anesthesia
- Cough relief
- Pain due to MI or pulmonary edema
- Pain unresponsive to nonopioid analgesics

When NOT to use opioid agonists and mixed agonists-antagonists

- History of opioid abuse.

OPIOID AGONISTS AND MIXED OPIOID AGONISTS-ANTAGONISTS

● Mechanism of action

- Opioid agonists bind to opiate receptors in the peripheral nervous system and CNS to alter the perception of and emotional response to pain
- Mixed opioid agonists-antagonists have an unknown mechanism of action but weakly antagonize the effects of opiates at the receptors

● Pharmacokinetics

- Absorption
  - Oral doses are absorbed readily from GI tract
  - I.V. administration produces the most rapid, reliable analgesic effect
  - Mixed opioid agonists-antagonists are absorbed rapidly from parenteral administration
- Distribution: Distributed widely
- Metabolism: Metabolized extensively in liver
- Excretion: Excreted in urine

● Drug examples

- Opioid analgesics: codeine, fentanyl (Sublimaze, Duragesic), hydromorphone (Dilaudid), levorphanol (Levo-Dromoran), meperidine (Demerol), methadone (Dolophine), morphine sulfate (Duramorph, MS Contin, MSIR), oxycodone (OxyContin, Roxicodone), propoxyphene (Darvon, DarvonN), sufentanil (Sufenta)
- Mixed opioid agonists-antagonists: buprenorphine (Buprenex), butorphanol (Stadol), nalbuphine (Nubain), pentazocine (Talwin)

● Indications

- Treat pain that's unresponsive to nonopioid analgesics; type and amount of analgesic depends on type and level of pain and patient's response to previous therapy
- Adjunct to anesthesia (butorphanol, fentanyl, meperidine, morphine, nalbuphine, and pentazocine)
- Relieve cough (codeine and hydromorphone)
- Treat pain caused by MI or acute pulmonary edema (morphine)
- During childbirth and postoperatively (mixed opioid agonists-antagonists)
- Local anesthesia via epidural route (fentanyl and morphine)
- Local anesthesia via transdermal patch (fentanyl)
- Temporary maintenance of opioid addiction (methadone)

● Contraindications and precautions

- Contraindicated in patients with a history of opioid abuse because they may induce withdrawal symptoms (mixed opioid agonists-antagonists)
- Used cautiously in patients with head injury, hepatic or renal disease, and CNS depression; pregnant and breast-feeding patients; and elderly or debilitated patients; dosage may need to be reduced for all these patients

Adverse reactions

- Orthostatic hypotension, sedation, constipation, respiratory depression, psychological dependence, nausea, flushing, and pupil constriction
- Tremors, palpitations, tachycardia, delirium, neurotoxicity, and seizures (meperidine)
- Nausea, vomiting, light-headedness, sedation, and euphoria (mixed agonists-antagonists)

Interactions

- Use with alcohol, sedating antihistamines, hypnotics, monoamine oxidase (MAO) inhibitors, tricyclic antidepressants, or sedatives causes additive CNS depression
- Mixed opioid agonists-antagonists may cause withdrawal symptoms in patients with physical dependence on opioid analgesics
- Use with nonopioid analgesics may enhance pain relief
- Tricyclic antidepressants, phenothiazines, and anticoagulants given with opioid agonists may cause severe constipation and urine retention

Nursing responsibilities

- Assess the patient's pain before and after administering the drug
- Assess the patient's blood pressure, pulse, and respiratory status before administering the drug and periodically throughout analgesic therapy
- Because regular analgesic administration may be more effective than as-needed doses, administer doses before pain becomes severe
- Know that prolonged use of an opioid analgesic or opioid agonist-antagonist may cause dependence and tolerance; however, this shouldn't preclude administration of adequate analgesia
  - Patients receiving opioids for pain relief rarely develop psychological dependence; but with long-term therapy, they may require progressively higher doses to relieve pain (because of increased drug tolerance)
  - To prevent withdrawal symptoms, discontinue opioid analgesics gradually after long-term use; signs and symptoms of withdrawal include tremors, agitation, nausea, and vomiting
  - Dependency shouldn't preclude administration of opioids for pain relief in patients with cancer or as palliative treatment in terminally ill patients
- Know that naloxone is the antidote for opioid overdose
- Instruct the patient to take oral analgesics with food to minimize GI irritation
- Administer I.V. forms slowly and in a diluted solution
- Teach the patient to change position slowly to minimize orthostatic hypotension
- Warn the patient to avoid activities requiring alertness until response to drug is known (see *Teaching about opioid analgesics,* page 76)
- Discuss ways to minimize dry mouth and constipation (such as sucking on hard candy and increasing fluid intake and consumption of bulk foods

---

Adverse reactions

- Orthostatic hypotension, sedation, constipation, respiratory depression, psychological dependence, pupil constriction
- Neurotoxicity, seizures (meperidine)

Key nursing actions

- Assess the patient's blood pressure, pulse, and respiratory status before administering the drug and periodically throughout analgesic therapy.
- Prolonged use of an opioid analgesic or opioid agonist-antagonist may cause dependence and tolerance, but shouldn't preclude administration of adequate analgesia.
- Know that naloxone is the antidote for opioid overdose.

Topics for patient discussion

- Medication prescribed
- Administration instructions
- Signs and symptoms, including adverse reactions

TIME-OUT FOR TEACHING

Teaching about opioid analgesics

Be sure to include these topics in your teaching plan for the patient receiving an opioid analgesic:
- medication prescribed, including name, dose, frequency, action, and adverse effects
- instructions for administering drug before pain becomes severe
- avoidance of alcohol and other central nervous system depressants
- measures to prevent constipation
- alternative pain management strategies
- signs and symptoms to discuss with practitioner, including adverse reactions and overdose
- medical follow-up needed.

high in fiber); suggest that the practitioner include a stool softener or laxative daily with the patient's pain regimen

Key facts about opioid antagonists

- Competitively block the effects of opioids without producing analgesic effects
- Metabolized in liver
- Excreted in urine

When to use opioid antagonists

- Opioid overdose
- Adjunct to therapy in treating drug abuse

When NOT to use opioid antagonists

- Use cautiously in patients physically dependent on opioids

OPIOID ANTAGONISTS

● Mechanism of action
- Competitively block the effects of opioids without producing analgesic effects
- Displace opioid attached to the opiate receptor

● Pharmacokinetics
- Absorption
  - Nalmefene and naloxone: administered I.V., I.M., or subcutaneously
  - Naltrexone: absorbed orally
- Distribution: Rapidly distributed to block more than 80% of the brain opioid receptors within 5 minutes after I.V. administration
- Metabolism: Metabolized by liver
- Excretion: Excreted in urine

● Drug examples
- Nalmefene (Revex), naloxone (Narcan), naltrexone (ReVia, Trexan)

● Indications
- Reverse CNS and respiratory depression in opioid overdose
- Adjunctive therapy to keep detoxified patients drug-free, similar to use of disulfiram in preventing resumption of alcohol (naltrexone)
- Treat opioid overdose (nalmefene and naloxone)

● Contraindications and precautions
- Used cautiously in patients physically dependent on opioids because of the risk of severe withdrawal symptoms

Adverse reactions
- Nausea, vomiting, tachycardia, hypotension, hypertension, arrhythmias, tremors, drowsiness, and hyperventilation
- Hyperventilation and tremors in unconscious patients returning to consciousness abruptly after naloxone administration

Interactions
- Use with an opioid reverses all opioid effects, including analgesia
- Withdrawal symptoms if given to a patient receiving an opioid agonist or addicted to opioids (naltrexone)

Nursing responsibilities
- Assess the patient's respiratory status, blood pressure, pulse, and LOC until the opioid wears off
- Monitor the duration of drug effects; repeat doses may be needed if effects of the opioid outlast those of the opioid antagonist
- Because an opioid antagonist reverses analgesia (as well as respiratory depression), the dosage should be adjusted according to the patient's pain level
- Know that patient's failure to improve markedly means that signs and symptoms result from disease or from use of CNS depressants other than opioids
- Administer the drug slowly, and monitor the patient's respiratory and pain status and LOC at all times; give only the amount required to reverse respiratory depression or increase mental alertness because total reversal of pain relief will put the patient in undue distress

GENERAL ANESTHETICS

RAPID-ACTING HYPNOTICS

Mechanism of action
- Stabilize neuronal membranes to produce progressive, reversible CNS depression

Pharmacokinetics
- Absorption: Administered I.V
- Distribution: Distributed rapidly
- Metabolism: Metabolized in liver
- Excretion: Excreted renally or hepatically

Drug examples
- Methohexital, midazolam hydrochloride (Versed), propofol (Diprivan), thiopental sodium (Pentothal)

Indications
- Induce and maintain anesthesia for short-term procedures
- Prolong anesthesia when used with gaseous anesthetics

Adverse reactions
- Nausea, vomiting, tachycardia, hypotension, hypertension, arrhythmias, hyperventilation, tremors

Key nursing actions
- Assess respiratory status, blood pressure, pulse, and LOC until the opioid wears off.
- Opioid antagonist dosage should be adjusted according to the patient's pain level.
- Give only the amount required to reverse respiratory depression or increase mental alertness.

Key facts about rapid-acting hypnotics
- Stabilize neuronal membranes to produce progressive, reversible CNS depression
- Metabolized in the liver
- Excreted renally or hepatically

When to use rapid-acting hypnotics
- Anesthesia induction and maintenance
- Anesthesia extension

Topics for patient discussion

- Type of anesthetic prescribed
- Possible psychomotor function impairment
- Signs and symptoms, including adverse reactions

Adverse reactions

- Respiratory depression, apnea, hypotension, tachycardia, nausea and vomiting, muscle twitching, tissue necrosis with extravasation

Key nursing actions

- Determine if the patient has allergies before the surgery.
- Assess cardiovascular, respiratory, and renal status and LOC before and after surgery.

Key facts about inhalation anesthetics

- Depress the CNS
- Metabolized in lungs and liver
- Excreted in urine

TIME-OUT FOR TEACHING

Teaching about general anesthetics

Be sure to include these topics in your teaching plan for the patient receiving a general anesthetic:
- type of anesthetic prescribed, including name, dose, frequency, action, and possible adverse effects
- withholding of food and fluids for at least 8 hours before surgery
- avoidance of alcohol and other central nervous system depressants for at least 24 hours after receiving anesthetic
- possible psychomotor function impairment for 24 hours or more after receiving anesthetic
- signs and symptoms to discuss with the practitioner, including adverse effects.

Contraindications and precautions
- Used cautiously in patients with cardiovascular or respiratory instability

Adverse reactions
- Respiratory depression, apnea, hypotension, tachycardia, nausea and vomiting, muscle twitching, and tissue necrosis with extravasation

Interactions
- Additive CNS depression when used with similar-acting drugs

Nursing responsibilities
- Find out if the patient has any allergies before the surgery or procedure
- Inform the patient about what to expect before, during, and after the surgery or procedure
- Explain to the patient that no food or fluids will be allowed for at least 8 hours before surgery (see *Teaching about general anesthetics*)
- Assess the patient's cardiovascular, respiratory, and renal status and LOC before and after the surgery or procedure

INHALATION ANESTHETICS

Mechanism of action
- Depress the CNS to produce loss of consciousness, loss of responsiveness to sensory stimulation, and muscle relaxation

Pharmacokinetics
- Absorption: Absorbed by lungs
- Distribution: Distributed to other tissues; rapidly distributed to organs with high blood flow
- Metabolism: Eliminated primarily by lungs; enflurane and halothane also metabolized by liver
- Excretion: Excreted in urine

Drug examples
- Desflurane (Suprane), enflurane (Ethrane), halothane (Fluothane), isoflurane (Forane), nitrous oxide

Indications
- Produce loss of consciousness, loss of responsiveness to sensory stimulation (including pain), and muscle relaxation
- Maintain anesthesia for surgery requiring precise, rapid control of the depth of anesthesia

Contraindications and precautions
- Contraindicated in patients with known hypersensitivity to the drug, liver disorders, or a history of malignant hyperthermia
- Used cautiously in elderly or debilitated patients because they're predisposed to an exaggerated response to these drugs

Adverse reactions
- Exaggerated response to normal dose (most common), postanesthesia nausea and vomiting, hypotension, arrhythmias, tachycardia, confusion, agitation, memory loss, ataxia, and hypothermia

Interactions
- Use with labetalol increases hypotensive effects
- Use with other CNS depressants increases CNS and respiratory depression and hypotension
- Use with xanthines (such as caffeine or theophylline) increases risk of arrhythmias
- Use with neuromuscular blockades (including succinylcholine) increases blockade effects and risk of malignant hyperthermia
- Enflurane given with isoniazid or aminoglycosides increases the risk of nephrotoxicity
- Desflurane given with midazolam or fentanyl decreases anesthetic requirements

Nursing responsibilities
- Find out if patient has any allergies to drugs before surgery
- Advise the patient not to eat or drink anything for at least 8 hours before surgery to prevent aspiration of stomach contents into the lungs during anesthesia
- Inform the patient that psychomotor functions may be impaired for 24 hours or more after inhalation anesthesia
- Monitor the patient for adverse reactions to the inhalation anesthetic during entire drug administration and recovery
- Keep atropine available at all times to reverse possible bradycardia
- Monitor the patient's temperature frequently; hypothermia commonly occurs with inhalation anesthesia
- If shivering (common during recovery) occurs, keep the patient warm with extra blankets or heat; administer oxygen, as prescribed, to compensate for the increased oxygen demand

When to use inhalation anesthetics
- Promotion of loss of consciousness, loss of responsiveness to sensory stimulation including pain, and muscle relaxation
- Anesthesia maintenance

When NOT to use inhalation anesthetics
- Hypersensitivity, liver disorders, history of malignant hyperthermia

Adverse reactions
- Exaggerated response to the normal dose (most common), postanesthesia nausea and vomiting, hypotension, arrhythmias, tachycardia, confusion, agitation, memory loss

Key nursing actions
- Keep atropine available at all times to reverse possible bradycardia.
- Monitor the patient's temperature frequently.
- Shivering is normal during recovery; if shivering occurs, keep the patient warm with extra blankets or heat and administer oxygen, as prescribed, to compensate for the increased oxygen demand.

Key facts about injectable analgesic anesthetics

- Depress the CNS
- Metabolized by liver
- Excreted in feces

When to use injectable analgesic anesthetics

- Rapid anesthesia or moderate sedation induction
- Pain

When NOT to use injectable analgesic anesthetics

- Hypersensitivity

Adverse reactions

- Respiratory depression, arrhythmias, bradycardia, skeletal and thoracic muscle rigidity, seizures, asystole, dry mouth, urine retention, shivering

Key nursing actions

- Continuously assess respiratory status.
- Only those experienced in endotracheal intubation should use these drugs.

Key facts about neuroleptanesthetics

- Produce dissociation from the environment during induction of anesthesia
- Metabolized in liver
- Excreted in feces

INJECTABLE ANALGESIC ANESTHETICS

● **Mechanism of action**
- Depress the CNS to produce loss of consciousness, loss of responsiveness to sensory stimulation, and muscle relaxation

● **Pharmacokinetics**
- Absorption: Administered I.V.
- Distribution: Distributed rapidly; onset of action is rapid and short-acting
- Metabolism: Metabolized by liver
- Excretion: Excreted in feces

● **Drug examples**
- Alfentanil (Alfenta), etomidate, remifentanil (Ultiva), sufentanil (Sufenta)

● **Indications**
- Induce rapid anesthesia (usually for situations requiring anesthesia of short duration, such as outpatient surgery) or moderate sedation
- Decrease pain

● **Contraindications and precautions**
- Contraindicated in patients hypersensitive to these drugs
- Used cautiously in patients with cardiovascular and respiratory instability

● **Adverse reactions**
- Respiratory depression, arrhythmias, bradycardia, and skeletal and thoracic muscle rigidity
- Possible seizures, asystole, dry mouth, urine retention, and shivering (alfentanil and fentanyl)

● **Interactions**
- Use of verapamil with etomidate may increase anesthetic effect and cause respiratory depression and apnea
- Use with other opioids, inhalation anesthetics, hypnotics, or sedatives increases effects of injection anesthetic

● **Nursing responsibilities**
- Continuously assess the patient's respiratory status for signs of respiratory depression
- Be aware that only persons experienced in endotracheal intubation should use these drugs; keep necessary equipment on hand
- Know that many injectable drugs are incompatible with other drugs or solutions

NEUROLEPTANESTHETICS

● **Mechanism of action**
- Produce dissociation from the environment during induction of anesthesia by directly acting on the cortex and limbic system

● **Pharmacokinetics**
- Absorption: Administered I.V.

- Distribution: Rapidly distributed
- Metabolism: Metabolized in liver
- Excretion: Excreted in feces

● **Drug examples**
  - Droperidol (Inapsine), ketamine (Ketalar)

● **Indications**
  - Sedate and induce analgesia before surgery or diagnostic procedures

● **Contraindications and precautions**
  - Ketamine contraindicated in patients with significant hypertension, severe cardiac decompensation, a history of psychiatric disorders, any condition in which a significant blood pressure increase would endanger the patient's life, or a history of stroke; also during surgery of the pharynx, larynx, or bronchial tree (unless used with a muscle relaxant)
  - Droperidol used with extreme caution in patients with heart failure, bradycardia, or electrolyte abnormalities

● **Adverse reactions**
  - Extrapyramidal signs and symptoms, QT interval prolongation, and torsade de pointes (droperidol)
  - Prolonged recovery, seizures, shivering, hypertension, hallucinations, and tachycardia (ketamine)

● **Interactions**
  - Use with CNS depressants causes additive or potentiating CNS effects
  - Epinephrine may paradoxically enhance droperidol-induced hypotension
  - Ketamine given with halothane increases risk of hypotension and decreased cardiac output

● **Nursing responsibilities**
  - Monitor vital signs and cardiopulmonary status before, during, and after injection
  - Minimize environmental stimulation to prevent untoward reactions on emergence from anesthesia
  - Inform the patient that mental alertness, coordination, and physical dexterity may be impaired for some time after general anesthesia

LOCAL ANESTHETICS

● **Mechanism of action**
  - Provide analgesic relief by blocking conduction of nerve impulses at the point of contact, causing expansion of the nerve-cell membrane and inability of the cell to depolarize, which is necessary for impulse transmission

● **Pharmacokinetics**
  - Absorption: Varies widely
  - Distribution: Distributed throughout body
  - Metabolism: Varies by drug
  - Excretion: Excreted in urine

When to use neuroleptanesthetics

- Analgesia induction

When NOT to use neuroleptanesthetics

- Hypertension
- Cardiac decompensation
- History of stroke
- Surgery of the pharynx, larynx, or bronchial tree

Adverse reactions

- Hallucinations, seizures, shivering, extrapyramidal signs and symptoms, QT interval prolongation, torsade de pointes

Key nursing actions

- Monitor vital signs and cardiopulmonary status.
- Minimize environmental stimulation.

Key facts about local anesthetics

- Provide analgesic relief by blocking the conduction of nerve impulses at the point of contact
- Metabolism varies
- Excreted in urine

When to use local anesthetics

- Pain
- Anesthesia, including spinal and epidural

When NOT to use local anesthetics

- Drug hypersensitivity
- Myasthenia gravis
- Severe shock
- Impaired cardiac conduction

Adverse reactions

- Anxiety, restlessness, arrhythmias, bradycardia, hypotension, chills

Key nursing actions

- Assess for return of motor function and sensation postoperatively.
- Ensure that the gag reflex has returned before feeding a patient whose throat has been anesthetized.

Drug examples
- Benzocaine (Dermoplast), bupivacaine hydrochloride (Marcaine), chloroprocaine hydrochloride (Nesacaine), cocaine hydrochloride, dibucaine (Nupercainal), lidocaine hydrochloride (Xylocaine Hydrochloride), mepivacaine (Carbocaine), procaine hydrochloride (Novocain), ropivacaine (Naropin), tetracaine hydrochloride (Pontocaine)

Indications
- Prevent or relieve pain from a medical procedure, disease, or injury
- Treat severe pain unrelieved by topical anesthetics or analgesics
- Spinal anesthesia (bupivacaine, procaine, and tetracaine)
- Epidural anesthesia (bupivacaine, lidocaine, and mepivacaine)
- Epidural analgesia and anesthesia (bupivacaine, lidocaine, and tetracaine)
- Anesthesia for itching, burning, or short procedures (cocaine, benzocaine, and dibucaine applied directly to skin or mucous membranes)

Contraindications and precautions
- Contraindicated in patients with known hypersensitivity to these drugs and in those with myasthenia gravis, severe shock, or impaired cardiac conduction
- Used cautiously in patients with hepatic disease, hypotension, heart block, and hyperthyroidism or other endocrine diseases
- Used cautiously in elderly or debilitated patients because of the risk of toxicity
- Benzocaine: Used cautiously in children because absorption through skin may cause unwanted effects
- Ropivacaine: Contraindicated during labor because pushing becomes difficult and prolongs labor time

Adverse reactions
- Anxiety, restlessness, arrhythmias, bradycardia, hypotension, chills, tremors, nervousness, confusion, and dizziness; the higher the dose, the higher the incidence of adverse reactions

Interactions
- Slow anesthetic absorption and prolongs anesthetic effects when used with epinephrine (deliberate drug combination)
- Increase CNS depression when used with other CNS depressants

Nursing responsibilities
- Know that at onset of drug action, the patient's ability to sense cold, warmth, pain, and touch decreases in the affected area; then, local motor function diminishes
- Postoperatively, assess for return of motor function and sensation in reverse order to that described above
- Advise the patient to expect transient lack of sensation in the anesthetized area after surgery
- Ensure that the gag reflex has returned before feeding a patient whose throat has been anesthetized

TOPICAL ANESTHETICS

- **Mechanism of action**
  - Benzocaine, butacaine, butamben, dyclonine, and procaine: Block nerve impulse transmission, causing nerve to expand and lose ability to depolarize
  - Benzyl alcohol: Stimulates nerve endings and interferes with pain perception
  - Ethyl chloride and menthol: Superficially freeze tissue, stimulating cold sensation receptors and blocking nerve endings in the frozen area
  - Dibucaine, lidocaine, and tetracaine: Block nerve impulse transmission across nerve cell membranes

- **Pharmacokinetics**
  - Absorption: No significant systemic absorption, unless with frequent or high-dose application to the eye or large areas of burned or injured skin
  - Distribution: Distributed locally
  - Metabolism
    - Tetracaine and other esters: Extensively metabolized in blood and liver
    - Dibucaine, lidocaine, and other amides: Metabolized primarily by liver
  - Excretion: Excreted in urine

- **Drug examples**
  - Benzocaine, benzyl alcohol, butacaine, butamben, dyclonine, ethyl chloride, lidocaine, menthol, procaine, tetracaine

- **Indications**
  - Relieve or prevent pain, especially minor pain, itching, and irritation
  - Anesthetize site before giving injection
  - Numb mucosal surfaces before inserting tube or catheter

- **Contraindications and precautions**
  - Contraindicated in patients with a known hypersensitivity to the drug or its group
  - Dibucaine shouldn't be used in large quantities, especially in denuded or blistered areas
  - Dyclonine used cautiously in areas with traumatized mucosa or localized sepsis
  - Lidocaine used cautiously in elderly patients and patients with large areas of broken skin or mucous membranes

- **Adverse reactions**
  - Hypersensitivity reaction (including rash, pruritus, and breathing difficulty)
  - Topical reactions (benzyl alcohol)
  - Frostbite at the application site (ethyl chloride)

Key facts about topical anesthetics

- Block nerve impulse transmission
- Stimulate the nerve endings and interfere with pain perception
- Stimulate the cold sensation receptors and block the nerve endings in the frozen area
- Metabolized in blood and liver
- Excreted in urine

When to use topical anesthetics

- Pain
- Anesthesia
- Surface numbing

When NOT to use topical anesthetics

- Drug hypersensitivity

Adverse reactions

- Hypersensitivity

Key nursing actions

- Assess the area where topical anesthetic is to be applied before, during, and after application.
- Don't apply a refrigerated topical anesthetic to broken skin or mucous membranes.

TOP 6

Items to study for your next test on drugs and pain

1. Mechanisms of action of opioid and nonopioid analgesics, opioid and opioid-agonist antagonists, and general and local anesthetics

2. Nursing responsibilities when administering analgesics

3. Effects of general anesthesia and local anesthesia on a patient who undergoes surgery

4. Nursing measures that may enhance the therapeutic response to analgesics.

5. Nursing responsibilities when caring for a patient receiving a general or local anesthetic

6. Appropriate teaching for the patient who is receiving an analgesic or anesthetic

● Interactions
- Increased risk of lidocaine toxicity if lidocaine is used with beta-adrenergic blockers or cimetidine

● Nursing responsibilities
- Assess the area where the topical anesthetic is to be applied before, during, and after drug administration
- Don't apply a refrigerated topical anesthetic (such as ethyl chloride) to broken skin or mucous membranes
- Watch for signs of localized frostbite in patients receiving a refrigerant (such as ethyl chloride) or for skin irritation with other topical anesthetics
- Discontinue the drug if a rash develops

NCLEX CHECKS

It's never too soon to begin your NCLEX® examination preparation. Now that you've reviewed this chapter, carefully read each of the following questions and choose the best answer. Then compare your responses with the correct answers.

1. A client is hospitalized with terminal cancer. For the past 3 weeks, he has been receiving morphine, 5 mg I.V., every 4 hours, and has experienced relief from pain. He now says pain is still present, even after receiving the drug. The nurse recognizes that this client:
- ☐ **1.** has become dependent on the drug.
- ☐ **2.** has developed a tolerance to the opioid.
- ☐ **3.** resents that the nurse is healthy and he isn't.
- ☐ **4.** is seeking attention for himself because of poor self-image.

2. Which symptoms should a nurse observe in an adult client developing salicylism?
- ☐ **1.** Rash and bronchial wheezing
- ☐ **2.** Respiratory depression and acidosis
- ☐ **3.** Respiratory alkalosis and tachypnea
- ☐ **4.** Bleeding from the gums and blood in the urine

3. A client in the intensive care unit was given an accidental overdose of morphine. He's unconscious and has slow, shallow respirations at a rate of 8 breaths/minute. What drug should be given?
- ☐ **1.** Flumazenil (Romazicon)
- ☐ **2.** Naloxone (Narcan)
- ☐ **3.** Naltrexone (ReVia)
- ☐ **4.** Norepinephrine (Levophed)

4. A client who's taking the NSAID naproxen (Naprosyn) for his osteoarthritis has recently started taking a thiazide diuretic for moderate hypertension. Which instruction is the most important for the nurse to give to this client?

☐ **1.** Stick to the therapeutic regimen.
☐ **2.** Watch for GI bleeding.
☐ **3.** Have regular blood pressure checks.
☐ **4.** Increase dietary fiber to avoid constipation.

5. During a thoracotomy, a client received halothane and nitrous oxide. After the surgery, the nurse monitors him closely. Which adverse reaction to inhalation anesthetics is most common?

☐ **1.** Respiratory distress
☐ **2.** Nausea and vomiting
☐ **3.** Hypersensitivity reaction
☐ **4.** Exaggerated response to a normal dose

6. A physician orders a topical anesthetic to relieve a child's pain from a knee abrasion. When instructing the child's parents about the drug, the nurse should tell them to be alert for:

☐ **1.** minor pain.
☐ **2.** arrhythmias.
☐ **3.** signs of infection.
☐ **4.** rash, pruritus, and breathing difficulty.

7. A physician orders an I.V. push of 0.6 mg naloxone (Narcan) for a client. The vial has a concentration of 0.4 mg/ml. How many milliliters of naloxone hydrochloride should the client receive per dose? Record your answer using one decimal place.

_____ milliliters

8. A nurse should question an order for celecoxib written for a client with which condition?

☐ **1.** A sprained knee
☐ **2.** Unstable angina
☐ **3.** Painful menses
☐ **4.** Arthritis of the hands

9. Which drug is most appropriate to give preoperatively to a client scheduled for a skin biopsy?

☐ **1.** Acetaminophen (Tylenol)
☐ **2.** Pentazocine (Talwin)
☐ **3.** Mepivacaine (Carbocaine)
☐ **4.** Thiopental sodium (Pentothal)

10. A nurse administering oxycodone (OxyContin) to a client should be most concerned about which finding?

☐ **1.** The client complains of dizziness when standing up.

☐ **2.** The client is asleep and has a respiratory rate of 6 breaths/minute.

☐ **3.** The client experiences nausea 15 minutes after taking the medication.

☐ **4.** The client states he's more tired than usual and takes a nap in the afternoon.

ANSWERS AND RATIONALES

1. CORRECT ANSWER: 2

Long-term use of central nervous system drugs can lead to tolerance, which means that increased doses of the drug are needed to achieve the same effect. Clients being treated with opioids for chronic pain may require higher doses of the drug for effective pain relief. Dependency usually isn't an issue in treating terminally ill cancer patients. Lack of pain relief doesn't necessarily indicate dependency. The nurse can't conclude that the client has a poor self-image or feels resentful based on the information given.

2. CORRECT ANSWER: 3

Salicylate (aspirin) levels directly stimulate the respiratory centers in the central nervous system, thereby resulting in tachypnea and respiratory alkalosis. Rash and bronchial wheezing are signs of an allergic reaction to salicylates. Respiratory depression and acidosis aren't commonly associated with high salicylate levels. Bleeding is an adverse reaction to salicylates.

3. CORRECT ANSWER: 2

Morphine is an opioid and the client needs an opioid receptor antagonist. Naloxone is a rapid-acting parenteral opiate antagonist. Flumazenil is a benzodiazepine antagonist. Naltrexone is available only in oral form and is too slow-acting for this client. Norepinephrine isn't involved in the mechanism of action of opioids and would be ineffective.

4. CORRECT ANSWER: 3

NSAIDs taken with thiazide diuretics can cause reduced antihypertensive and diuretic effects, so blood pressure must be checked regularly and the client should be alert for signs of fluid retention. Although it's important for the nurse to encourage the client to stick to the therapeutic regimen, stressing the importance of regular blood pressure checks takes priority. Using naproxen with oral anticoagulants or corticosteroids (not diuretics) may increase the risk of GI bleeding. Using naproxen with other drugs has no effect on bowel pattern, so the client need not increase dietary fiber.

5. CORRECT ANSWER: 4

Because the client is receiving two inhaled drugs, the most common adverse reaction would be an exaggerated response to the normal dose, most likely because of predisposing medical conditions before surgery. Hypersensitivity is a potential adverse reaction that's more common with injection anesthetics. Although nausea, vomiting, and respiratory distress may occur postoperatively, they aren't as common as an exaggerated response.

6. CORRECT ANSWER: 4

Rash, pruritus, and breathing difficulty indicate a hypersensitivity reaction and can be caused by a topical anesthetic. Minor pain should be relieved with, not caused by, the use of topical anesthetics. Arrhythmias are common with inhalation or injection anesthetics. The risk of infection is always present with an injury or surgery.

7. CORRECT ANSWER: 1.5

To calculate how many milliliters the client should receive per dose, use this formula:

$$0.6 \text{ mg}: X \text{ ml} : 0.4 \text{ mg}: 1 \text{ ml}$$
$$0.4 \text{ mg} \times X \text{ ml} = 1 \text{ ml} \times 0.6 \text{ mg}$$

To solve for X, divide both sides by 0.4 mg:

$$X = 1.5 \text{ ml}$$

8. CORRECT ANSWER: 2

Celecoxib increases the risk of thromboembolic events, including MI, and shouldn't be given to client with a history of heart disease. Celecoxib is appropriate for a client with a sprained knee, painful menses, or arthritis of the hands.

9. CORRECT ANSWER: 3

Mepivacaine is a local anesthetic that can be used to anesthetize the area of a skin biopsy preoperatively. Acetaminophen may be appropriate for the client to take after the procedure; it won't provide adequate pain relief before. Pentazocine is a mixed opioid agonist-antagonist and may provide some pain relief, but it isn't the most appropriate medication for this client. Thiopental sodium is an injectable anesthetic; a skin biopsy doesn't call for the use of general anesthesia.

10. CORRECT ANSWER: 2

Respiratory depression is a serious adverse reaction associated with opioid agonists. A respiratory rate of 6 breaths/minute is too slow and requires immediate intervention. Orthostatic hypotension and nausea are common adverse reactions to oxycodone, but aren't cause for immediate concern. To help prevent these effects, the nurse should administer the medication with food, and remain with the client when he's standing up. Drowsiness is also a common adverse reaction seen with oxycodone; it isn't an immediate concern.

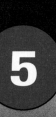

Drugs and mood alteration

5

PRETEST

1. Which medication is commonly used to treat bipolar affective disorder?
☐ 1. Propofol (Diprivan)
☐ 2. Temazepam (Restoril)
☐ 3. Lithium (Eskalith)
☐ 4. Haloperidol (Haldol)

CORRECT ANSWER: 3

2. A common adverse effect of an antipsychotic is:
☐ 1. extrapyramidal symptoms.
☐ 2. tachycardia.
☐ 3. diarrhea.
☐ 4. nausea.

CORRECT ANSWER: 1

3. Which teaching point is important for a client taking an antimanic drug?
☐ 1. Limit salt consumption.
☐ 2. Drink at least 2 qt (2 L) of water daily.
☐ 3. Blood tests aren't necessary while taking the drug.
☐ 4. The drug dose will never change.

CORRECT ANSWER: 2

4. Barbiturates work by enhancing the effects of which neurotransmitter?

☐ 1. Acetylcholine

☐ 2. Dopamine

☐ 3. Glutamate

☐ 4. Gamma-aminobutyric acid

CORRECT ANSWER: 4

5. Which medication is commonly used as an anxiolytic?

☐ 1. Pentobarbital (Nembutal)

☐ 2. Alprazolam (Xanax)

☐ 3. Fluphenazine (Prolixin)

☐ 4. Loxapine (Loxitane)

CORRECT ANSWER: 2

LEARNING OBJECTIVES

After studying this chapter, you should be able to:

- Identify medications commonly used as mood-altering drugs.
- Describe the mechanism of action and indications for sedative-hypnotics, anxiolytics, antipsychotics, antidepressants, and antimanics.
- Describe precautions the nurse must take when administering mood-altering drugs.
- List the common adverse effects of the different types of sedative-hypnotics, anxiolytics, antipsychotics, antidepressants, and antimanics.
- Identify nursing responsibilities and patient teaching needed when administering mood-altering drugs.

CHAPTER OVERVIEW

Sedative-hypnotics, anxiolytics, antipsychotics (or neuroleptics), and antidepressants all depress the central nervous system (CNS). The degree of CNS depression is dose dependent. Sedative-hypnotics and anxiolytics are prescribed for their calming effect and ability to reduce anxiety. These drugs can produce physiologic and psychological dependence and tolerance; many are controlled substances, having the potential for abuse, and are generally prescribed for short-term use.

Antipsychotics are used to manage schizophrenia and psychotic depression and to treat bipolar disorder (characterized by periods of euphoria and excessive activity, depression, or both) unresponsive to lithium. These drugs are useful for controlling psychotic symptoms, including thought disturbances, hallucinations, and delusions.

Antidepressants are used to treat depression, a mood disorder characterized by sadness, hopelessness, worthlessness, agitation, or anxiety. These drugs inhibit the reuptake of norepinephrine, leaving more available to the CNS. The antimanic agents lithium carbonate and lithium citrate are the treatment of choice for bipolar disorder, although certain anticonvulsants also may be used.

ANATOMY AND PHYSIOLOGY

● Anatomy
- Psychosocial and biological factors play key roles in psychopathology
- Abnormal neurotransmission can occur among several neurotransmitters: acetylcholine, dopamine, gamma-aminobutyric acid (GABA), glutamate, serotonin, and norepinephrine
- Neuronal signaling occurs in the CNS

● Physiology
- Neurotransmitters released from presynaptic neuron relay impulses across synapse to receptors on postsynaptic neuron
- Binding of neurotransmitters to respective receptors produces physiologic responses that indirectly affect behavior

● Function
- Psychopharmacology alters neurotransmission in the CNS, which influences behavior
- Psychoactive drugs aren't intended to cure psychiatric disorders; rather, they provide symptomatic relief of psychotic disorders

SEDATIVE-HYPNOTICS AND ANXIOLYTICS
BARBITURATES

● Mechanism of action
- Exact mechanism unknown; may cause generalized CNS depression by mimicking or enhancing effects of GABA in brain

---

Pharmacokinetics
- Absorption: Rapidly absorbed in GI tract
- Distribution: Rapidly and widely distributed
- Metabolism: Metabolized by the liver
- Excretion: Excreted in feces

Drug examples
- Rapidacting barbiturates: thiopental (Pentothal)
- Short-acting barbiturates: pentobarbital (Nembutal), secobarbital (Seconal sodium)
- Longacting barbiturates: phenobarbital (Luminal)

Indications
- Induce anesthesia (rapid-acting barbiturates)
- Treat insomnia and as adjuncts to anesthesia (short-acting barbiturates)
- Treat insomnia and seizures (long-acting barbiturates)

Contraindications and precautions
- Contraindicated in pregnant patients, patients with uncontrolled pain, and those with a history of acute intermittent porphyria or preexisting CNS depression
- Used cautiously in suicidal patients, those with a history of drug addiction, and elderly patients (may require a decreased dosage)

Adverse reactions
- Hangover feeling, slurred speech, and paradoxical excitement in the elderly and those in severe pain; drowsiness; lethargy; depression; hypotension; hypoventilation; decreased respiratory rate; dizziness; nausea; vomiting; headache; and allergic reaction
- Possibly rapid tolerance to drug

Interactions
- May increase metabolism and decrease effectiveness of many concurrently used drugs (such as warfarin, beta-adrenergic blockers, corticosteroids, tricyclic antidepressants, theophylline, and hormonal contraceptives)
- Use with herbal preparations (such as valerian and kava) causes additive CNS effects
- Use with valproic acid increases drug's serum levels
- Use with monoamine oxidase (MAO) inhibitors decreases metabolism and increases drug's adverse effects
- Concurrent use with acetaminophen increases risk of liver toxicity

Nursing responsibilities
- Administer I.V. doses slowly because rapid administration may cause respiratory and cardiovascular depression; have emergency resuscitation equipment available
- Assess the patient's sleep patterns; barbiturates reduce rapid-eye-movement sleep
- Base patient evaluation on decreased insomnia without excessive daytime sedation
- Know that many sedative-hypnotics are controlled substances

When to use barbiturates
- Anesthesia
- Insomnia
- Seizures

When NOT to use barbiturates
- Pregnancy
- Uncontrolled pain
- History of acute intermittent porphyria or CNS depression

Adverse reactions
- Hangover feeling, slurred speech, paradoxical excitement, drowsiness, lethargy, hypoventilation, nausea, vomiting

Key nursing actions
- Administer I.V. doses slowly.
- Assess patient's sleep patterns.
- Know that many sedative-hypnotics are controlled substances.
- Limit amount of medication available to patient.
- Know that long-term use of these drugs may cause physical and psychological dependence.
- Monitor patient's respiratory status.

Topics for patient discussion

- Therapy regimen
- Signs and symptoms of possible adverse reactions
- Activity restrictions
- Safety measures
- Avoidance of alcohol and OTC antihistamines and other CNS depressants
- Notification of practitioner before using other prescription drugs
- Possibility of dependence and tolerance
- Need for compliance with therapy and medical follow-up

TIME-OUT FOR TEACHING

Teaching about sedative-hypnotics

Include these topics in your teaching plan for the patient receiving a sedative-hypnotic:
- medication therapy regimen, including drug name, dose, frequency, duration, and possible adverse effects
- signs and symptoms of possible adverse effects and when to notify the practitioner
- activity restrictions, such as motor vehicle operation or other hazardous activities
- safety measures

- avoidance of alcohol and self-medication with over-the-counter (OTC) products containing alcohol, antihistamines, or other central nervous system depressants
- notification of the practitioner before using other prescription drugs, such as opioids or pain relievers
- possibility of dependence and tolerance
- compliance with therapy and medical follow-up.

- Limit the amount of medication available to the patient to prevent hoarding of drug, especially when risk of suicide exists
- Know that the long-term use of sedative-hypnotics may cause tolerance and physical and psychological dependence
- Inform the patient that the dosage should be decreased gradually after longterm use to prevent withdrawal symptoms
- Caution the patient to avoid driving and other activities requiring alertness until drug response is known (see *Teaching about sedative-hypnotics*)
- Warn the patient to avoid alcohol and other CNS depressants
- Monitor the patient's respiratory status to detect respiratory depression
- Institute safety precautions to prevent injury
- Monitor serum drug levels to help minimize toxicity

BENZODIAZEPINES

Mechanism of action
- Cause generalized CNS depression by mimicking or enhancing the effects of GABA by antagonizing a protein that inhibits GABA binding to its receptors

Pharmacokinetics
- Absorption: Well absorbed in GI tract
- Distribution: Highly protein-bound; widely and rapidly distributed into tissues, especially the brain
- Metabolism: Metabolized by the liver
- Excretion: Excreted in urine

Drug examples
- Alprazolam (Xanax, Xanax XR), chlordiazepoxide (Librium), clonazepam (Klonopin), clorazepate (Tranxene), diazepam (Valium), estazolam (Pro-

Key facts about benzodiazepines

- Cause generalized CNS depression by mimicking or enhancing the effects of GABA
- Metabolized by the liver
- Excreted in the urine

Som), flurazepam (Dalmane), lorazepam (Ativan), midazolam (Versed), quazepam (Doral), temazepam (Restoril), triazolam (Halcion)

Indications
- Relaxation before surgery and for I.V. anesthesia
- Promote skeletal muscle relaxation
- Treat insomnia, anxiety, seizure disorders, and alcohol withdrawal symptoms

Contraindications and precautions
- Contraindicated in pregnant or breast-feeding patients; patients with uncontrolled pain, preexisting CNS depression, or acute angle-closure glaucoma; and patients who are suicidal or who have a history of substance abuse
- Used cautiously in elderly patients (may require a decreased dosage) and in those with renal or hepatic impairment

Adverse reactions
- Commonly causes drowsiness, ataxia, temporary memory impairments, and reactions of rage, excitement, or hostility
- Possible increased depression, confusion, muscle weakness, dry mouth, vertigo, nausea, and vomiting

Interactions
- Use with herbal preparations (such as valerian, chamomile, and kava) causes additive CNS effects
- Use with antihistamines, barbiturates, MAO inhibitors, other cyclic antidepressants, or alcohol increases CNS depression

Nursing responsibilities
- Administer I.V. doses slowly to prevent respiratory depression or apnea
- Don't discontinue a drug abruptly after long-term administration; may result in withdrawal symptoms
- Administer with food to minimize GI upset
- Monitor renal and liver function tests periodically
- Assess patient's anxiety before therapy and frequently thereafter
- Instruct the patient to notify the practitioner if dose becomes ineffective after a few weeks—but *not* to increase the dosage unless instructed to do so

NONBARBITURATES

Mechanism of action
- Cause generalized CNS depression

Pharmacokinetics
- Absorption: Rapidly absorbed
- Distribution: Widely distributed into tissues
- Metabolism: Metabolized by the liver
- Excretion: Excreted in feces

When to use benzodiazepines

- Anxiety
- Alcohol withdrawal
- Preoperative sedation
- Insomnia
- Seizures
- Skeletal muscle relaxation

When NOT to use benzodiazepines

- Pregnancy
- Uncontrolled pain
- Preexisting CNS depression
- Acute angle-closure glaucoma

Adverse reactions

- Commonly drowsiness; ataxia; temporary memory impairments; reactions of rage, excitement, or hostility
- Possibly confusion, dry mouth, nausea

Key nursing actions

- Administer I.V. doses slowly.
- Instruct patient to notify practitioner if dose becomes ineffective after a few weeks.
- Advise patient not to increase dosage unless instructed by practitioner.
- Don't discontinue abruptly.

Key facts about nonbarbiturate sedative-hypnotics and anxiolytics

- Cause generalized CNS depression
- Metabolized by the liver
- Excreted in the feces

When to use nonbarbiturate sedative-hypnotics and anxiolytics

- Insomnia
- Preoperative sedation
- General anesthesia

When NOT to use nonbarbiturate sedative-hypnotics and anxiolytics

- Pregnancy
- Uncontrolled pain
- Preexisting CNS depression

Adverse reactions

- Drowsiness, respiratory depression, nausea, vomiting

Key nursing actions

- Use Z-track method of injection (hydroxyzine).
- Administer after meals (chloral hydrate).
- Know that long-term use may cause dependence.

Key facts about phenothiazines

- Block the neurotransmitter dopamine in the limbic system, inhibiting transmission of neural impulses
- Inhibit the chemoreceptor trigger zone in the medulla of the brain
- Metabolized by the liver
- Excreted mostly in the urine

● **Drug examples**
- Buspirone (BuSpar), chloral hydrate, diphenhydramine (Benadryl, Sominex), hydroxyzine (Atarax, Vistaril), meprobamate (Miltown), promethazine (Anergan 50, Phenergan), propofol (Diprivan), ramelteon (Rozerem), zaleplon (Sonata), zolpidem (Ambien)

● **Indications**
- Short-term treatment of simple insomnia
- Sedation before surgery and during electroencephalogram studies
- General anesthetic (propofol)

● **Contraindications and precautions**
- Contraindicated in pregnant patients and in those with uncontrolled pain or preexisting CNS depression
- Used cautiously in suicidal patients, elderly patients (may require a decreased dosage), and those with a history of drug addiction

● **Adverse reactions**
- Drowsiness, respiratory depression, nausea, vomiting, and hangover effect

● **Interactions**
- Concurrent use with alcohol, antidepressants, antihistamines, or phenothiazines may potentiate CNS depression; can be lethal
- Use with herbal preparations (such as valerian or kava) may have additive effects
- Use with I.V. furosemide may cause sweating, flushing, and variable blood pressure

● **Nursing responsibilities**
- Use a Z-track injection method to prevent tissue irritation when administering hydroxyzine I.M.
- Administer chloral hydrate after meals to minimize GI irritation
- Know that diphenhydramine is an ingredient in over-the-counter hypnotics
- Keep in mind that these drugs aren't for long-term treatment of insomnia; efficacy in promoting sleep decreases after 14 days
- Know that long-term use may cause drug dependence; withdrawal symptoms may occur if drug is stopped suddenly

ANTIPSYCHOTICS

PHENOTHIAZINES

● **Mechanism of action**
- Block dopamine in the limbic system, inhibiting transmission of neural impulses (antipsychotic action)
- Inhibits the medulla's chemoreceptor trigger zone

● **Pharmacokinetics**
- Absorption: Readily absorbed orally and parenterally; absorbed over weeks with long-acting depot I.M. administration

- Distribution: Widely distributed; highly protein-bound
- Metabolism: Metabolized by the liver
- Excretion: Excreted mostly in urine

● **Drug examples**
- Chlorpromazine (Thorazine), fluphenazine (Prolixin), mesoridazine (Serentil), perphenazine (Trilafon), prochlorperazine (Compazine), thiethylperazine (Torecan), thioridazine (Mellaril), thiothixene (Navane), trifluoperazine

● **Indications**
- Treat psychosis, schizophrenia, schizoaffective disorder, depression with psychotic features, and psychotic symptoms associated with organic brain syndrome (fluphenazine, mesoridazine, perphenazine, prochlorperazine, thioridazine, thiothixene, and trifluoperazine)
- Treat nausea and vomiting (chlorpromazine, perphenazine, prochlorperazine, and thiethylperazine)

● **Contraindications and precautions**
- Contraindicated in patients with angle-closure glaucoma or CNS depression; pregnant patients in their first trimester; patients who are comatose or likely to experience significant CNS depression from other substances or medications; and those at risk for suicide
- Must be withheld 48 hours before and 24 hours after myelography with metrizamide because phenothiazines may reduce the seizure threshold
- Used cautiously in elderly patients and those with acute myocardial infarction (MI), heart disease, benign prostatic hyperplasia, orthostatic hypotension, or respiratory distress (including asthma and emphysema)
- Thioridazine, which prolongs the QT interval, contraindicated in patients with cardiac arrhythmias and those taking fluvoxamine, propranolol, pindolol, fluoxetine, or any other drug that prolongs the QT interval

● **Adverse reactions**
- Extrapyramidal symptoms (such as akathisia, dystonia, and parkinsonism), tardive dyskinesia, neuroleptic malignant syndrome, sedation, blurred vision, dry mouth, constipation, blood dyscrasias, photosensitivity reaction (may cause temporary blue-gray skin pigmentation on exposed surfaces), sunburn, and heat intolerance

● **Interactions**
- Potentiates effects of alcohol and CNS depressants
- Concurrent use with antihypertensives and nitrates causes additive hypotension
- Concurrent use with lithium increases the risk of toxicity
- Use with antacids decreases drug absorption
- Use with neuroleptics decreases the seizure threshold; increased doses of anticonvulsants may be needed
- Concurrent use with anticholinergics (including antihistamines, antiparkinsonians, and antidepressants) may increase anticholinergic adverse effects

When to use phenothiazines

- Psychosis, schizophrenia, schizoaffective disorder, depression with psychotic features, psychotic symptoms associated with organic brain syndrome
- Nausea and vomiting

When NOT to use phenothiazines

- Angle-closure glaucoma
- CNS depression
- Pregnancy (first trimester)
- Coma
- Risk of suicide

Adverse reactions

- Extrapyramidal symptoms, tardive dyskinesia, neuroleptic malignant syndrome, sedation, blurred vision, dry mouth, constipation, blood dyscrasias, photosensitivity reaction, sunburn, heat intolerance

Key nursing actions

- Tell patient that phenothiazines may discolor urine to pink or red-brown.
- Instruct patient to call practitioner before taking over-the-counter or herbal preparations.
- Monitor QT interval in patient taking thioridazine.

Key facts about butyrophenones

- Block the neurotransmitter dopamine in the limbic system, inhibiting the transmission of neural impulses
- Inhibit the chemoreceptor trigger zone in the medulla of the brain
- Metabolized by the liver
- Excreted mostly in the urine

When to use butyrophenones

- Nausea and vomiting during surgery and diagnostic procedures
- As adjunct to anesthesia
- Psychosis, Tourette syndrome, behavioral problems in children with explosive hyperexcitability, hyperactivity in hyperactive children

When NOT to use butyrophenones

- Angle-closure glaucoma
- CNS depression

Adverse reactions

- Extrapyramidal symptoms, tardive dyskinesia, neuroleptic malignant syndrome, sedation, blurred vision, dry mouth, constipation, blood dyscrasias, photosensitivity reaction, sunburn, heat intolerance

● **Nursing responsibilities**
- Inform the patient that phenothiazines may discolor urine pink or red-brown; offer reassurance that this color change is harmless
- Instruct the patient to consult the practitioner before taking over-the-counter or herbal preparations during drug therapy
- Monitor the QT interval in the patient taking thioridazine
- Monitor the patient for the onset of involuntary movements

BUTYROPHENONES

● **Mechanism of action**
- Block dopamine in the limbic system, inhibiting transmission of neural impulses (antipsychotic action)
- Inhibit the medulla's chemoreceptor trigger zone

● **Pharmacokinetics**
- Absorption: Readily absorbed orally and parenterally; absorbed over weeks with long-acting depot I.M. administration
- Distribution: Widely distributed; highly protein-bound
- Metabolism: Metabolized by the liver
- Excretion: Excreted mostly in urine

● **Drug examples**
- Droperidol (Inapsine), haloperidol (Haldol)

● **Indications**
- Treat nausea and vomiting during surgery and diagnostic procedures and as an adjunct to anesthesia in combination with fentanyl (droperidol)
- Treat psychosis, Tourette syndrome, and behavioral problems in children with combative, explosive hyperexcitability and hyperactivity in hyperactive children (haloperidol)

● **Contraindications and precautions**
- Contraindicated in patients with angle-closure glaucoma and CNS depression
- Must be withheld 48 hours before and 24 hours after myelography with metrizamide because butyrophenones may reduce the seizure threshold
- Used cautiously in patients with acute MI, heart disease, benign prostatic hyperplasia, and orthostatic hypotension
- Droperidol contraindicated in patients with known or suspected QT prolongation

● **Adverse reactions**
- Extrapyramidal symptoms, tardive dyskinesia, neuroleptic malignant syndrome, sedation, blurred vision, dry mouth, constipation, blood dyscrasias, photosensitivity reaction (may cause temporary blue-gray skin pigmentation on exposed surfaces), sunburn, and heat intolerance

Interactions

- Potentiates effects of alcohol and CNS depressants
- Concurrent use with antihypertensives and nitrates causes additive hypotension
- Use of antacids decreases drug absorption
- Neuroleptics decrease the seizure threshold; increased doses of anticonvulsants may be needed

Nursing responsibilities

- Instruct the patient to avoid driving or performing other hazardous activities until CNS effects are known
- Advise the patient to avoid alcohol or other CNS depressants during drug therapy because of possible additive effects and hypotension

ATYPICAL ANTIPSYCHOTICS

Mechanism of action

- Block dopamine in the limbic system, inhibiting transmission of neural impulses (antipsychotic action)
- Inhibit the medulla's chemoreceptor trigger zone

Pharmacokinetics

- Absorption: Readily absorbed orally and parenterally; absorbed over weeks with long-acting depot I.M. administration
- Distribution: Widely distributed; highly protein-bound
- Metabolism: Metabolized by the liver
- Excretion: Excreted mostly in urine

Drug examples

- Clomipramine (Anafranil), clozapine (Clozaril), loxapine (Loxitane), molindone (Moban), olanzapine (Zyprexa), quetiapine (Seroquel), risperidone (Risperdal), ziprasidone (Geodon)

Indications

- Manage psychotic disorders, such as schizophrenia and schizoaffective disorders
- Treat obsessive-compulsive disorder (clomipramine)
- Treat bipolar disorder (olanzapine and risperidone)
- Reduce risk of recurrent suicidal behavior in patients with schizophrenia and schizoaffective disorders (clozapine)

Contraindications and precautions

- Contraindicated in patients with angle-closure glaucoma and CNS depression
- Must be withheld 48 hours before and 24 hours after myelography with metrizamide because atypical antipsychotics may reduce the seizure threshold
- Used cautiously in patients with acute MI, heart disease, benign prostatic hyperplasia, and orthostatic hypotension

---

Key nursing actions

- Tell patient to avoid driving or other hazardous activities until CNS effects of drug are known.
- Advise patient to avoid alcohol and other CNS depressants during therapy.

Key facts about atypical antipsychotics

- Block the neurotransmitter dopamine in the limbic system, inhibiting the transmission of neural impulses
- Inhibit the chemoreceptor trigger zone in the medulla of the brain
- Metabolized by the liver
- Excreted mostly in the urine

When to use atypical antipsychotics

- Psychotic disorders, such as schizophrenia and schizoaffective disorders
- Obsessive-compulsive disorder
- Bipolar disorder
- Risk of recurrent suicidal behavior

When NOT to use atypical antipsychotics

- Angle-closure glaucoma
- CNS depression

Adverse reactions

- Extrapyramidal symptoms, tardive dyskinesia, neuroleptic malignant syndrome, sedation, blurred vision, dry mouth, constipation, blood dyscrasias, photosensitivity reaction, sunburn, heat intolerance

Key nursing actions

- Assess patient's mental status.
- Monitor patient for extrapyramidal symptoms and other adverse reactions.
- If patient is recovering from anesthesia with droperidol or fentanyl, decrease opioid analgesic dosages to one-quarter to one-third of normal.
- After parenteral doses, monitor patient for orthostatic hypotension.
- Know that patient receiving long-term antipsychotic therapy should undergo regular evaluation of red and white blood cell counts.
- Don't give antacids within 1 hour of administering these drugs.
- Know that drug should be discontinued gradually.
- Teach patient to:
  – comply with therapy
  – avoid alcohol and other CNS depressants
  – avoid driving and hazardous activities until CNS effects of drug are known
  – use sunscreen and wear protective clothing.

● **Adverse reactions**
- Extrapyramidal symptoms, tardive dyskinesia, neuroleptic malignant syndrome, sedation, blurred vision, dry mouth, constipation, blood dyscrasias, photosensitivity reaction (may cause temporary blue-gray skin pigmentation on exposed surfaces), sunburn, and heat intolerance
- Agranulocytosis, which requires close monitoring of white blood cell count (clozapine)
- Possible cataract development and increased liver function test values (quetiapine)
- Possible increased QT interval and prolactin levels (ziprasidone and risperidone)

● **Interactions**
- Use may potentiate the effects of alcohol and CNS depressants
- Concurrent use with antihypertensives and nitrates causes additive hypotension
- Use with antacids decreases drug absorption
- Use with neuroleptics decreases the seizure threshold; increased doses of anticonvulsants may be needed

● **Nursing responsibilities**
- Assess the patient's mental status; loss of contact with reality may signal noncompliance with drug therapy
- Monitor the patient for extrapyramidal symptoms and other adverse effects such as tardive dyskinesia, which is irreversible
- Decrease opioid analgesic dosages to one-quarter to one-third of normal if the patient is recovering from anesthesia with droperidol or fentanyl to prevent further CNS depression
- Monitor the patient for orthostatic hypotension after parenteral doses
- Know that the patient who receives long-term antipsychotic therapy should undergo regular evaluation of red and white blood cell counts to detect blood dyscrasias
- Know that the drug should be discontinued gradually
- Teach the patient about the importance of complying with therapy because these drugs may take several weeks to produce desired effects (see *Teaching about antipsychotics*)
- Warn the patient not to consume alcohol or take other CNS depressants while taking these drugs
- Caution the patient to avoid driving and other activities requiring alertness until response to drug is known
- Instruct the patient not to take antacids within 1 hour of taking drug
- Discuss ways to minimize dry mouth and constipation
- Urge the patient to use a sunscreen and protective clothing (to prevent photosensitivity reaction) and to avoid temperature extremes (to prevent heat intolerance)
- Base patient evaluation on improved interaction with others and greater participation in activities of daily living (or on resolution of nausea and vomiting with antiemetic use)

TIME-OUT FOR TEACHING

Teaching about antipsychotics

Include these topics in your teaching plan for the patient receiving an antipsychotic:

- medication therapy regimen, including drug name, dose, frequency, duration, and possible adverse effects
- signs and symptoms of possible adverse effects, including extrapyramidal effects and tardive dyskinesia, and when to notify the practitioner
- time required for the drug to reach maximum effectiveness
- safety measures
- avoidance of central nervous system depressants
- need for compliance with therapy and medical follow-up.

ANTIDEPRESSANTS

TRICYCLIC, QUADRACYCLIC, SECOND-GENERATION, AND MISCELLANEOUS ANTIDEPRESSANTS AND SSRIs

● **Mechanism of action**
  - Tricyclic and second-generation antidepressants: Increase the amount of norepinephrine or serotonin (or both) through reuptake inhibition, thus normalizing the hyposensitive receptor site associated with depression
  - Selective serotonin reuptake inhibitors (SSRIs): Block the reuptake of serotonin into presynaptic cells, thereby increasing serotonin levels at the synapse

● **Pharmacokinetics**
  - Absorption: Well absorbed in GI tract
  - Distribution: Widely distributed in tissues
  - Metabolism: Metabolized by the liver
  - Excretion: Excreted primarily in urine

● **Drug examples**
  - Tricyclic and quadracyclic antidepressants: amitriptyline (Elavil), amoxapine (Asendin), clomipramine (Anafranil), desipramine (Norpramin), doxepin (Sinequan), imipramine (Tofranil), mirtazapine (Remeron), nortriptyline (Pamelor), protriptyline (Vivactil)
  - Second-generation and miscellaneous antidepressants: bupropion (Wellbutrin), duloxetine (Cymbalta), fluoxetine (Prozac, Prozac Weekly, Sarafem), maprotiline, nefazodone (Serzone), trazodone (Desyrel), venlafaxine (Effexor)
  - SSRIs: citalopram (Celexa), escitalopram (Lexapro), fluoxetine (Prozac), fluvoxamine (Luvox), paroxetine (Paxil), sertraline (Zoloft)

● **Indications**
  - Treat endogenous depression
    - Tricyclic antidepressants are the drugs of choice for episodes of major depression

---

Topics for patient discussion

- Therapy regimen
- Signs and symptoms of possible adverse reactions
- Time required for drug to reach maximum effectiveness
- Safety measures
- Avoidance of alcohol and other CNS depressants
- Need for compliance with therapy and medical follow-up

Key facts about tricyclic, second-generation, and miscellaneous antidepressants and SSRIs

- Tricyclic and second-generation antidepressants increase the amount of norepinephrine, serotonin, or both through reuptake inhibition, thus normalizing the receptor site associated with depression
- SSRIs block the reuptake of serotonin into the presynaptic cells, thus increasing serotonin levels at the synapse
- Metabolized by the liver
- Excreted mostly in the urine

When to use tricyclic, second-generation, and miscellaneous antidepressants and SSRIs

- Endogenous depression; episodes of major depression
- Enuresis
- Anxiety
- Neurogenic pain (unlabeled use)
- Generalized anxiety disorder
- Obsessive-compulsive disorder
- Depression
- Bulimia nervosa
- Smoking cessation
- Premenstrual dysphoric disorder

– Second-generation antidepressants treat same major depressive episodes as tricyclic antidepressants; have same degree of effectiveness but fewer adverse effects

- Treat enuresis (imipramine)
- Treat anxiety (doxepin)
- Treat neurogenic pain—unlabeled use (amitriptyline, doxepin, imipramine, nortriptyline, and trazodone)
- Treat generalized anxiety disorder, depression, obsessive-compulsive disorder, and bulimia nervosa (SSRIs)
- Smoking cessation (fluoxetine and bupropion)
- Treat premenstrual dysphoric disorder (fluoxetine)
- Treat obsessive-compulsive disorder (clomipramine; first drug approved for this use)
- Management of diabetic neuropathic pain (duloxetine)

● Contraindications and precautions

- Concurrent use of antidepressants and MAO inhibitors contraindicated
- Should be discontinued 48 hours before and 24 hours after myelography involving metrizamide to prevent lowering the seizure threshold
- Increased risk in older patients for adverse effects from tricyclic antidepressants; SSRIs better tolerated
- Contraindicated in those with active liver disease (nefazodone)
- SSRIs used cautiously in elderly patients and those with hepatic or renal failure

● Adverse reactions

- Tricyclic and quadracyclic antidepressants may cause orthostatic hypotension, tachycardia, blurred vision, dry mouth, constipation, seizure, and rash; may exacerbate heart failure or existing bundle-branch block
- Second-generation antidepressants may cause seizures, insomnia, and nausea; some may cause anticholinergic effects
- Bupropion is distinguishable from all other tricyclic antidepressants because it doesn't cause drowsiness and has fewer cardiovascular and anticholinergic adverse effects
- SSRIs may cause insomnia, somnolence, drowsiness, fatigue, tremor, asthenia, or seizures; may also cause sexual disturbances, such as delayed ejaculation and anorgasmia

● Interactions

- Effectiveness of antihypertensives may be reduced
- Concurrent use with alcohol, antihistamines, or other CNS depressants causes additive CNS depression
- Antidepressant use with MAO inhibitors may cause hypertensive crisis and seizures
- SSRIs and MAO inhibitors or other serotonergic agents (such as clomipramine or buspirone) may cause serotonin syndrome

– Symptoms include fever, agitation, hypertension, hyperthermia, rigidity, and myoclonus
– Seizures, coma, or death may result
- Patient should wait 5 weeks before starting MAO inhibitor therapy after beginning fluoxetine; 2-week "washout" period should follow discontinuation of other SSRIs before MAO inhibitor therapy begins
- Patient shouldn't use these drugs with St. John's wort because the herb may cause additive CNS depression
- Tricyclic antidepressants cause photosensitivity; advise wearing protective clothing and using sunblock with prolonged exposure to sunlight
- Bupropion should be used cautiously with other drugs that affect hepatic metabolism
- Use of paroxetine with tryptophan can produce adverse reactions, such as headache, nausea, sweating, and dizziness
- Trazodone may produce additive effects when combined with other drugs

● **Nursing responsibilities**
- Know that these drugs should be discontinued gradually
- Teach the patient about the importance of complying with therapy
  – Tricyclics may take up to 30 days to reach their full therapeutic response
  – Amitriptyline may produce a therapeutic effect within 10 to 14 days
  – SSRIs may begin to take effect in 1 to 4 weeks
- Warn the patient to avoid alcohol and nonprescription drugs to prevent adverse drug interactions
- Caution the patient to avoid driving and other activities requiring alertness until drug effects are known
- Instruct the patient taking fluoxetine or paroxetine to take the drug early in the day to avoid interference with sleep; for patient using any other tricyclic antidepressant, daily dose should be taken at bedtime to avoid sedation or anticholinergic effects
- Tell the patient not to crush controlled-release tablets, but to swallow them whole

Key nursing actions

- Know that these drugs should be discontinued gradually.
- Know that these drugs may take several weeks to produce desired effects.
- Teach patient to:
  - avoid alcohol and nonprescription drugs
  - avoid driving and other hazardous activities until CNS effects of drug are known
  - take fluoxetine or paroxetine early in day
  - take daily dose of other tricyclic antidepressants at bedtime
  - not crush controlled-release tablets, but to swallow them whole.

MONOAMINE OXIDASE (MAO) INHIBITORS

● **Mechanism of action**
- Impairs inactivation of norepinephrine or serotonin (or both), prolonging its presence in CNS synapses and increasing its concentrations in the body

● **Pharmacokinetics**
- Absorption: Well absorbed from GI tract
- Distribution: Widely distributed
- Metabolism: Metabolized by the liver
- Excretion: Excreted mainly in feces

● **Drug examples**
- Phenelzine (Nardil), tranylcypromine (Parnate)

Key facts about MAO inhibitors

- Impair inactivation of norepinephrine, serotonin, or both, thus prolonging their presence in CNS synapses and increasing their concentrations in the body
- Metabolized by the liver
- Excreted mainly in the feces

When to use MAO inhibitors

- Atypical depression
- Panic disorder with associated agoraphobia

When NOT to use MAO inhibitors

- Hypersensitivity to drug or their components
- Pheochromocytomas, heart failure, liver disease or abnormal liver function test results, renal impairment, confirmed or suspected stroke, cardiovascular disease, hypertension, history of headaches
- With other MAO inhibitors, tricyclic antidepressants, anesthetics, CNS depressants, antihypertensives, caffeine, cheeses, or other foods high in tyramine

Adverse reactions

- Hypertensive crisis
- Restlessness, insomnia, dizziness, drowsiness, headache, orthostatic hypotension, anorexia, blurred vision, peripheral edema, constipation, dry mouth, nausea, and vomiting

● Indications
- Treatment of panic disorders with agoraphobia, eating disorders, post-traumatic stress syndrome, pain disorders, atypical depression, phobic anxieties, neurodermatitis, hypochondriasis, and refractory narcolepsy

● Contraindications and precautions
- Contraindicated in patients with known hypersensitivity to drug or its components and in those with pheochromocytoma, heart failure, liver disease or abnormal liver function test results, renal impairment, confirmed or suspected stroke, cardiovascular disease, hypertension, or history of headaches
- Concurrent administration with other MAO inhibitors, tricyclic antidepressants, anesthetics, CNS depressants, antihypertensives, caffeine, cheeses, or other foods high in tyramine contraindicated
- Used cautiously in pregnant and breast-feeding patients; patients with diabetes, epilepsy, or hyperthyroidism; elderly patients; and those who may be suicidal or have a history of drug dependence
- Safety and efficacy not established in children younger than age 16

● Adverse reactions
- Hypertensive crisis; can lead to death
- Restlessness, insomnia, dizziness, drowsiness, headache, orthostatic hypotension, weakness, joint pain, urine retention, anorexia, blurred vision, peripheral edema, constipation, dry mouth, nausea, and vomiting

● Interactions
- These drugs interact with most other drugs
- Concurrent use with amphetamines, antidepressants, dopamine, epinephrine, guanethidine, levodopa, methyldopa, nasal decongestants, norepinephrine, reserpine, tyramine-containing foods, and vasoconstrictors may cause hypertensive crisis
- Concurrent use with opioid analgesics may cause hypertension, hypotension, coma, or seizures; MAO inhibitors should be discontinued several weeks before surgery
- Concurrent use with high doses of tranylcypromine may cause dependence and addiction
- Serious, potentially fatal serotonin syndrome may occur with concurrent use of St. John's wort

● Nursing responsibilities
- Don't administer the drug in the evening; it may cause insomnia
- Assess the patient's mental status for mood changes and suicidal tendencies
- Advise the patient that it may take 1 to 4 weeks for antidepressant effects to occur
- Be alert for suicide attempts when depression begins to lift and energy improves
- Discontinue these drugs gradually

TIME-OUT FOR TEACHING

Teaching about MAO inhibitors

Include these topics in your teaching plan for the patient receiving a mono-amine oxidase (MAO) inhibitor:
- medication therapy regimen, including drug name, dose, frequency, duration, and possible adverse effects
- signs and symptoms of possible adverse effects and when to notify the practitioner
- signs and symptoms of hypertensive crisis
- dietary restrictions
- need to inform other health care providers about MAO therapy
- need for compliance with therapy and medical follow-up.

- Teach the patient about the importance of complying with therapy; drug may take several weeks to produce desired effects (see *Teaching about MAO inhibitors*)
- Caution the patient to avoid alcohol and foods containing tyramine (red wine, beer, aged cheeses, yeast, avocados, bananas, yogurt, smoked or pickled fish, chocolate, overripe fruit, and beverages containing caffeine) to prevent hypertensive crisis
- Monitor the patient for signs and symptoms of hypertensive crisis: increased blood pressure, severe headache, palpitations, neck stiffness or soreness, nausea, and vomiting
- Instruct the patient to carry identification describing the disorder and drug regimen

ANTIMANICS

● **Mechanism of action**
- Compete with calcium, magnesium, potassium, and sodium in body tissues and at the binding site; alter sodium transport in nerve and muscle cells
- Affect the synthesis, storage, release, and reuptake of central monoamine neurotransmitters; specific mechanism unknown
- May produce antimanic effects by increasing norepinephrine reuptake and serotonin sensitivity

● **Pharmacokinetics**
- Absorption: Readily absorbed from GI tract
- Distribution: Widely distributed in most body tissues
- Metabolism: Not metabolized
- Excretion: Excreted unchanged in urine

● **Drug examples**
- Lithium carbonate (Eskalith, Lithobid, Lithonate, Lithotabs), lithium citrate (Lithium Citrate Syrup)

When to use lithium

- Mania
- Bipolar affective disorders

When NOT to use lithium

- Renal or cardiovascular disease
- Breast-feeding
- Severe dehydration
- Severe sodium depletion
- Severe debilitation

Adverse reactions

- Hand tremors, transient muscle weakness, hypertonia, nausea, vomiting, bloating, diarrhea, anorexia, abdominal pains, mild thirst, polyuria, polydipsia, nephrogenic diabetes insipidus

Key nursing actions

- Know that long-term therapeutic range is 0.6 to 1.2 mEq/L.
- Know that tolerance for lithium is high in acute phase of mania and decreases as mania subsides.
- Assess for suicidal tendencies, and institute suicide precautions, as necessary.
- Assess patient for signs and symptoms of lithium toxicity, including vomiting, diarrhea, slurred speech, decreased coordination, drowsiness, muscle weakness, and twitching.
- Teach patient to:
- drink 2 to 3 L of fluid daily; maintain adequate salt intake; avoid excessive amounts of coffee, tea, and cola; and avoid activities that cause excess sodium loss
- consult practitioner before taking nonprescription drugs.

● Indications

- Treat mania and bipolar affective disorders (also known as *bipolar disorder*)

● Contraindications and precautions

- Contraindicated in patients with renal or cardiovascular disease, breast-feeding patients, and those with severe dehydration, sodium depletion, or debilitation because the risk of toxicity is increased
- Used cautiously in elderly patients and those with thyroid disease or diabetes mellitus
- Used during pregnancy only when benefits outweigh risks to fetus

● Adverse reactions

- Mild nausea and general discomfort during first few days; symptoms usually subside with continued treatment or temporary reduction or cessation of drug
- Reactions of the CNS, GI tract, and kidneys, including hand tremors, transient muscle weakness, hypertonia, nausea, vomiting, bloating, diarrhea, anorexia, abdominal pains, mild thirst, polyuria, polydipsia, and nephrogenic diabetes insipidus
- Possible hypothyroidism
- Lithium toxicity (characterized by confusion, lethargy, slurred speech, increased reflexes, and seizures)

● Interactions

- Concurrent use of diuretics, fluoxetine, methyldopa, or nonsteroidal anti-inflammatory drugs increases lithium reabsorption by the kidney or inhibits lithium excretion, either of which increases the risk of lithium toxicity
- Use of acetazolamide, aminophylline, or sodium bicarbonate or an increased sodium intake may increase renal excretion of lithium, reducing its effectiveness
- Lithium interferes with norepinephrine and may reduce the effects of antihypertensives
- Use with antipsychotics (such as phenothiazines and haloperidol) may increase lithium levels and cause neurotoxicity; may also cause acute encephalopathic syndrome (weakness, lethargy, fever, confusion, disorientation, and adverse extrapyramidal reactions)

● Nursing responsibilities

- Monitor serum lithium levels to evaluate drug effectiveness and prevent toxicity
- Know that the therapeutic range for long-term lithium use ranges from 0.6 to 1.2 mEq/L
- Be aware that tolerance for lithium is high in the acute phase of mania and then decreases as the mania subsides; effective lithium levels range from 1 to 1.5 mEq/L during acute mania and require dosage adjustment afterward

- Assess for suicidal tendencies; institute suicide precautions as necessary
- Administer drug with food to minimize GI irritation
- Monitor the patient's renal function before drug therapy begins and regularly thereafter because lithium is excreted renally
- Know that lithium toxicity can occur despite normal lithium levels; assess the patient for signs and symptoms of toxicity (vomiting, diarrhea, slurred speech, decreased coordination, drowsiness, muscle weakness, and twitching)
- Know that lithium depletes sodium reabsorption, causing sodium depletion in the body, which in turn increases the risk of lithium toxicity
- Instruct the patient to drink 2 to 3 qt (2 to 3 L) of fluid daily; maintain adequate salt intake; avoid excessive amounts of coffee, tea, and cola (have a diuretic effect); and avoid activities that cause excess sodium loss to help avoid lithium toxicity.
- Instruct the patient to consult the practitioner or pharmacist before taking nonprescription drugs to prevent adverse drug interactions
- Know that lithium can cause drowsiness, blackouts, and confusion; caution the patient to avoid hazardous activities or driving until CNS effects are known

NCLEX CHECKS

It's never too soon to begin your NCLEX® preparation. Now that you've reviewed this chapter, carefully read each of the following questions and choose the best answer. Then compare your responses with the correct answers.

1. A client taking a barbiturate such as pentobarbital (Nembutal) should be taught to:
- ☐ **1.** decrease the drug gradually rather than stop it abruptly.
- ☐ **2.** decrease the dose if drowsiness occurs.
- ☐ **3.** drink alcohol only in moderation.
- ☐ **4.** avoid driving a car while taking the drug.

2. Which drugs are thought to work by stimulating the inhibitory neurotransmitter GABA?
- ☐ **1.** Barbiturates
- ☐ **2.** Benzodiazepines
- ☐ **3.** SSRIs
- ☐ **4.** Tricyclic antidepressants

3. Which description of the anxiolytic buspirone (BuSpar) is accurate?
- ☐ **1.** It has a rapid onset of action.
- ☐ **2.** It has a high potential for abuse.
- ☐ **3.** It has more adverse reactions than benzodiazepines.
- ☐ **4.** It doesn't interact with alcohol.

TOP 7

Items to study for your next test on drugs and mood alteration

1. Medications commonly used as sedative-hypnotics, anxiolytics, antipsychotics, antidepressants, and antimanics
2. Mechanism of action of sedative-hypnotics, anxiolytics, antipsychotics, antidepressants, and antimanics
3. Indications for sedative-hypnotics, anxiolytics, antipsychotics, antidepressants, and antimanics
4. Precautions the nurse must take when administering sedative-hypnotics, anxiolytics, antipsychotics, antidepressants, or antimanics
5. Common adverse effects of sedative-hypnotics, anxiolytics, antipsychotics, antidepressants, and antimanics
6. Nursing responsibilities when administering sedative-hypnotics, anxiolytics, antipsychotics, antidepressants, or antimanics
7. Appropriate teaching for a patient receiving a sedative-hypnotic, an anxiolytic, an antipsychotic, an antidepressant, or an antimanic

4. A client with schizophrenia has been taking chlorpromazine (Thorazine) for several months and wants to attend a picnic on the 4th of July. The nurse would be most concerned about which of the drug's adverse reactions?

- ☐ **1.** Constipation
- ☐ **2.** Hypotension
- ☐ **3.** Increased appetite
- ☐ **4.** Photosensitivity

5. A client began taking haloperidol (Haldol) yesterday for schizophrenia. Today, he says that his neck feels stiff and he's having trouble walking. The nurse notes that his eyes are rolled slightly upward. Which change would the nurse expect the physician to make to this client's drug regimen?

- ☐ **1.** Change the drug to fluoxetine (Prozac).
- ☐ **2.** Add diazepam (Valium) to the regimen.
- ☐ **3.** Change the drug to fluphenazine (Prolixin).
- ☐ **4.** Add benztropine (Cogentin) 1 mg twice daily.

6. A postmenopausal client with major depression is started on fluoxetine (Prozac) therapy. What's the most important point to include in her discharge instructions?

- ☐ **1.** The daily dose of fluoxetine can be taken either in the morning or in the evening.
- ☐ **2.** A rash or itching may develop when the drug is first started, but it will go away.
- ☐ **3.** There are no restrictions about driving or other hazardous activities because the drug is nonsedating.
- ☐ **4.** Over-the-counter (OTC) or other prescription drugs are safe because few drug interactions occur with fluoxetine.

7. Which information is most important to tell a client who's being discharged with a prescription for amitriptyline (Elavil)?

- ☐ **1.** The drug will help reduce the symptoms of depression.
- ☐ **2.** Anxiety will disappear completely once the drug becomes effective.
- ☐ **3.** Pulmonary function studies should be performed periodically.
- ☐ **4.** Long-term use of the drug causes extrapyramidal adverse reactions.

8. When teaching a client about MAO inhibitors, the nurse should instruct the client to avoid foods containing which substance?

- ☐ **1.** Pyridoxine
- ☐ **2.** Riboflavin
- ☐ **3.** Thiamine
- ☐ **4.** Tyramine

9. A client started taking lithium for bipolar disorder. Which signs or symptoms signal to the nurse that the client's serum level of lithium is too high?

- ☐ **1.** Rash
- ☐ **2.** Hypothyroidism
- ☐ **3.** Fine hand tremor
- ☐ **4.** Elevated white blood cell count

10. A physician prescribes lithium for a client diagnosed with bipolar disorder. Which topics should the nurse cover when teaching this client? Select all that apply.

☐ **1.** Potential for addiction
☐ **2.** Signs and symptoms of drug toxicity
☐ **3.** Potential for tardive dyskinesia
☐ **4.** Information about a low-tyramine diet
☐ **5.** Need to monitor blood levels consistently
☐ **6.** Time frame (7 to 21 days) in which mood changes will take place

ANSWERS AND RATIONALES

1. CORRECT ANSWER: 1
Barbiturates should be tapered gradually. Stopping the drug abruptly may cause withdrawal symptoms, such as nausea, vomiting, muscle twitches, hallucinations, or seizures. Drowsiness is an expected adverse reaction of barbiturates. Dose adjustment isn't necessary. The client shouldn't drink alcohol during drug therapy because alcohol will potentiate CNS depressant effects. Driving a car isn't contraindicated during drug therapy; however, the client needs to know the drug's effects on mental alertness before operating a motor vehicle.

2. CORRECT ANSWER: 2
Benzodiazepines, which stimulate GABA, are used primarily as sedative-hypnotics. Examples of benzodiazepines include diazepam, flurazepam, and lorazepam. Barbiturates are general CNS depressants. SSRIs inhibit the neurotransmitter serotonin, not GABA. Tricyclic antidepressants inhibit norepinephrine and serotonin.

3. CORRECT ANSWER: 4
Buspirone is unlike other anxiolytics because it doesn't interact with alcohol or other central nervous system depressants. It has a slow onset of action, is less sedating, has fewer adverse reactions than benzodiazepines, and has a lower chance of being abused than other anxiolytics.

4. CORRECT ANSWER: 4
Thorazine may cause photosensitivity. Attending a July 4th picnic may expose the client to bright sunlight, which would put the client at risk for sunburn. Constipation shouldn't be a concern for this client. Hypotension is an occasional adverse reaction that usually occurs early in treatment. Increased appetite is also an occasional adverse reaction, but isn't of concern in this instance.

5. CORRECT ANSWER: 4
The client's symptoms are extrapyramidal reactions induced by the antipsychotic haloperidol. Adding an anticholinergic such as benztropine will reverse extrapyramidal reactions. Fluoxetine isn't effective for psychosis. There are no indications that the client would benefit from diazepam, a benzodiazepine. Fluphenazine has the same risk of extrapyramidal reactions as haloperidol.

6. CORRECT ANSWER: 2

Some of the less serious adverse effects of fluoxetine, such as rash and itching, occur when the drug is first taken, but these are easily controlled with antihistamines or corticosteroids and usually subside with continued therapy. The drug should be taken in the morning; evening doses may cause insomnia. Fluoxetine is less sedating than many other psychotropic drugs; however, some clients experience dizziness and drowsiness when first starting the drug, so driving and performing other hazardous activities should be avoided. The drug interacts with many other drugs, so the client should be encouraged to check with the prescriber before taking any OTC medications.

7. CORRECT ANSWER: 1

Amitriptyline is a tricyclic antidepressant that increases the levels of serotonin and norepinephrine in the neurons, thereby reducing the symptoms of depression. It usually isn't possible to be completely anxiety-free. Liver and renal function and blood counts, not pulmonary function, should be monitored for clients on long-term therapy. Extrapyramidal adverse reactions occur from long-term use of phenothiazines, not amitriptyline.

8. CORRECT ANSWER: 4

Clients receiving MAO inhibitors should avoid foods containing tyramine because of the risk of a hypertensive crisis. Tyramine is contained in foods such as aged cheese, coffee, avocados, bananas, ales, red wines, and other undistilled beverages. The need for a restrictive diet makes the use of MAO inhibitors difficult. These drugs may also interact adversely with other drugs, further limiting their use. MAO inhibitors usually are prescribed in dire situations when other drugs don't work. The intake of thiamine, riboflavin, and pyridoxine (water-soluble vitamins) isn't limited with MAO inhibitors.

9. CORRECT ANSWER: 3

Although all of the symptoms are potential adverse reactions to lithium, only hand tremor occurs as a result of increased serum lithium levels. Rash, hypothyroidism, and elevated white blood cell count aren't dose-related and can occur even with low lithium serum levels.

10. CORRECT ANSWER: 2, 5, 6

Client teaching should cover the signs and symptoms of drug toxicity as well as the need to report them to the physician. The client should be taught the importance of monitoring blood levels for lithium on a regular basis to avoid toxicity. The nurse should explain that 7 to 21 days may pass before the client notes a change in his mood. Lithium doesn't have addictive properties. Tardive dyskinesia isn't a concern for clients taking lithium. Information on a low-tyramine diet is necessary for clients taking MAO inhibitors, not lithium.

6

Drugs and the musculoskeletal system

PRETEST

1. Antarthritics work by:
- [ ] 1. blocking pain receptors.
- [ ] 2. inhibiting prostaglandin synthesis and reducing inflammation.
- [ ] 3. interfering with muscle contraction at the neuromuscular junction.
- [ ] 4. decreasing the serum urate levels.

CORRECT ANSWER: 2

2. Allopurinol (Zyloprim) is used to:
- [ ] 1. prevent recurrent gout attacks.
- [ ] 2. treat malignant hyperthermia.
- [ ] 3. treat psoriasis.
- [ ] 4. treat spasticity associated with multiple sclerosis.

CORRECT ANSWER: 1

3. Which adverse reaction commonly occurs with the use of skeletal muscle relaxants?
- [ ] 1. Tachycardia
- [ ] 2. Hyperventilation
- [ ] 3. Constipation
- [ ] 4. Hypertension

CORRECT ANSWER: 3

4. A nurse should tell a client to expect to see a therapeutic response to methotrexate (Rheumatrex) in:

☐ 1. 6 hours.
☐ 2. 5 days.
☐ 3. 3 to 6 weeks.
☐ 4. 12 weeks.

CORRECT ANSWER: 3

5. A nurse shouldn't administer which drug to a client taking an antigout drug?

☐ 1. Acetaminophen
☐ 2. Morphine
☐ 3. Antacids
☐ 4. Aspirin

CORRECT ANSWER: 4

LEARNING OBJECTIVES

After studying this chapter, you should be able to:

● Describe the mechanisms of action of drugs commonly used to treat the musculoskeletal system.

● List indications and adverse reactions to antigout drugs, antarthritics, and skeletal muscle relaxants.

● Identify the nurse's responsibilities when administering musculoskeletal system drugs.

● Discuss patient teaching related to antigout drugs, antarthritics, and skeletal muscle relaxants.

CHAPTER OVERVIEW

Drugs used to treat the musculoskeletal system include antigout drugs, antarthritics (sometimes called *gold salts*), and skeletal muscle relaxants. Gout is a musculoskeletal disorder of purine metabolism that causes uric acid to accumulate in the blood. The uric acid may precipitate into joints, skin, and other tissues, producing inflammation and tenderness. Antigout drugs work by either decreasing uric acid production or enhancing renal excretion of the uric acid.

Rheumatoid arthritis, a chronic, systemic disease that causes joint inflammation, is treated with various anti-inflammatories. Although nonsteroidal anti-inflammatory drugs (NSAIDs) are generally effective for mild to moderate rheumatoid arthritis, antarthritics are indicated for severe rheumatoid arthritis unresponsive to other drug therapies.

Skeletal muscle relaxants are used to decrease spasticity caused by various spinal cord lesions or to relieve painful musculoskeletal problems.

ANATOMY AND PHYSIOLOGY

● Anatomy
- Includes bones, joints, ligaments, tendons, and muscles
- Includes three muscle types
  - Smooth muscle
  - Cardiac muscle
  - Skeletal muscle
    - Is attached to the skeleton
    - Contracts rapidly and vigorously for short periods
    - Consists of myofibrils, threadlike structures composed of thick and thin filaments
      - Thick filaments contain myosin
      - Thin filaments contain actin

● Physiology
- Skeletal muscle movement
  - Is under voluntary control
  - Involves impulses transmitted from the central nervous system (CNS) by motor nerves, which result in contraction
- Muscle innervation
  - Involves sensory neurons from the somatic (voluntary) nervous system and at least one motor nerve in each muscle
  - Sensory (afferent) neurons
    - Receive impulses concerning the degree of muscle contraction
    - Transmit these impulses to the CNS, coordinating muscle activity
  - Motor (efferent) neurons
    - Convey impulses from the CNS to the muscle, triggering muscle contraction

A&P highlights

- The musculoskeletal system consists of bones, joints, ligaments, tendons, and muscles.
- There are three types of muscle: smooth, cardiac, and skeletal.
- Skeletal muscle is under voluntary control.
- Each skeletal muscle is innervated by sensory neurons from the somatic nervous system and at least one motor nerve.
- Muscle contraction occurs when thick and thin filaments slide over each other, forming structures called cross-bridges.
- The musculoskeletal system moves body parts or the body as a whole.
- The musculoskeletal system is responsible for voluntary and reflex movements.
- Contractions generate body heat.
- Spasticity is caused by injury to muscles, joints, tendons, or ligaments or by CNS damage.

- Muscle contraction
  - Occurs when thick and thin filaments slide over each other, forming structures called *cross-bridges*
  - Involves diffusion of calcium ions into surrounding structures of the filaments, changing the position of these structures and keeping the thick and thin filaments from binding together
- Spasticity
  - Is caused by injury to muscles, joints, tendons, or ligaments or by CNS damage (such as cerebral palsy, multiple sclerosis, poliomyelitis, spinal cord injury or tumors, or tetanus)
  - Occurs when an excessive number of motor impulses pass to the periphery from the spinal cord
  - Results from an increase in excitatory influences or a decrease in inhibitory influences

● **Function**
- Moving body parts or the body as a whole
- Performing voluntary and reflex movements
- Generating body heat through contraction

ANTIGOUT DRUGS

● **Mechanism of action**
- Allopurinol (Zyloprim): decreases uric acid production
- Colchicine: reduces the inflammatory process by interfering with polymorphonuclear leukocyte activity
- Probenecid (Probalan) and sulfinpyrazone (Anturane): enhance renal excretion of uric acid, thereby reducing serum urate level

● **Pharmacokinetics**
- Absorption: Well absorbed from GI tract
- Distribution: Highly protein-bound
- Metabolism: Metabolized by the liver
- Excretion: Excreted primarily by the kidneys

● **Drug examples**
- Allopurinol, colchicine, probenecid, sulfinpyrazone

● **Indications**
- Treat active gout, especially if adequate doses are given early in attack (colchicine; used I.V. if rapid response needed during acute attacks)
- Prevent recurrent attacks of gout or gouty arthritis (allopurinol, probenecid, and sulfinpyrazone)
  - Allopurinol isn't intended for asymptomatic hyperuricemia
  - Probenecid should be used only after acute gouty attack has subsided; however, if acute gouty attack occurs during therapy, drug may be continued

---

Key facts about antigout drugs

- Decrease uric acid production
- Reduce inflammatory process
- Enhance renal excretion of uric acid
- Metabolized by the liver
- Excreted primarily by the kidneys

When to use antigout drugs

- Active gout
- Prevention of recurrent attacks of gout or gouty arthritis
- After acute gouty attack

When NOT to use antigout drugs

- Hypersensitivity to these drugs or to sulfonamides or phenylbutazone or other pyrazoles
- Blood dyscrasias
- Salicylate therapy, uric acid kidney stones, children younger than age 2
- Active peptic ulcer disease, symptoms of GI inflammation or ulceration
- Serious GI, renal, hepatic, or cardiac disorders

Contraindications and precautions

- Probenecid contraindicated in patients taking salicylates, patients hypersensitive to probenecid or sulfonamides (probenecid is a sulfonamide), those with blood dyscrasias or uric acid renal calculi, and in children younger than age 2
- Sulfinpyrazone contraindicated in patients with active peptic ulcer disease, symptoms of GI inflammation or ulceration, hypersensitivity to phenylbutazone or other pyrazoles, or blood dyscrasias
- Allopurinol contraindicated in patients with previous severe reaction to the drug
- Colchicine contraindicated in patients hypersensitive to the drug and those with blood dyscrasias or serious GI, renal, hepatic, or cardiac disorders
- Allopurinol, probenecid, and sulfinpyrazone used cautiously in patients with GI, renal, and hepatic disease

Adverse reactions

- GI disturbances (diarrhea, nausea, vomiting, and abdominal pain), bone marrow depression
- Rash, drowsiness, acute gouty attacks, and renal calculi (allopurinol)
- Rash, headache, and uric acid renal calculi (probenecid)
- Headache and uric acid renal calculi (sulfinpyrazone)
- Myopathy, neuropathy, and malabsorption of vitamin B_{12} (colchicine)

Interactions

- Probenecid and sulfinpyrazone cause sustained increases in serum levels of many drugs (such as penicillin, antineoplastics, ketoprofen, and dapsone)
- Allopurinol increases the risk of azathioprine and mercaptopurine toxicity, enhances effects of oral hypoglycemics, and increases the half-life of anticoagulants, thereby increasing the risk of bleeding
- Use of sulfinpyrazone with aspirin may increase uric acid levels

Nursing responsibilities

- Give the drug with food or milk to reduce adverse GI effects
- Assess the involved joints for pain and immobility
- Make sure the patient maintains a fluid intake of 64 to 96 oz daily to avoid renal calculi
- Teach the patient the importance of complying with therapy; explain that irregular administration of antigout drugs may cause elevated uric acid levels and trigger a gout attack
- Instruct the patient to follow the practitioner's recommendations concerning weight loss, dietary measures, and alcohol restriction
- Caution the patient not to take aspirin with antigout drugs; this could trigger a gout attack (see *Teaching about antigout drugs*, page 114)
- Monitor blood urea nitrogen levels and renal function in long-term therapy

Adverse reactions

- Diarrhea, nausea, vomiting, abdominal pain, bone marrow depression

Key nursing actions

- Give drugs with food or milk.
- Assess joints for pain and immobility.
- Teach patient to:
  - maintain fluid intake of 64 to 96 oz daily
  - follow practitioner's recommendations concerning weight loss, dietary measures, and alcohol restriction
  - avoid taking aspirin with antigout drugs.

Topics for patient discussion

- Therapy regimen
- Signs and symptoms to discuss with practitioner
- Avoidance of products containing aspirin
- Dietary restrictions
- Safety measures
- Need for compliance with therapy
- Need to report use of any over-the-counter or herbal products
- Need for follow-up care

Key facts about antarthritics

- Inhibit prostaglandin synthesis, thereby reducing inflammation
- Excreted mainly in the urine, and the remainder in the feces

When to use antarthritics

- Rheumatoid arthritis
- Crohn's disease
- Psoriasis
- Acute lymphocytic leukemia

When NOT to use antarthritics

- Severe renal or hepatic dysfunction, uncontrolled diabetes mellitus, heart failure, systemic lupus erythematosus, recent radiation therapy
- Hypersensitivity to any murine protein
- Pregnancy, breast-feeding, alcoholism, alcoholic or other chronic liver disease, immunodeficiency disease, blood dyscrasias

TIME-OUT FOR TEACHING

Teaching about antigout drugs

Include these topics in your teaching plan for the patient receiving an antigout drug:
- medication regimen, including the drug's name, dose, frequency, duration, and possible adverse effects
- signs and symptoms to discuss with the practitioner
- avoidance of products containing aspirin
- dietary restrictions
- safety measures
- compliance with therapy
- need to notify the practitioner of any over-the-counter or herbal drugs
- follow-up care, including laboratory tests and practitioner visits.

ANTARTHRITICS

● Mechanism of action
- Inhibit prostaglandin synthesis, thereby reducing inflammation

● Pharmacokinetics
- Absorption: Absorbed subcutaneously, from the GI tract (auranofin [Ridaura]), or administered I.V. (aurothioglucose [Solganal], gold sodium thiomalate [Myochrysine])
  - Auranofin: absorbed from GI tract
  - Aurothioglucose and gold sodium thiomalate: administered I.V.
- Distribution: Distributed mainly intracellularly
- Metabolism: Unknown
- Excretion: Mainly excreted in urine; remainder, in feces

● Drug examples
- Adalimumab (Humira), anakinra (Kineret), auranofin (Ridaura), aurothioglucose (Solganal), etanercept (Enbrel), gold sodium thiomalate (Myochrysine), infliximab (Remicade), leflunomide (Arava), methotrexate (Rheumatrex), soluble interleukin-1 (IL-1ra)

● Indications
- Treat rheumatoid arthritis
- Treat Crohn's disease (infliximab)
- Treat psoriasis and acute lymphocytic leukemia (methotrexate)

● Contraindications and precautions
- Contraindicated in patients with severe renal or hepatic dysfunction, uncontrolled diabetes mellitus, heart failure, systemic lupus erythematosus (SLE), or recent radiation therapy
- Used cautiously in patients with GI, renal, and hepatic disease
- Infliximab
  - Contraindicated in patients hypersensitive to any murine protein
  - Used with extreme caution in patients with heart failure
  - Latent tuberculosis (TB) infection should be treated before starting drug

- Methotrexate
  - Contraindicated in pregnant or breast-feeding patients
  - Contraindicated in alcoholics, and those with alcoholic liver disease or other chronic liver disease, immunodeficiency disease, or blood dyscrasias
- Adalimumab and etanercept
  - Contraindicated in patients with infections, TB, SLE, demyelinating disease, or heart failure

Adverse reactions

- Toxic adverse effects (such as pruritus, rash, metallic taste, stomatitis, diarrhea, and bone marrow suppression marked by thrombocytopenia, aplastic anemia, and agranulocytosis) dizziness, dermatitis, abdominal pain, and photosensitivity reactions when used to treat rheumatoid arthritis
- Hypertension, dizziness, alopecia, and respiratory tract infection (leflunomide)
- Nausea and vomiting, respiratory tract infection, headache, and hypersensitivity reactions (including urticaria, dyspnea, and hypotension occurring within 2 hours of drug infusion) (infliximab)
- Liver toxicity, nausea and vomiting, bone marrow depression, and drug-induced lung disease (methotrexate)
- Injection site reactions and infections (adalimumab and etanercept)

Interactions

- Antarthritics cause additive bone marrow depression when used concurrently with drugs that cause bone marrow depression
- Food delays methotrexate absorption; administer drug on empty stomach

Nursing responsibilities

- Know that most patients require concurrent therapy with glucocorticoids, NSAIDs, or salicylates, especially during the first few months of therapy
- Monitor for signs and symptoms of toxicity, including pruritus, rash, metallic taste, stomatitis, and diarrhea; if toxicity occurs, the practitioner may prescribe dimercaprol (BAL In Oil) to enhance antarthritic excretion
- Instruct the patient to report signs and symptoms of toxicity promptly
- Teach the patient about the importance of maintaining good oral hygiene to prevent stomatitis
- Instruct the patient to use sunscreen and wear protective clothing to prevent photosensitivity reactions
- Monitor the patient receiving methotrexate (given in a once-weekly dose) for 30 minutes after administration for vasomotor response
- Know that the therapeutic response to methotrexate usually occurs within 3 to 6 weeks of the start of therapy, and the patient may continue to improve for another 12 weeks or more
- Know that leflunomide requires a loading dose and frequent liver tests to assess for toxicity
- Be aware that a tuberculin skin test will likely be ordered before starting infliximab therapy because TB has occurred in those receiving drug

---

Adverse reactions

- Dizziness, rash, dermatitis, stomatitis, diarrhea, abdominal pain, metallic taste, bone marrow suppression, photosensitivity reaction

Key nursing actions

- Know signs and symptoms of toxicity: pruritus, rash, metallic taste, stomatitis, and diarrhea.
- Be aware that leflunomide requires loading dose and frequent liver tests.
- Know that tuberculin test will likely be ordered before start of infliximab therapy.
- Teach patient to:
- report signs and symptoms of toxicity promptly
- maintain good oral hygiene
- use sunscreen and wear protective clothing.

Key facts about skeletal muscle relaxants

- Work directly by acting on the neuromuscular junction or indirectly by acting on the CNS
- Block polysynaptic pathways in the spinal cord, inhibiting nerve-impulse transmission
- Interfere with calcium release in muscle fibers, thus interfering with muscle contraction at the neuromuscular junction
- Metabolized by the liver
- Excreted in urine

When to use skeletal muscle relaxants

- Spasticity associated with spinal cord injury
- As adjunct in acute, painful musculoskeletal conditions
- Malignant hyperthermia
- Acute muscle spasms

When NOT to use skeletal muscle relaxants

- Hypersensitivity to these drugs
- Spasticity to maintain posture and balance
- Acute intermittent porphyria
- Arrhythmias
- Pregnancy, breast-feeding, hepatic disease

Adverse reactions

- Transient dizziness, drowsiness, ataxia, nausea, GI upset

SKELETAL MUSCLE RELAXANTS

- **Mechanism of action**
  - Act directly on the neuromuscular junction or indirectly on the CNS
    - Centrally acting drugs (baclofen, carisoprodol, chlorzoxazone, cyclobenzaprine, diazepam, and methocarbamol): block polysynaptic pathways in the spinal cord, inhibiting nerve-impulse transmission
    - Direct-acting drugs (dantrolene): interfere with calcium release in muscle fibers, interfering with muscle contraction at neuromuscular junction

- **Pharmacokinetics**
  - Absorption: Absorbed from GI tract
  - Distribution: Widely distributed
  - Metabolism: Metabolized by the liver
  - Excretion: Excreted in urine

- **Drug examples**
  - Direct-acting: dantrolene (Dantrium)
  - Centrally acting: baclofen (Lioresal), carisoprodol (Soma), chlorphenesin (Maolate), chlorzoxazone (Parafon Forte DSC), cyclobenzaprine (Flexeril), diazepam (Valium), metaxalone (Skelaxin), methocarbamol (Robaxin), orphenadrine (Norflex), tizanidine (Zanaflex)

- **Indications**
  - Treat acute muscle spasms
  - Treat spasticity associated with spinal cord injury, multiple sclerosis, and stroke (baclofen and dantrolene)
  - Adjunctive therapy in acute, painful musculoskeletal conditions (carisoprodol, chlorzoxazone, cyclobenzaprine, diazepam, and methocarbamol)
  - Prevent and treat malignant hyperthermia (dantrolene)

- **Contraindications and precautions**
  - Used cautiously in patients with renal or hepatic impairment
  - Baclofen and oral dantrolene contraindicated in patients who use spasticity to maintain posture and balance
  - Carisoprodol contraindicated in pregnant and breast-feeding patients and patients with acute intermittent porphyria or drug hypersensitivity
  - Metaxalone contraindicated in patients with hemolytic or other anemias
  - Orphenadrine contraindicated in patients with glaucoma, achalasia, bladder neck obstruction, and myasthenia gravis
  - Orphenadrine used cautiously in patients with coronary artery disease and arrhythmias

- **Adverse reactions**
  - Transient dizziness, drowsiness, ataxia, nausea, GI upset, arrhythmias, constipation, vomiting, and bradycardia
  - Possible physical and psychological dependence with long-term use

Interactions

- Concurrent use with other CNS depressants or alcohol causes increased sedation, impaired motor function, and respiratory distress
- Concurrent use of baclofen or cyclobenzaprine with monoamine oxidase inhibitors may cause hypertensive crisis, seizures, high body temperature, and death
- Concurrent use of cyclobenzaprine with antidepressants or antihistamines causes additive anticholinergic effects
- Prolonged anesthesia occurs when fentanyl (Sublimaze) and baclofen are administered together
- Tricyclic antidepressants administered with baclofen increase muscle relaxation

Nursing responsibilities

- Give drug with meals or milk to prevent GI distress
- Assess involved joints for pain and immobility
- Instruct the patient to avoid activities requiring alertness until drug response is known
- Instruct the patient to avoid alcohol and CNS depressants
- Keep emergency equipment nearby to treat respiratory depression
- Don't discontinue skeletal muscle relaxants (especially baclofen, carisoprodol, and cyclobenzaprine) abruptly; may cause hallucinations, seizures, or acute exacerbations of spasticity
- Monitor the patient for orthostatic hypotension

NCLEX CHECKS

It's never too soon to begin your NCLEX® preparation. Now that you've reviewed this chapter, carefully read each of the following questions and choose the best answer. Then compare your responses with the correct answers.

1. A client is experiencing malignant hyperthermic crisis. Which peripherally acting skeletal muscle relaxant is used to treat this condition?

☐ **1.** Baclofen (Lioresal)
☐ **2.** Cyclobenzaprine (Flexeril)
☐ **3.** Dantrolene (Dantrium)
☐ **4.** Diazepam (Valium)

2. While monitoring a client for adverse reactions to his antigout medication, the nurse should pay particular attention to adverse reactions involving which body system?

☐ **1.** Cardiovascular
☐ **2.** GI
☐ **3.** Renal
☐ **4.** Respiratory

Key nursing actions

- Give these drugs with meals or milk.
- Assess involved joints for pain and immobility.
- Keep emergency equipment nearby to treat respiratory depression.
- Don't discontinue these drugs abruptly.
- Teach patient to:
  - avoid activities requiring alertness until CNS effects of drug are known.
  - avoid alcohol and CNS depressants.

TOP 5

Items to study for your next test on drugs and the musculoskeletal system

1. Mechanisms of action of antigout drugs, antarthritics, and skeletal muscle relaxants
2. Indications for antigout drugs, antarthritics, and skeletal muscle relaxants
3. Common adverse effects of antigout drugs, antarthritics, and skeletal muscle relaxants
4. Nursing responsibilities when administering antigout drugs, antarthritics, and skeletal muscle relaxants
5. Patient teaching related to antigout drugs, antarthritics, and skeletal muscle relaxants

3. The antarthritic aurothioglucose (Solganal) is ordered to treat a client's rheumatoid arthritis. Aurothioglucose relieves the symptoms of rheumatoid arthritis by:

☐ **1.** acting as an analgesic.
☐ **2.** relaxing skeletal muscles.
☐ **3.** reversing arthritic deformities.
☐ **4.** decreasing liposomal enzyme release.

4. A client takes probenecid (Probalan) for treatment of gouty arthritis. The client asks the nurse why he has been instructed avoid using aspirin with this drug. The nurse responds that aspirin:

☐ **1.** increases uric acid excretion.
☐ **2.** interferes with uric acid excretion.
☐ **3.** decreases the effects of probenecid.
☐ **4.** increases the effects of probenecid.

5. While admitting a client, the nurse notes the client is allergic to diazepam (Valium). The physician has ordered clonazepam (Klonopin), 1.5 mg (by mouth) three times daily, for this client. The best action would be to:

☐ **1.** give the drug as ordered.
☐ **2.** withhold the drug and notify the physician.
☐ **3.** give a trial dose of 0.75 mg and monitor the client for effect.
☐ **4.** give the drug but watch closely for adverse reactions.

6. A client is prescribed an antarthritic for her rheumatoid arthritis. The nurse is teaching the client about signs and symptoms of toxicity. Which signs and symptoms should the nurse include in her teaching? Select all that apply.

☐ **1.** Rash
☐ **2.** Itching
☐ **3.** Diarrhea
☐ **4.** Shortness of breath
☐ **5.** Metallic taste
☐ **6.** Headaches

7. A nurse begins preparing discharge instructions for a client taking allopurinol (Zyloprim). Which information should the nurse include?

☐ **1.** Drink at least eight 8-oz glasses of water per day.
☐ **2.** You don't need to restrict your alcohol intake more than normal.
☐ **3.** Take aspirin if you have pain.
☐ **4.** Take this medication 2 hours before meals.

8. Which route is the best way to administer aurothioglucose (Solganal)?

☐ **1.** By mouth
☐ **2.** Subcutaneous (subQ)
☐ **3.** I.V.
☐ **4.** I.M.

9. A nurse is caring for a client taking baclofen (Lioresal) for muscle spasms and appropriately questions an order for which drug?
- [ ] **1.** Aspirin
- [ ] **2.** Fentanyl (Sublimaze)
- [ ] **3.** Acetaminophen (Tylenol)
- [ ] **4.** Ibuprofen (Motrin)

10. A client with rheumatoid arthritis and Crohn's disease may benefit most from which drug?
- [ ] **1.** Etanercept (Enbrel)
- [ ] **2.** Sulfinpyrazone (Anturane)
- [ ] **3.** Metaxalone (Skelaxin)
- [ ] **4.** Infliximab (Remicade)

ANSWERS AND RATIONALES

1. CORRECT ANSWER: 3
Diazepam, baclofen, dantrolene, and cyclobenzaprine are all used for muscle spasm and spasticity. However, I.V. dantrolene is the only drug used to treat malignant hyperthermic crisis. Dantrolene may be given by mouth prophylactically (2 to 3 days before anesthesia) for clients with a history of malignant hyperthermia or a family history of the disorder.

2. CORRECT ANSWER: 2
Clients typically take antigout medication with food because GI distress is the most common adverse reaction to antigout medications. Cardiovascular, renal, and respiratory adverse reactions rarely occur with antigout drugs.

3. CORRECT ANSWER: 4
Antarthritics, such as aurothioglucose, relieve the symptoms of rheumatoid arthritis by decreasing liposomal enzyme release, thereby altering immune response. Antarthritics don't act as analgesics, relax skeletal muscles, or reverse rheumatoid arthritis deformation.

4. CORRECT ANSWER: 3
Aspirin decreases but doesn't inactivate the action of probenecid. Aspirin has no effect on the rate of uric acid excretion.

5. CORRECT ANSWER: 2
Cross-allergies among benzodiazepines are common, so clonazepam (a benzodiazepine) shouldn't be given to a client who's allergic to diazepam (another benzodiazepine). Withholding the drug and notifying the physician are the most appropriate actions. Because of the possibility of an allergic reaction, the drug shouldn't be given. It's illegal to give trial doses without an order.

6. CORRECT ANSWER: 1, 2, 3, 5
Signs and symptoms of antarthritic toxicity include bone marrow suppression, diarrhea, stomatitis, pruritus (itching), rash, and a metallic taste. Shortness of breath and headaches aren't signs or symptoms of toxicity.

7. CORRECT ANSWER: 1

The client taking antigout medication should drink 64 to 96 ounces of fluid daily to avoid the formation of renal calculi. The client should limit his alcohol intake to help prevent acute gout attacks. Aspirin can cause increased uric acid levels, so the client shouldn't take aspirin for pain. Antigout medications can cause GI upset, so it's recommended to take them with food or milk.

8. CORRECT ANSWER: 3

Aurothioglucose is administered I.V.; it isn't administered by any other route.

9. CORRECT ANSWER: 2

Because baclofen and fentanyl given together prolong anesthesia, the nurse should question the physician about the order. A different analgesic will need to be ordered. None of the other drugs is a concern for a client taking baclofen.

10. CORRECT ANSWER: 4

Infliximab, an antarthritic, is also used to treat Crohn's disease. Etanercept is also an antarthritic, but it isn't the best choice for this client. Sulfinpyrazone is an antigout drug. Metaxalone is a skeletal muscle relaxant.

7

Drugs and the respiratory system

PRETEST

1. Leukotriene receptor modifiers work by:
- [ ] 1. inhibiting cyclic adenosine monophosphate (cAMP) breakdown and blocking adenosine receptors.
- [ ] 2. blocking inflammatory action that causes signs and symptoms of asthma.
- [ ] 3. preventing release of or counteracting biochemical mediators that cause inflammation.
- [ ] 4. stimulating the production of cAMP.

CORRECT ANSWER: 2

2. A client using a nasal decongestant may experience:
- [ ] 1. rebound congestion.
- [ ] 2. hypotension.
- [ ] 3. edema.
- [ ] 4. anorexia.

CORRECT ANSWER: 1

3. What action should the client take after using an inhaled corticosteroid?
- [ ] 1. Wait 2 hours before eating.
- [ ] 2. Have blood levels drawn.
- [ ] 3. Drink 2 to 3 qt (2 to 3 L) of fluid per day.
- [ ] 4. Rinse his mouth with water.

CORRECT ANSWER: 4

4. Which medication is most effective for a client with a nonproductive cough that occurs more frequently at night?

- ☐ 1. Acetylcysteine (Mucomyst)
- ☐ 2. Benzonatate (Tessalon)
- ☐ 3. Phenylephrine
- ☐ 4. Theophylline (Slo-Bid)

CORRECT ANSWER: 2

5. A nurse must monitor the serum level of which drug?

- ☐ 1. Albuterol (Proventil)
- ☐ 2. Montelukast (Singulair)
- ☐ 3. Theophylline (Slo-Bid)
- ☐ 4. Methylprednisolone (Medrol)

CORRECT ANSWER: 3

LEARNING OBJECTIVES

After studying this chapter, you should be able to:

- Describe the mechanism of action of commonly prescribed respiratory system drugs.
- Describe the rationale for using bronchodilators, leukotriene receptor modifiers, antitussives, expectorants, mucolytics, and decongestants.
- Name common adverse effects of the various types of respiratory system drugs.
- Describe the nursing responsibilities and patient teaching required for patients receiving drugs to treat the respiratory system.

CHAPTER OVERVIEW

Bronchodilators are used to prevent or terminate bronchospasm caused by pulmonary disease, allergy, exercise, or emotional factors. Leukotriene receptor modifiers are used to decrease bronchial inflammation and airway edema. These drugs are useful for prophylactic and long-term treatment of bronchial asthma.

Antitussives, expectorants, mucolytics, and nasal decongestants are used to control cough, facilitate secretion removal, and liquefy tenacious mucus in the airways. Antitussives, which can be opioid or nonopioid, are used to suppress dry, nonproductive cough. Expectorants increase secretions in the respiratory tract and may decrease viscosity of thick mucus secretions to allow for expectoration in chronic obstructive pulmonary disease (COPD), pneumonia, and other disorders. Mucolytics break down chemical bonds in tenacious mucus and allow for its removal by coughing or suctioning. Acetylcysteine, a mucolytic, also may be given to decrease hepatotoxicity in acetaminophen overdose. Nasal decongestants shrink swollen mucous membranes, promoting nasal drainage and improving nasal ventilation and breathing.

ANATOMY AND PHYSIOLOGY

● **Anatomy**
- Upper airway structures: nose, pharynx, larynx
- Lower airway structures: trachea and bronchi
  - Primary bronchi
    - Branch from the trachea and lead into the lungs
    - Divide into smaller secondary bronchi
  - Secondary bronchi
    - Branch into even smaller tertiary bronchi
    - Eventually become bronchioles
  - Bronchioles
    - Terminate in alveolar sacs composed of alveoli—tiny, grapelike clusters of air sacs surrounded by an extensive network of capillaries (see *Bronchioles and alveoli*, page 124)
- Lungs
  - Are paired, cone-shaped organs that fill the pleural division of the thoracic cavity
  - Extend from the root of the neck to the diaphragm

● **Physiology**
- Uses diaphragm and intercostal muscles to produce the normal inspiratory and expiratory movements of the lungs and ribs, which allows for ventilation
- Moves oxygen and carbon dioxide between the alveoli, blood, and tissues (gas exchange)
  - Depends on the concentrations and pressures of these gases
  - Diffuses gas from an area with high partial pressure to one with low partial pressure

A&P highlights

- The respiratory system consists of the upper and lower airways and the lungs.
- Upper airways include the nose, pharynx, and larynx.
- Lower airways include the trachea and bronchi.
- Lungs are paired, cone-shaped organs that fill the pleural division of the thoracic cavity and extend from the root of the neck to the diaphragm.
- The diaphragm and intercostal muscles produce the normal inspiratory and expiratory movements of the lungs and ribs.
- Movement of oxygen and carbon dioxide between the alveoli, blood, and tissues depends on the concentrations and pressures of these gases; they diffuse from an area with a high partial pressure of the gas to one with a low partial pressure.

Bronchioles and alveoli

This illustration shows bronchioles branching into progressively smaller tubes that eventually become alveolar ducts. The alveoli are the basic functional units of the respiratory system; gas exchange (exchange of oxygen and carbon dioxide) between the lungs and bronchi occurs here.

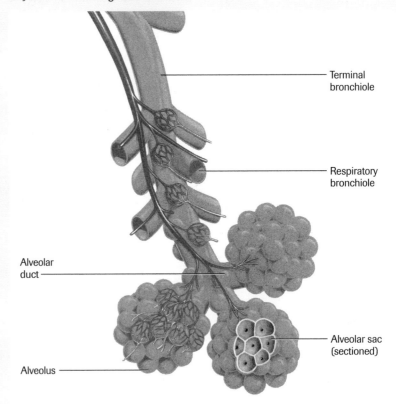

Terminal bronchiole

Respiratory bronchiole

Alveolar duct

Alveolar sac (sectioned)

Alveolus

● **Function**
  • Supplies body tissues with oxygen and removes carbon dioxide
  • Distributes air to the lungs via the bronchi
  • Performs gas exchange via the alveoli, exchanging oxygen and carbon dioxide by diffusion

BRONCHODILATORS

ADRENERGIC-AGONIST BRONCHODILATORS

● **Mechanism of action**
  • Produce bronchodilation by stimulating production of cyclic adenosine monophosphate (cAMP)

● **Pharmacokinetics**
  • Absorption: Absorbed from respiratory tract; well absorbed from GI tract

---

Key facts about adrenergic-agonist bronchodilators

• Produce bronchodilation by stimulating cAMP production
• Metabolized by the liver
• Excreted in the urine and feces

- Distribution: Not widely distributed
- Metabolism: Metabolized by the liver
- Excretion: Excreted in urine and feces

Drug examples
- Short-acting drugs: albuterol (AccuNeb, Proventil), bitolterol mesylate (Tornalate), ephedrine (Pretz-D), epinephrine (Primatene Mist), isoproterenol (Isuprel), levalbuterol (Xopenex), metaproterenol (Alupent), pirbuterol (Maxair), terbutaline (Brethine)
- Long-acting drugs: formoterol (Foradil), ipratropium and albuterol (Combivent), salmeterol (Serevent Diskus)

Indications
- Treat acute bronchospasm (short-acting drugs)
- Prevention of and maintenance therapy for bronchospasms in select patients with COPD, asthma, and exercise-induced asthma
- Manage bronchospasms during anesthesia (isoproterenol)

Contraindications and precautions
- Contraindicated in patients with uncontrolled arrhythmias, hypertension, coronary artery disease, or history of stroke
- Used cautiously in patients with diabetes, hyperthyroidism, or a history of seizures

Adverse reactions
- Anxiety, nervousness, tremor, palpitations, tachycardia, hypertension, arrhythmias, dry mouth, and bronchospasms
- Hypokalemia in dialysis patients (albuterol)
- Increased severity of any asthma episodes that occur (long-acting drugs)

Interactions
- Concurrent use with theophylline preparations causes additive effects
- Use with betaadrenergic blockers decrease drug's bronchodilating effects
- Caffeine increases drug's adverse effects

Nursing responsibilities
- Monitor the patient's blood pressure, pulse, respiratory rate, and breath sounds
- Administer the prescribed drug around the clock as ordered
- Monitor the patient's respiratory status for development of bronchospasm
- Don't administer long-acting drug more often than prescribed; serious adverse effects, including death, can occur
- Don't administer drug during an acute asthma attack
- If inhalation drug has been prescribed, teach the patient how to use it
- Instruct the patient to maintain a fluid intake of 2 to 3 qt (2 to 3 L)/day to make secretions less viscous (see *Teaching about inhaled bronchodilators,* page 126)
- Advise the patient to consult the practitioner before taking any nonprescription drugs to prevent adverse drug interactions
- Instruct the patient to avoid respiratory irritants, such as smoke, dust, and strong scents

When to use adrenergic–agonist bronchodilators
- Bronchospasms

When NOT to use adrenergic–agonist bronchodilators
- Uncontrolled arrhythmias, hypertension, coronary artery disease

Adverse reactions
- Anxiety, nervousness, tremor, palpitations, tachycardia, hypertension, arrhythmia
- Hypokalemia in dialysis patient

Key nursing actions
- Monitor patient's blood pressure, pulse, respiratory rate, and breath sounds.
- Administer drug around the clock, as ordered.
- Don't administer a long-acting drug more often than prescribed.
- Teach patient to:
 - maintain fluid intake of 2 to 3 L/day
 - consult practitioner before taking nonprescription drugs
 - avoid respiratory irritants.

Topics for patient discussion

- Therapy regimen
- Signs and symptoms to discuss with the practitioner
- Proper method for administration
- Peak flow monitoring
- Information about the disease
- Concomitant use of inhaled bronchodilator and inhaled anti-inflammatory
- Avoidance of possible allergens or irritants
- Emergency measures
- Compliance with therapy
- Follow-up care

Key facts about methylxanthine bronchodilators

- Produce bronchodilation by inhibiting cAMP breakdown and blocking adenosine receptors
- Metabolized primarily by the liver
- Excreted in the urine

When to use methylxanthine bronchodilators

- Bronchospasm
- Asthma, bronchitis, emphysema, neonatal apnea

When NOT to use methylxanthine bronchodilators

- Status asthmaticus
- Hypersensitivity to any xanthine or ethylenediamine
- Peptic ulcer disease
- Untreated seizure disorders
- Infection or irritation of the rectum or lower colon

TIME-OUT FOR TEACHING

Teaching about inhaled bronchodilators

Include these topics in your teaching plan for the patient receiving an inhaled bronchodilator:

- medication regimen, including the drug's name, dose, frequency, duration, and possible adverse effects
- signs and symptoms to discuss with the practitioner, including adverse effects
- proper method for administration, including care of a metered-dose inhaler
- peak flow monitoring, if indicated
- information about the patient's disease, including signs and symptoms of exacerbations
- fluid needs
- concomitant use of an inhaled bronchodilator and an inhaled anti-inflammatory
- avoidance of possible allergens or irritants
- emergency measures
- compliance with therapy, including taking the drug as prescribed
- follow-up care, including laboratory tests and practitioner visits.

- Discuss with the patient the importance of avoiding products containing caffeine

METHYLXANTHINE BRONCHODILATORS

● **Mechanism of action**
- Produce bronchodilation by inhibiting cAMP breakdown and blocking adenosine receptors

● **Pharmacokinetics**
- Absorption: Absorbed rapidly and completely from GI tract
- Distribution: Not well distributed in fat tissues; dosage is based on patient's ideal or actual body weight, whichever is less
- Metabolism: Metabolized primarily by the liver
- Excretion: Excreted in urine

● **Drug examples**
- Aminophylline, caffeine, theophylline (Elixophyllin, Slo-Bid, S0-Phyllin), dyphylline (Dilor)

● **Indications**
- Prevent or treat bronchospasm
- Treat asthma, bronchitis, emphysema, and neonatal apnea

● **Contraindications and precautions**
- Shouldn't be used for patients with status asthmaticus; these are conventional bronchodilators, not emergency drugs
- Contraindicated in patients with xanthine hypersensitivity, peptic ulcer disease, or untreated seizure disorders

- Used cautiously in neonates, elderly patients, and those with heart disease, hypoxemia, hepatic disease, hypertension, heart failure, or alcoholism; also during labor and in breast-feeding patients
- Aminophylline contraindicated in patients who are hypersensitive to ethylenediamine and those with an infection or irritation of the rectum or lower colon

Adverse reactions
- Headache, irritability, restlessness, anxiety, insomnia, dizziness, nausea, vomiting, abdominal cramping, epigastric pain, anorexia, and diarrhea

Interactions
- Use with beta-adrenergic blockers partially antagonizes the effect of drug, altering its rate of metabolism and increasing the concentration
- Use with sympathomimetics or cardiac glycosides potentiates drug's adverse effects
- Use with diuretics potentiates drug's diuretic effects
- Phenobarbital, phenytoin, rifampin, cigarette smoking, and charcoal-broiled foods may shorten the drug's halflife, reducing its effectiveness
- Methylxanthines increase lithium clearance, reducing the effectiveness of lithium
- Use with erythromycin may increase the drug's half-life, increasing the risk of methylxanthine toxicity
- Smoking increases theophylline elimination and decreases the serum concentration and effectiveness
- Use with caffeinated beverages or caffeinelike substances may result in additive adverse reactions or signs and symptoms of methylxanthine toxicity
- Grapefruit juice can increase the serum levels of theophylline, increasing the risk of toxicity

Nursing responsibilities
- Assess for signs and symptoms of toxicity, such as arrhythmias and seizures
- Monitor serum drug levels to detect toxicity (therapeutic serum theophylline level should range from 10 to 20 mcg/ml)
- Instruct the patient to reduce consumption of xanthine-containing foods and beverages (such as cola, coffee, and chocolate) to prevent toxicity
- Emphasize the importance of routine laboratory studies to determine serum drug levels
- Administer time-released forms on an empty stomach

CORTICOSTEROIDS

Mechanism of action
- Prevent release of or counteract biochemical mediators (kinins, serotonin, histamine) that cause the tissue inflammation responsible for edema and airway narrowing

---

Adverse reactions
- Headache, irritability, restlessness, anxiety, insomnia, dizziness, nausea, vomiting, abdominal cramping, epigastric pain, anorexia, diarrhea

Key nursing actions
- Assess for signs and symptoms of toxicity.
- Know that therapeutic serum theophylline level ranges from 10 to 20 mcg/ml.
- Instruct patient to reduce consumption of xanthine-containing foods and beverages.
- Emphasize importance of routine lab studies.

Key facts about anti-inflammatory inhalants

- Prevent the release of or counteract the biochemical mediators that cause the tissue inflammation responsible for edema and airway narrowing
- Metabolized primarily by the liver
- Excreted in the feces and urine

When to use anti-inflammatory inhalants

- Chronic bronchitis
- Bronchial asthma
- Allergic rhinitis
- As adjuncts for perennial asthma
- As prophylaxis for exercise-induced asthma

When NOT to use anti-inflammatory inhalants

- Acute bronchospasms

Adverse reactions

- Oral candidiasis

Key nursing actions

- Know that cromolyn is ineffective during acute bronchospasm attacks.
- Teach patient to:
- use bronchodilator several minutes before corticosteroid inhaler
- rinse mouth after using inhaled steroids
- use and care for inhaler properly.

● Pharmacokinetics

- Absorption: Rapidly absorbed I.V.; poor systemic absorption after inhalation
- Distribution: Not widely distributed into tissues; highly protein-bound
- Metabolism: Metabolized primarily by the liver
- Excretion: Eliminated in feces and urine

● Drug examples

- Beclomethasone (Beconase AQ), budesonide (Pulmicort), cromolyn sodium (Intal Aerosol Spray), dexamethasone (Decadron Phosphate Respihaler), flunisolide (AeroBid), fluticasone (Flovent), methylprednisolone (Medrol, Solu-Medrol), prednisone (Deltasone), triamcinolone (Azmacort)

● Indications

- Treat chronic bronchitis (beclomethasone)
- Control bronchial asthma in patients with steroid-dependent asthma (budesonide, dexamethasone, flunisolide, and triamcinolone)
- Treat allergic rhinitis; adjunctive treatment for severe perennial asthma; and prophylactic treatment for exercise-induced asthma (budesonide and cromolyn sodium)

● Contraindications and precautions

- Contraindicated for patients with acute bronchospasms
- Used with extreme caution in patients with clinical tuberculosis or viral respiratory infections, systemic infections, hypertension, diabetes, peptic ulcer disease, or glaucoma

● Adverse reactions

- Mouth irritation, oral candidiasis, and upper respiratory infections

● Interactions

- Hormonal contraceptives, ketoconazole, and macrolide antibiotics increase the activity of corticosteroids
- Barbiturates, cholestyramine, and phenytoin decrease the effectiveness of corticosteroids

● Nursing responsibilities

- Instruct the patient who's receiving a bronchodilator and a corticosteroid inhaler to use the bronchodilator several minutes before the corticosteroid; doing so ensures penetration of the corticosteroid into the airways
- Instruct the patient to rinse his mouth after using inhaled steroids
- Inform the patient who's receiving cromolyn that this drug is ineffective during acute bronchospasm attacks; explain that frequent daily use over a prolonged period helps decrease the severity or frequency of attacks
- Instruct the patient on the proper use and care of the inhaler and spacer
- Give oral doses with food to minimize GI upset
- Don't abruptly discontinue use; drug must be tapered

LEUKOTRIENE RECEPTOR MODIFIERS

- **Mechanism of action**
  - Selectively compete for leukotriene receptor sites, thereby blocking inflammatory action that causes the signs and symptoms of asthma

- **Pharmacokinetics**
  - Absorption: Rapidly absorbed in GI tract
  - Distribution: Highly protein-bound
  - Metabolism: Metabolized by the liver
  - Excretion: Excreted in urine and feces

- **Drug examples**
  - Montelukast (Singulair), zafirlukast (Accolate), zileuton (Zyflo)

- **Indications**
  - Prophylactic and long-term treatment of bronchial asthma in adults and children; montelukast approved for use in children as young as 12 months

- **Contraindications and precautions**
  - Shouldn't be used for treatment of status asthmaticus or acute asthma attacks
  - Contraindicated in patients with previous allergy to any leukotriene modifier
  - Used cautiously in pregnant patients

- **Adverse reactions**
  - Headache, dizziness, nausea, diarrhea, abdominal pain, nasal congestion, fever, rash, and generalized fatigue
  - Possible Churg-Strauss syndrome in patients who are decreasing oral steroid dose while using zafirlukast

- **Interactions**
  - Warfarin used with zafirlukast may result in increased bleeding; monitor prothrombin time closely, and adjust warfarin dose accordingly
  - Calcium-channel blockers and cyclosporine increase the effects of zafirlukast and may cause toxicity
  - Concurrent use of erythromycin and theophylline may decrease the effectiveness of these drugs
  - Phenobarbital and rifampin may decrease the bioavailability and effects of montelukast when taken concurrently

- **Nursing responsibilities**
  - Administer zafirlukast 1 hour before or 2 hours after meals for best absorption
  - Know that montelukast is best absorbed when given at night
  - Instruct the patient about the use of rescue medication for acute attacks or when a short-acting inhaled medication is needed
  - Advise the patient to take drug continually for optimal effects

Key facts about leukotriene receptor modifiers

- Block the inflammatory action that causes the signs and symptoms of asthma by competing for leukotriene receptor sites
- Metabolized by the liver
- Excreted in urine and feces

When to use leukotriene receptor modifiers

- Bronchial asthma

When NOT to use leukotriene receptor modifiers

- Status asthmaticus
- Acute asthma attacks
- Previous allergy

Adverse reactions

- Headache, dizziness, nausea, diarrhea, nasal congestion, rash, generalized fatigue

Key nursing actions

- Administer zafirlukast 1 hour before or 2 hours after meals; administer montelukast at night.
- Teach the patient about using rescue medications for acute attacks.

Key facts about antitussives

- Suppress the cough reflex
- Anesthetize cough receptors of vagal afferent fibers throughout bronchi, alveoli, and pleura
- Metabolized by the liver
- Excreted in the urine

When to use antitussives

- Nonproductive cough
- Cough that interferes with sleep or daily activities

When NOT to use antitussives

- Hypersensitivity to these drugs
- Pregnancy
- Breast-feeding

Adverse reactions

- Drowsiness, drying of respiratory secretions, constipation, dizziness

Key nursing actions

- Maintain airway patency.
- Assess breath sounds, cough, and bronchial secretions.
- Administer codeine cautiously if patient is receiving CNS depressant.
- Teach patient to:
  - maintain fluid intake of 2 to 3 L/day
  - minimize talking, stop smoking, use chewing gum or sugarless candy
  - consult practitioner if cough lasts more than 1 week or fever or chest pain occurs
  - avoid liquids within 30 minutes of taking drug
  - check with practitioner before taking over-the-counter or herbal products.

ANTITUSSIVES

Mechanism of action
- Suppress the cough reflex by acting on medulla's cough center
- Act by anesthetizing cough receptors of vagal afferent fibers throughout the bronchi, alveoli, and pleura (benzonatate only)

Pharmacokinetics
- Absorption: Well absorbed through GI tract
- Distribution: Unknown
- Metabolism: Metabolized by the liver
- Excretion: Excreted in urine

Drug examples
- Opioid antitussives: codeine phosphate, codeine sulfate (Codeine), hydrocodone (Hycodan)
- Nonopioid antitussives: benzonatate (Tessalon), dextromethorphan (Robitussin DM), diphenhydramine (Benadryl, Benylin)

Indications
- Treat nonproductive cough and cough that interferes with sleep or daily activities

Contraindications and precautions
- Contraindicated in patients who are hypersensitive, pregnant, or breast-feeding
- Used cautiously in patients with benign prostatic hyperplasia, debilitation, thoracotomy, laparotomy, or a history of drug or alcohol abuse

Adverse reactions
- Opioid antitussives: Drowsiness, drying of respiratory secretions, and constipation
- Nonopioid antitussives: Drowsiness, dizziness, headache, nasal congestion, GI upset, and constipation

Interactions
- These drugs may potentiate antitussive effects when used with alcohol, sedatives, monoamine oxidase (MAO) inhibitors, anticholinergics, or tranquilizers
- MAO inhibitors may cause excitation, extremely elevated temperature, hypertension, or hypotension when taken with codeine or hydrocodone

Nursing responsibilities
- Instruct the patient taking benzonatate to swallow drug whole
- Maintain airway patency; provide suction if necessary
- Assess the patient's breath sounds, evaluate cough for characteristics (such as productive or nonproductive) and frequency, and assess characteristics of bronchial secretions
- Instruct the patient to maintain a fluid intake of 2 to 3 qt (2 to 3 L)/day
- Advise the patient with nonproductive cough to minimize talking, stop smoking, maintain adequate environmental humidity, and use chewing

TIME-OUT FOR TEACHING

Teaching about antitussives

Include these topics in your teaching plan for the patient receiving an antitussive:

- medication regimen, including the drug's name, dose, frequency, duration, and possible adverse effects
- signs and symptoms to discuss with the practitioner, including persistent cough and adverse effects
- safety measures

- fluid needs
- possible physical dependency if an opioid drug is used
- avoidance of alcohol and other over-the-counter products
- compliance with therapy, including taking the drug as prescribed
- follow-up care, including laboratory tests and practitioner visits.

gum or sugarless candy to reduce coughing (see *Teaching about antitussives*)

- Instruct the patient to consult the practitioner if cough lasts more than 1 week or is accompanied by fever, chest pain, rash, nausea, or headache
- Instruct the patient not to consume liquids within 30 minutes of taking an antitussive because liquids may negate soothing local effects
- Instruct the patient to check with the practitioner before taking any over-the-counter or herbal medications
- Administer codeine with caution to a patient who's receiving a central nervous system (CNS) depressant because this combination can be fatal; closely monitor the patient's level of consciousness and respiratory status

EXPECTORANTS

Mechanism of action

- Decrease the viscosity of tenacious secretions by increasing fluid in the respiratory tract (efficacy is questionable)

Pharmacokinetics

- Absorption: Absorbed through GI tract
- Distribution: Unknown
- Metabolism: Metabolized by the liver
- Excretion: Excreted primarily in urine

Drug examples

- Guaifenesin (Humibid L.A., Liquibid, Mucinex, Robitussin, Tussin)

Indications

- Treat cough associated with common cold and upper respiratory tract infections (questionable efficacy), including minor bronchial irritations, bronchitis, influenza, sinusitis, emphysema, and bronchial asthma
- Relieve dry, hacking cough

When NOT to use expectorants

- Hypersensitivity to these drugs

Adverse reactions

- Vomiting, diarrhea, nausea, drowsiness, abdominal pain

Key nursing actions

- Maintain airway patency.
- Assess breath sounds, cough, and bronchial secretions.
- Teach patient to:
- maintain fluid intake of 2 to 3 L/day
- check with practitioner before taking over-the-counter or herbal products
- avoid taking guaifenesin for persistent cough associated with smoking, asthma, emphysema, or excessive secretions.

Key facts about mucolytics

- Decrease mucus viscosity by breaking or altering chemical bonds of glycoprotein complexes in the mucus
- Metabolized by the liver
- Excretion method unknown

When to use mucolytics

- Abnormal, viscid, or thick and hard mucus
- As antidote for acetaminophen overdose

When NOT to use mucolytics

- Hypersensitivity to these drugs

Adverse reactions

- Stomatitis, nausea, vomiting, drowsiness, severe rhinorrhea, bronchospasms

---

● Contraindications and precautions
- Contraindicated in patients with hypersensitivity
- Used cautiously in patients with ineffective cough reflex or respiratory insufficiency and those who are pregnant or breastfeeding

● Adverse reactions
- Vomiting (if taken in large doses), diarrhea, nausea, drowsiness, and abdominal pain

● Interactions
- Use with anticoagulants may increase the risk of bleeding

● Nursing responsibilities
- Maintain airway patency; provide suction if necessary
- Assess the patient's breath sounds, evaluate cough for characteristics (such as productive or nonproductive) and frequency, and assess characteristics of bronchial secretions
- Instruct the patient to maintain a fluid intake of 2 to 3 qt (2 to 3 L)/day; increased fluid intake may enhance effects of expectorants by making secretions less viscous
- Tell the patient to check with the practitioner before taking any over-the-counter or herbal medications
- Caution the patient not to take guaifenesin for a persistent cough associated with smoking, asthma, emphysema, or excessive secretions

MUCOLYTICS

● Mechanism of action
- Decrease mucus viscosity by breaking or altering the chemical bonds of glycoprotein complexes in mucus

● Pharmacokinetics
- Absorption: Absorbed from pulmonary epithelium
- Distribution: About 50% protein-bound
- Metabolism: Metabolized by the liver
- Excretion: Unknown

● Drug examples
- Acetylcysteine (Mucomyst), dornase alfa (Pulmozyme)

● Indications
- Treat abnormal, viscid, or thick and hard mucus
- Antidote for acetaminophen overdose

● Contraindications and precautions
- Acetylcysteine contraindicated in patients with known hypersensitivity
- Acetylcysteine and dornase alfa used cautiously in elderly, debilitated, pregnant, or breastfeeding patients and in those with asthma

● Adverse reactions
- Stomatitis, nausea, vomiting, drowsiness, and severe rhinorrhea
- Bronchospasms, especially in asthmatic patients

Interactions
- Activated charcoal decreases acetylcysteine's effectiveness

Nursing responsibilities
- Maintain airway patency; provide suction if necessary
- Assess the patient's breath sounds, evaluate cough for characteristics (such as productive or nonproductive) and frequency, and assess characteristics of bronchial secretions
- Tell the patient to maintain a fluid intake of 2 to 3 qt (2 to 3 L)/day
- Tell the patient to check with the practitioner before taking any over-the-counter or herbal medications
- Warn the patient about acetylcysteine's "rotten egg" smell
- Be prepared to administer a beta$_2$-adrenergic agonist by aerosol if the patient experiences bronchospasms

DECONGESTANTS

Mechanism of action
- Act directly on alpha-adrenergic receptors in the nasal mucosa and elsewhere, causing contraction of sphincters and constriction of secretory cells
- Indirectly result in norepinephrine release, which, together with the direct action on receptors, causes vasoconstriction and nasal decongestion

Pharmacokinetics
- Absorption: Readily absorbed in GI tract when taken orally; otherwise, absorbed from respiratory tract
- Distribution: Widely distributed throughout body
- Metabolism: Metabolized by the liver
- Excretion: Excreted in urine

Drug examples
- Ephedrine (Pretz-D), fluticasone (Flonase), oxymetazoline (Afrin), phenylephrine (Afrin Children's, Neo-Synephrine), pseudoephedrine hydrochloride (Sudafed), pseudoephedrine sulfate (Drixoral)

Indications
- Temporary relief of nasal congestion due to common cold, hay fever or other upper respiratory tract allergies, and sinusitis
- Promote nasal or sinus drainage

Contraindications and precautions
- Contraindicated in patients taking an MAO inhibitor and those hypersensitive to drug's ingredients
- Used cautiously in elderly patients (older than age 60 more likely to experience adverse reactions); patients with thyroid disease, cardiovascular disease, coronary artery disease, hypertension, intraocular pressure, or peripheral vascular disease; and those who have difficulty urinating because of an enlarged prostate
- Pseudoephedrine contraindicated in patients with hypertension because of risk of cardiac arrest

---

Key nursing actions
- Maintain patent airway.
- Assess breath sounds, cough, and bronchial secretions.
- Be prepared to administer beta$_2$-adrenergic agonist if bronchospasm occurs.
- Teach patient to:
  - maintain fluid intake of 2 to 3 L/day
  - check with practitioner before taking over-the-counter or herbal products
  - be aware of "rotten egg" smell of acetylcysteine.

Key facts about decongestants
- Cause contraction of sphincters and constriction of secretory cells
- Cause vasoconstriction and nasal decongestion
- Metabolized by the liver
- Excreted in the urine

When to use decongestants
- Temporary relief of nasal decongestion
- Nasal or sinus drainage

When NOT to use decongestants
- MAO inhibitor therapy
- Hypersensitivity to these drugs
- Hypertension

Adverse reactions

- Arrhythmias, palpitations, tachycardia, bradycardia, hypertension, headache, dizziness, light-headedness, drowsiness, insomnia, nervousness, giddiness, psychological disturbances, hypersensitivity reactions, including rash, urticaria, and leukopenia

Key nursing actions

- Notify practitioner if insomnia, dizziness, weakness, tremor, or irregular heartbeat occurs.
- Monitor blood pressure, pulse rate, and ECG.
- Teach patient to:
- use medication properly
- avoid sharing medication
- take medication as prescribed.

● Adverse reactions

- Arrhythmias, palpitations, tachycardia, bradycardia, hypertension, headache, dizziness, light-headedness, drowsiness, insomnia, nervousness, giddiness, psychological disturbances, and hypersensitivity reactions (including rash, urticaria, and leukopenia)
- Toxicity and rebound congestion from increasing the dosage frequency or amount of dose
- Rebound congestion with prolonged use
  – Topical (nasal) drugs shouldn't be used for more than 3 days
  – Oral drugs shouldn't be used for more than 7 days

● Interactions

- Nasal decongestants given with other sympathomimetic amines may increase CNS stimulation
- MAO inhibitors given concurrently with a nasal decongestant may cause severe hypertension or hypertensive crisis
- Giving pseudoephedrine with alkalinizing agents may decrease urinary excretion of pseudoephedrine, increasing its effects

● Nursing responsibilities

- Teach the patient the proper method for using decongestant sprays, inhalers, and drops
- Instruct the patient not to share the container with other people and not to allow the tip of the container to touch the nasal passage to avoid contamination
- Notify the practitioner if the patient experiences insomnia, dizziness, weakness, tremor, or irregular heartbeat
- Monitor the patient's blood pressure, pulse rate, and electrocardiogram during therapy
- Tell the patient not to exceed the prescribed frequency of dosage or amount of each dose; doing so may increase the risk of toxicity and cause rebound congestion

NCLEX CHECKS

It's never too soon to begin your NCLEX® preparation. Now that you've reviewed this chapter, carefully read each of the following questions and choose the best answer. Then compare your responses with the correct answers.

1. A client is receiving theophylline (Slo-Bid). Which assessment finding indicates the client is responding positively to the drug?
- ☐ **1.** Easy, unlabored respirations
- ☐ **2.** Heart rate of 92 beats/minute
- ☐ **3.** Urine output of 450 ml/shift
- ☐ **4.** Blood pressure of 138/82 mm Hg

2. A nurse is checking for adverse reactions in a client who has just been given metaproterenol (Alupent) for asthma. Which reaction is most likely to occur with this drug?

☐ **1.** Edema, moon face
☐ **2.** Tachycardia, shaking
☐ **3.** Bleeding peptic ulcer, vomiting
☐ **4.** Moderate hypotension, dizziness

3. A nurse is instructing a client about the use of albuterol (Proventil) and beclomethasone (Beconase AQ) inhalation therapy at home. The nurse should teach the client to:

☐ **1.** use the corticosteroid followed by the bronchodilator.
☐ **2.** use the bronchodilator followed by the corticosteroid.
☐ **3.** alternate the order of use each time to prevent tolerance.
☐ **4.** rinse the mouth both before and after use to prevent gum breakdown.

4. A client comes into the ambulatory care clinic with an upper respiratory tract infection evidenced by nasal stuffiness, low-grade fever, and a productive cough. He reports difficulty coughing up the mucus. The chest examination is consistent with bronchitis. He would like cough syrup. Which ingredient commonly included in cough syrups is most appropriate for the client?

☐ **1.** Codeine
☐ **2.** Dextromethorphan (Robitussin DM)
☐ **3.** Diphenhydramine (Benadryl)
☐ **4.** Guaifenesin (Robitussin)

5. A client who had an upper respiratory tract infection has been using oxymetazoline (Afrin) nasal spray twice daily for 10 days. Although the client gets some relief after using it, he says he has to use more and more, and if he doesn't use it, the congestion comes back. What's the most likely explanation for this problem?

☐ **1.** He has used the oxymetazoline for too long.
☐ **2.** The twice-daily dosing interval is too short for oxymetazoline.
☐ **3.** A viral infection has probably become a secondary bacterial infection.
☐ **4.** He has developed a tolerance to the pharmacologic effect of oxymetazoline.

6. A nurse is assessing the serum theophylline (Slo-Bid) level in a client with asthma. Which serum theophylline level represents the therapeutic range for treating asthma?

☐ **1.** 1 to 5 mcg/ml
☐ **2.** 5 to 10 mcg/ml
☐ **3.** 10 to 20 mcg/ml
☐ **4.** 20 to 25 mcg/ml

TOP 5

Items to study for your next test on drugs and the respiratory system

1. Mechanisms of action of bronchodilators, anti-inflammatory inhalants, antitussives, expectorants, mucolytics, and decongestants

2. Rationale for using bronchodilators, anti-inflammatory inhalants, antitussives, expectorants, mucolytics, and decongestants

3. Common adverse effects of bronchodilators, anti-inflammatory inhalants, antitussives, expectorants, mucolytics, and decongestants

4. Nursing responsibilities when administering bronchodilators, anti-inflammatory inhalants, antitussives, expectorants, mucolytics, and decongestants

5. Patient teaching related to bronchodilators, anti-inflammatory inhalants, antitussives, expectorants, mucolytics, and decongestants

7. A physician has ordered acetylcysteine (Mucomyst) for a client who has acute poisoning. The nurse knows that besides its use as a mucolytic, acetylcysteine is also used to treat the toxic effects of which drug?

☐ **1.** Acetaminophen (Tylenol)

☐ **2.** Atropine

☐ **3.** Codeine

☐ **4.** Lorazepam (Ativan)

8. Albuterol (Proventil) inhalation therapy is ordered for a client with chronic obstructive pulmonary disease. Which instruction should the nurse include in the teaching plan for this client?

☐ **1.** Watch for voice changes.

☐ **2.** Test your urine for protein weekly using a dipstick.

☐ **3.** Count your pulse before, during, and after treatment.

☐ **4.** Use your inhaler as often as needed throughout the day.

9. A nurse is teaching a client who's taking bronchodilators. Which statement by the client indicates that the client requires further instruction?

☐ **1.** "I can use albuterol (Proventil) for an asthmatic crisis."

☐ **2.** "I can use metaproterenol (Alupent) for an asthmatic crisis."

☐ **3.** "I can use pirbuterol (Maxair) for an asthmatic crisis."

☐ **4.** "I can use salmeterol (Serevent) for an asthmatic crisis."

10. Which information should a nurse include when teaching a client who's taking montelukast (Singulair)? Select all that apply.

☐ **1.** Keep rescue medication available for acute attacks.

☐ **2.** You may experience headaches, dizziness, nausea, and vomiting with this drug.

☐ **3.** This drug may cause an oral fungal infection (thrush).

☐ **4.** This drug may alter your blood glucose levels.

☐ **5.** Take this drug at bedtime for the best response.

ANSWERS AND RATIONALES

1. CORRECT ANSWER: 1

Theophylline, like other methylxanthines, is commonly used to treat chronic obstructive pulmonary disease and asthma. The goal of treatment is a normal respiratory rate and easy, unlabored respirations. Theophylline has no effect on urine output. The drug may increase heart rate and blood pressure, but these aren't indications that the drug is effective.

2. CORRECT ANSWER: 2

Metaproterenol stimulates beta receptors to dilate the bronchioles and stimulates the cardiovascular system. These actions result in tachycardia and shaking. Edema and moon face are usually seen with corticosteroid therapy. Bleeding ulcer and vomiting are usually associated with nonsteroidal anti-inflammatory therapy. Bronchodilators can cause hypertension rather than hypotension.

3. CORRECT ANSWER: 2

Albuterol, a bronchodilator, should be used first to open the airways so that the steroid (beclomethasone) can better penetrate the lungs. Taking the steroid first would reduce the therapeutic effects of the steroid. Alternating the order of use would also reduce the therapeutic effect. Gum breakdown isn't a concern with the use of these drugs.

4. CORRECT ANSWER: 4

Guaifenesin is an expectorant that helps decrease secretions in the client's airways, which reduces the urge to cough. Codeine, dextromethorphan, and diphenhydramine are antitussives, which reduce the frequency of the cough but don't help expectorate secretions from a productive cough.

5. CORRECT ANSWER: 1

The client is describing classic rebound congestion (also known as *rhinitis medicamentosa*) that occurs when topical decongestants are used for more than 3 days. Twice daily is the correct dosing interval for this drug. There are no signs of bacterial infection. The client's signs and symptoms don't indicate pharmacologic tolerance, which would involve receptor changes.

6. CORRECT ANSWER: 3

To treat a respiratory disease such as asthma, the therapeutic serum theophylline level should range from 10 to 20 mcg/ml. A lower serum level may not produce a therapeutic response; a higher level may lead to adverse reactions.

7. CORRECT ANSWER: 1

Acetaminophen toxicity is treated with orally administered acetylcysteine. Atropine toxicity can be treated with bethanechol (Urecholine), and codeine toxicity is treated with naloxone (Narcan). Treatment for lorazepam toxicity is symptomatic.

8. CORRECT ANSWER: 3

Albuterol is a potent sympathomimetic that may cause excessive sympathetic nervous system stimulation, manifested by a fast, pounding heartbeat; nervousness; tremors; and restlessness. Therefore, the client should count his pulse before, during, and after treatment. The drug has no effect on voice quality or urine protein levels. The drug should be taken as ordered, not as needed or more often than every 4 hours. Frequent use of this drug may lead to a loss of effectiveness or severe paradoxical bronchoconstriction.

9. CORRECT ANSWER: 4

The client requires further teaching if he states that he can use salmeterol for an asthmatic crisis. This drug is a long-acting bronchodilator. It's used to prevent wheezing from chronic asthma, not as a rescue drug during an asthmatic attack. Albuterol, metaproterenol, and pirbuterol are short-acting drugs that can be used to relieve acute wheezing.

10. CORRECT ANSWER: 1, 2, 5
Leukotriene receptor modifiers are used for the long-term treatment of asthma and won't help in an acute attack. The client should keep rescue medication on hand for acute attacks. Headaches, dizziness, nausea, and vomiting are commonly reported adverse reactions to these drugs. Oral fungal infections and altered blood glucose levels are typically associated with corticosteroids. Montelukast has been shown to have increased effectiveness if taken at bedtime.

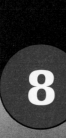

8

Drugs and the cardiovascular system

PRETEST

1. Which drug is most appropriate for a client with heart failure who's waiting for a heart transplant?

- ☐ 1. Digoxin (Lanoxin)
- ☐ 2. Milrinone (Primacor)
- ☐ 3. Telmisartan (Micardis)
- ☐ 4. Metoprolol (Lopressor)

CORRECT ANSWER: 2

2. Nitrates exert their antianginal effect by:

- ☐ 1. producing vasodilation, decreasing preload and afterload, and reducing myocardial oxygen consumption.
- ☐ 2. reducing myocardial oxygen demands by slowing the heart rate and deceasing the force of myocardial contractions.
- ☐ 3. preventing the passage of calcium ions across the myocardial cell membrane, dilating coronary arteries and preventing coronary artery vasospasm.
- ☐ 4. inhibiting the response to beta-adrenergic stimulation, thereby decreasing cardiac output.

CORRECT ANSWER: 1

3. One of the most common signs of digoxin toxicity is:
- ☐ 1. lethargy.
- ☐ 2. constipation.
- ☐ 3. dyspnea.
- ☐ 4. vision disturbances.

CORRECT ANSWER: 4

4. One of the most important assessments a nurse needs to make before administering a beta-adrenergic blocker for hypertension is to check the client's:
- ☐ 1. potassium level.
- ☐ 2. mental status.
- ☐ 3. heart rate.
- ☐ 4. urine output.

CORRECT ANSWER: 3

5. A client is about to begin antilipemic therapy with lovastatin (Mevinolin). To enhance the drug's absorption, the nurse should advise the client to take the drug at what time?
- ☐ 1. At bedtime
- ☐ 2. Upon arising
- ☐ 3. With the evening meal
- ☐ 4. With morning and evening meals

CORRECT ANSWER: 3

LEARNING OBJECTIVES

After studying this chapter, you should be able to:

- Understand the different indications for inotropics, antiarrhythmics, antihypertensives, antianginals, and antilipemics.
- Describe the general mechanisms of action of cardiac drugs and antilipemics.
- Name common adverse effects of cardiac drugs and antilipemics.
- Identify nursing responsibilities when administering cardiac drugs and antilipemics.
- Discuss appropriate teaching for the patient receiving a cardiac drug or an antilipemic.

CHAPTER OVERVIEW

Because inotropic drugs increase the force of myocardial contraction, they're used to treat symptoms of heart failure and manage atrial arrhythmias. These drugs increase stroke volume and cardiac output, slow conduction, and cause diuresis by increasing blood flow to the kidneys. Digoxin, the major inotropic drug, has a very narrow therapeutic margin. Inamrinone and milrinone, also inotropic drugs, are used in critically ill patients to increase cardiac output and decrease preload and afterload.

Antiarrhythmics are used to suppress or regulate atrial and ventricular conduction disturbances resulting from myocardial infarction (MI) and other causes. Most antiarrhythmics have proarrhythmic properties, meaning they can precipitate or aggravate an arrhythmia.

Antihypertensives lower blood pressure by inhibiting the central or peripheral nervous system, the renin-angiotensin mechanism, or sodium and chloride reabsorption in the renal tubules. They're prescribed based on the cause of hypertension.

Antianginals reduce myocardial oxygen demand and increase blood flow to ischemic areas of the myocardium. They terminate acute anginal attacks and prevent angina from occurring. Acute angina is managed with a short-acting nitrate, such as nitroglycerin sublingual (S.L.) tablets or spray. Nitroglycerin may be used I.V. for unrelieved chest pain during acute MI. Angina prevention is managed with one or more drugs, including nitrates, beta-adrenergic blockers, and calcium channel blockers.

Antilipemics are used to prevent and treat atherosclerosis. Because of the adverse effects of these drugs, dietary modification, weight loss, exercise, and smoking cessation are considered first-line treatment. Antilipemic therapy may be indicated if these measures are ineffective.

ANATOMY AND PHYSIOLOGY

● **Anatomy**
  - Heart
    – Made of upper chambers (atria) that communicate with lower chambers (ventricles) via atrioventricular (AV) valves
  - Blood vessels (arteries, arterioles, capillaries, venules, and veins)
  - Various circulations (cardiac, pulmonary, systemic, hepatic, and fetal [in pregnant women])
● **Physiology**
  - Cardiac cycle
    – Is a sequence of events that occur as the heart pumps blood through vessels to the body
    – Occurs during course of a single systole (contraction) and diastole (relaxation) of the atria and ventricles
    – Produces heart sounds and a pulse
  - Cardiac conduction system

A&P highlights

● The cardiovascular system consists of the heart and blood vessels and includes the cardiac circulation, pulmonary circulation, systemic circulation, and hepatic circulation.
● The heart pumps blood through the blood vessels.
● Events that occur during a single systole and diastole of the atria and ventricles make up the cardiac cycle; they also produce heart sounds and a pulse.
● The cardiac conduction system sends impulses and controls the heartbeat.
● Blood pressure refers to the pressure of the blood in the systemic circulation.
● Starling's law, baroreceptors and chemoreceptors in major arteries, and hormones secreted by the kidneys control cardiac output and blood pressure.
● The cardiovascular system moves blood throughout the body, helps maintain proper body pH and electrolyte composition, and helps regulate body temperature.

– Consists of the sinoatrial (SA) node and internodal tracts, AV node, bundle of His, and Purkinje fibers
– Generates and sends impulses that cause synchronized contractions of the atria and ventricles
– Controls the heartbeat
• Blood pressure
– Pressure of blood in the systemic circulation
  · Highest when blood is ejected during systole (systolic pressure)
  · Lowest during diastole (diastolic pressure)
– Factors affecting blood pressure and cardiac output
  · Starling's law (force of heart muscle contraction is proportional to its initial length)
  · Baroreceptors and chemoreceptors in major arteries
  · Hormones secreted by the kidneys
• Fluid transfer
– Involves cyclic flow of fluid from the interstitial space to the capillaries and back into the interstitial space
– Depends on capillary hydrostatic pressure, capillary permeability, osmotic pressure, and open lymphatic channels
– If disturbed, may lead to edema (excess fluid in interstitial space)

● **Function**
• Moves blood throughout body
• Helps maintain proper body pH and electrolyte composition
• Helps regulate body temperature

INOTROPIC DRUGS
CARDIAC GLYCOSIDES

● **Mechanism of action**
• Inhibit the sodium-potassium activation of adenosine triphosphate, which regulates the amount of sodium and potassium inside the cell
• Promote movement of calcium from extracellular to intracellular cytoplasms and strengthens myocardial contractility (positive inotropic action)
• Act on the central nervous system (CNS) to enhance vagal tone, slowing contractility through the SA and AV nodes (negative chronotropic action)

● **Pharmacokinetics**
• Absorption: Absorbed well from GI tract
• Distribution: Distributed widely throughout body; poorly protein-bound
• Metabolism: Metabolized by the liver and GI flora
• Excretion: Excreted unchanged in urine

● **Drug examples**
• Digoxin (Digitek, Lanoxicaps, Lanoxin)

● **Indications**
• Treat heart failure

Key facts about cardiac glycosides

• Promote calcium movement
• Strengthen myocardial contractility
• Enhance vagal tone
• Metabolized by the liver and GI flora
• Excreted unchanged in the urine

When to use cardiac glycosides

• Heart faillure
• Atrial fibrillation
• Atrial flutter
• Paroxysmal atrial tachycardia

- Control ventricular rate in atrial fibrillation, atrial flutter, and paroxysmal atrial tachycardia

Contraindications and precautions

- Contraindicated in uncontrolled ventricular arrhythmias, idiopathic hypertrophic subaortic stenosis, constrictive pericarditis, complete heart block, and sick sinus syndrome
- Used cautiously in patients with acute MI because it increases the risk of arrhythmias

Adverse reactions

- Bradycardia, nausea, vomiting, diarrhea, headaches, complete heart block, and vision changes
- Possible digoxin toxicity (anorexia, nausea, vomiting, vision disturbances, confusion, bradycardia, heart block, premature ventricular contractions, and tachyarrhythmias)
    - Increased risk in patients with hypercalcemia, hypokalemia, hypomagnesemia, hypothyroidism, or renal failure
    - Increased risk in elderly patients because they're more sensitive to drug's effects; anorexia may be an early warning sign

Interactions

- Potassium-wasting diuretics and other drugs causing potassium loss increase risk of digoxin toxicity
- Amiodarone, calcium, propafenone, omeprazole, cyclosporine, macrolides (erythromycin, clarithromycin), quinidine, spironolactone, tetracyclines, and verapamil increase serum digoxin levels; may cause toxicity
- Beta-adrenergic blockers, calcium channel blockers, succinylcholine, thyroid medications, and diuretics may cause bradycardia and other arrhythmias
- Antacids, barbiturates, cholestyramine, kaolin and pectin, metoclopramide, rifampin, and sulfasalazine decrease GI absorption of digoxin

Nursing responsibilities

- Assess the patient's apical pulse, serum drug and electrolyte levels, and renal function before administering digoxin; withhold the drug and notify the practitioner if the pulse rate is less than 60 beats/minute or the minimum specified by the practitioner
- Monitor the patient's serum digoxin level continuously and watch for signs and symptoms of toxicity, especially in elderly patients and during digitalization
- Don't alternate dosage forms because bioavailability of capsules doesn't equal that of tablets or elixir
- Know that digoxin immune Fab is used as an antidote in extreme toxicity
- Be aware that hypokalemia places the patient at risk for digoxin toxicity
- Instruct the patient how to take the prescribed drug; warn him *not* to take a double dose after missing a dose

---

When NOT to use cardiac glycosides

- Uncontrolled ventricular arrhythmias
- Idiopathic hypertrophic subaortic stenosis
- Constrictive pericarditis
- Complete heart block

Adverse reactions

- Bradycardia, nausea, vomiting, diarrhea, digoxin toxicity

Key nursing actions

- Before administering digoxin, assess patient's apical pulse, serum drug and electrolyte levels, and renal function; withhold drug and notify practitioner if pulse rate is below 60 beats/minute or minimum specified by practitioner.
- Continuously monitor serum digoxin level and watch for signs and symptoms of toxicity.
- Don't alternate dosage forms.
- Know that digoxin immune fab is an antidote for toxicity.
- Know that reduced dosage is needed in patients with renal impairment.

Topics for patient discussion

- Therapy regimen
- Signs and symptoms of possible adverse reactions and when to notify practitioner
- Procedure for taking and monitoring pulse
- Dietary restrictions
- Weight monitoring
- Need for compliance with therapy
- Follow-up care

TIME-OUT FOR TEACHING

Teaching about cardiac glycosides

Include these topics in your teaching plan for the patient receiving a cardiac glycoside:

- medication therapy regimen, including the drug's name, dose, frequency, duration, and possible adverse effects
- signs and symptoms of possible adverse effects, especially heart failure and toxicity, and when to notify the practitioner
- procedure for taking and monitoring pulse
- dietary restrictions and allowances
- weight monitoring
- need for compliance with therapy, including taking the drug as prescribed and instructions for missed doses
- follow-up care, including laboratory tests and practitioner visits.

- Advise the patient to consult the practitioner before discontinuing the drug
- Teach the patient to count his pulse before taking each dose; instruct him to notify the practitioner if his pulse rate is below 60 or above 100 beats/ minute
- Teach the patient how to recognize signs and symptoms of digoxin toxicity and heart failure (see *Teaching about cardiac glycosides*)
- Know that because digoxin is excreted unchanged by the kidneys, the dosage must be reduced in patients with renal impairment
- Monitor the patient receiving I.V. infusion of inotropic drugs for worsening or new arrhythmias, hypertension, and hypotension

PHOSPHODIESTERASE INHIBITORS

Key facts about phosphodiesterase inhibitors

- Increase myocardial contractility
- Decrease systemic vascular resistance
- Improve cardiac output
- Metabolized by the liver or kidneys
- Excreted primarily in the uine

● Mechanism of action

- Increase myocardial contractility and decrease systemic vascular resistance and venous return, resulting in improved cardiac output

● Pharmacokinetics

- Absorption: Administered I.V.
- Distribution: Distributed rapidly
- Metabolism: Metabolized by the liver (inamrinone) or kidneys (milrinone)
- Excretion: Excreted primarily in urine

● Drug examples

- Inamrinone (Inocor), milrinone (Primacor)

● Indications

- Short-term management of heart failure in patients who are closely monitored and don't respond adequately to digoxin preparations, diuretics, or vasodilators
- Long-term management in patients waiting for heart transplant

When to use phosphodiesterase inhibitors

- Heart failure
- Waiting for heart transplant

Contraindications and precautions
- Inamrinone contraindicated in patients who are hypersensitive to inamrinone or bisulfates or who have had an acute MI
- Milrinone contraindicated in patients with hypersensitivity to drug
- Shouldn't be used in patients with severe obstructive aortic or pulmonic valvular disease; may aggravate outflow tract obstruction in hypertrophic subaortic stenosis
- Requires correcting hypokalemia with potassium supplements before use because of the increased risk of arrhythmias

Adverse reactions
- Arrhythmias (ventricular) and hypotension (most common) because of drug's vasodilating effects
- Possible thrombocytopenia, headache, nausea, vomiting, anorexia, fever, chest pain, and hypokalemia

Interactions
- Use of inamrinone with disopyramide may cause excessive hypotension
- Use of inamrinone with digoxin may enhance AV conduction and increase ventricular response rate; therefore, concomitant therapy is recommended for patients with atrial flutter or fibrillation

Nursing responsibilities
- Monitor the patient's hemodynamic status closely, including pulmonary artery pressure and cardiac output; dosage is determined by patient response
- Monitor the patient's heart rate, heart rhythm, and blood pressure frequently to detect arrhythmias or hypotension
- Administer the drug I.V., using an infusion pump; slow or stop the infusion if the patient's blood pressure drops
- Monitor the patient receiving I.V. infusion of inotropic drugs for worsening or new arrhythmias, hypertension, and hypotension

ANTIARRHYTHMICS

CLASS I ANTIARRHYTHMICS

Mechanism of action
- All Class I drugs and subclasses: Block sodium channels (local anesthetic effect) and slow conduction of electrical impulses
- Class IA drugs: Slow depolarization and prolong repolarization
- Class IB drugs: Normalize depolarization and shorten repolarization
- Class IC drugs: Slow depolarization and normalize repolarization

Pharmacokinetics
- Absorption: Usually well absorbed in GI tract after oral administration
- Distribution: Highly protein-bound
- Metabolism: Metabolized by the liver
- Excretion: Excreted in urine

When NOT to use phosphodiesterase inhibitors

- Hypersensitivity to these drugs or bisulfates
- Acute MI
- Severe obstructive aortic or pulmonic valvular disease

Adverse reactions

- Arrhythmias (ventricular), hypotension, thrombocytopenia, headache, nausea, vomiting, anorexia, chest pain

Key nursing actions

- Closely monitor patient's hemodynamic status.
- Monitor patient's heart rate, heart rhythm, and blood pressure frequently.
- Administer drug I.V., using an infusion pump; slow or stop infusion if patient's blood pressure drops.

Key facts about class I antiarrhythmics

- Block sodium channels and slow conduction of electrical impulses
- Slow or normalize depolarization and shorten, normalize, or prolong repolarization
- Metabolized by the liver
- Excreted in the urine

When to use class I antiarrhythmics

- Ventricular arrhythmias
- Ventricular ectopy
- Ventricular tachycardia

When NOT to use class I antiarrhythmics

- Complete atrioventricular block
- Hypersensitivity to these drugs

Adverse reactions

- Hypotension, heart failure, nausea, vomiting, diarrhea, palpitations

Key nursing actions

- Before giving lidocaine, always check label to prevent administering form containing epinephrine or preservatives.
- Administer I.V. bolus for ventricular arrhythmias, followed by continuous I.V. infusion, as ordered.
- Don't administer Class IA drugs with food unless prescribed.
- Administer mexiletine or tocainide with food or antacids.
- Be aware that disopyramide has anticholinergic effects.
- Monitor QT interval when administering procainamide.

● Drug examples
- Class IA: disopyramide (Norpace), procainamide (Pronestyl), quinidine
- Class IB: lidocaine (Xylocaine), mexiletine (Mexitil), tocainide
- Class IC: flecainide (Tambocor), propafenone (Rythmol)

● Indications
- Treat life-threatening ventricular arrhythmias (Class IA and IC drugs and lidocaine)
- Treat symptomatic non-life-threatening arrhythmias (Class IA drugs and mexiletine)
- Suppress the frequency of ventricular ectopy and reduce the frequency and duration of abrupt, selflimiting ventricular tachycardia (tocainide)

● Contraindications and precautions
- Contraindicated in patients with complete AV block (because of risk of asystole) and those hypersensitive to antiarrhythmics or similar drugs
- Used cautiously in patients with acute MI or heart failure

● Adverse reactions
- Class IA: Diarrhea, nausea, vomiting, abdominal cramping, and anorexia
- Class IB: Drowsiness, light-headedness, paresthesia, hypotension, and bradycardia; possible lidocaine toxicity (seizures and respiratory and cardiac arrest)
- Class IC: Palpitations, shortness of breath, chest pain, heart failure, and cardiac arrest; possible bronchospasms with propafenone use

● Interactions
- Concurrent use with antihypertensives causes additive hypotension
- Concurrent use with other antiarrhythmics may cause increased toxicity
- Theophylline plasma levels increase when given with mexiletine
- Propafenone increases the serum concentration and effects of metoprolol and propranolol
- Quinidine and Class IC drugs may increase serum levels of digoxin or digitoxin

● Nursing responsibilities
- Before giving lidocaine, always check the label to prevent administering a form that contains epinephrine or preservatives; such solutions are used for local anesthesia only
- Know that lidocaine has a short duration of action
- Administer an I.V. bolus for ventricular arrhythmias, followed by a continuous I.V. infusion, as ordered
- Don't administer Class IA antiarrhythmics with food unless prescribed; food may affect reabsorption
- Administer mexiletine or tocainide with food or antacids to reduce GI distress
- Institute safety precautions to prevent injury
- Be aware that disopyramide has anticholinergic effects

– Observe for urine retention, constipation, dry mouth, and blurred vision
– Instruct the patient to follow a high-fiber diet or use a bulk laxative for constipation
- Monitor electrocardiograms (ECGs) continuously at the start of therapy; also monitor vital signs frequently
- Monitor for early signs of lidocaine toxicity (nervousness, confusion, dizziness, and tinnitus)
- Monitor the QT interval when administering procainamide; prepare to stop infusion if interval increases by 50% over baseline

CLASS II ANTIARRHYTHMICS

Mechanism of action
- Decrease sympathetic activity at the SA and AV nodes, decreasing automaticity and prolonging the refractory period

Pharmacokinetics
- Absorption: Well absorbed after oral administration; esmolol only available I.V.
- Distribution: Not widely distributed
- Metabolism: Extensive first-pass metabolism by the liver; esmolol metabolized by red blood cells
- Excretion: Excreted in urine and feces

Drug examples
- Acebutolol (Sectral), esmolol (Brevibloc), propranolol (Inderal)

Indications
- Treat sinus tachycardia and atrial fibrillation or flutter

Contraindications and precautions
- Contraindicated in patients with persistent severe bradycardia, second- and third-degree heart block, overt cardiac failure, and cardiogenic shock
- Used cautiously in patients at risk for heart failure and those with impaired hepatic function, bronchospastic disease (including asthma), diabetes, hyperthyroidism, or peripheral vascular disease

Adverse reactions
- Fatigue, hypotension, heart failure, bradycardia, arrhythmias, bronchospasm, and GI distress

Interactions
- Class II antiarrhythmics may increase hypotensive effects when used with alpha-adrenergic stimulants, indomethacin, nonsteroidal anti-inflammatories (NSAIDs), diuretics, phenothiazines, or calcium channel blockers
- Esmolol increases the risk of digoxin toxicity
- Concurrent administration with verapamil increases the risk of hypotension, bradycardia, AV heart block, and asystole

Key facts about class II antiarrhythmics
- Decrease sympathetic activity at the SA and AV nodes, decreasing automaticity and prolonging the refractory period
- Undergo extensive first-pass metabolism by the liver
- Excreted in the urine, and feces

When to use class II antiarrhythmics
- Sinus tachycardia
- Atrial fibrillation or flutter

When NOT to use class II antiarrhythmics
- Persistent severe bradycardia
- Second- or third-degree heart block
- Overt cardiac failure
- Cardiogenic shock

Adverse reactions
- Fatigue, hypotension, heart failure, bradycardia, arrhythmias, heart block, bronchospasm, GI distress

Topics for patient discussion

- Medication therapy regimen
- Signs and symptoms of possible adverse effects and when to notify the practitioner
- Procedure for taking and monitoring pulse
- Dietary restrictions
- Weight monitoring
- Safety measures
- Need for compliance with therapy
- Medical follow-up

Key nursing actions

- Instruct patient to watch for signs and symptoms of fluid retention.
- Advise patient to limit fluid and salt intake to minimize fluid retention.
- Inform patient that drug should be discontinued gradually; abrupt discontinuation may exacerbate angina symptoms or precipitate MI.
- Monitor ECG continuously when beginning therapy.

Key facts about class III antiarrhythmics

- Prolong the action potential and the absolute refractory period
- Metabolized extensively by the liver
- Excreted in bile

When to use class III antiarrhythmics

- Recurrent ventricular fibrillation
- Unstable ventricular tachycardia
- Atrial fibrillation
- Maintenance of normal sinus rhythm

 TIME-OUT FOR TEACHING

Teaching about class II antiarrhythmics

Include these topics in your teaching plan for the patient receiving a class II antiarrhythmic:

- medication therapy regimen, including the drug's name, dose, frequency, duration, and possible adverse effects
- signs and symptoms of possible adverse effects and when to notify the practitioner
- procedure for taking and monitoring pulse
- dietary restrictions, including fluid and sodium restrictions as appropriate
- weight monitoring
- safety measures
- measures to ensure compliance with therapy
- medical follow-up.

Nursing responsibilities

- Instruct the patient to watch for signs and symptoms of fluid retention, such as weight gain, peripheral edema, or shortness of breath (see *Teaching about class II antiarrhythmics*)
- Advise the patient to limit fluid and salt intake to minimize fluid retention
- Inform the patient that the drug should be discontinued gradually, under practitioner's supervision, over 2 weeks
- Warn the patient that discontinuing the drug abruptly may exacerbate angina symptoms or precipitate MI in those with coronary artery disease
- Institute safety precautions to prevent injury
- Monitor the ECG continuously when beginning therapy
- Administer the drug with meals to minimize GI upset

CLASS III ANTIARRHYTHMICS

Mechanism of action
- Prolong the action potential and absolute refractory period

Pharmacokinetics
- Absorption: Absorption slow and variable after oral administration
- Distribution: Widely distributed in fat tissues and liver; highly protein-bound
- Metabolism: Metabolized extensively by the liver
- Excretion: Excreted in bile; amiodarone has longest half-life of all antiarrhythmics

Drug examples
- Amiodarone (Cordarone), ibutilide (Corvert), sotalol (Betapace AF)

Indications
- Treat recurrent ventricular fibrillation
- Treat unstable ventricular tachycardia

- Treat atrial fibrillation
- Maintenance of normal sinus rhythm in patients who have been converted from atrial fibrillation or atrial flutter (sotalol)

● **Contraindications and precautions**
- Contraindicated in breast-feeding patients and those with hypokalemia, heart block, long QT syndrome, severe sinus node dysfunction, or bradycardia-induced syncope
- Used cautiously in patients with heart failure, diabetes, or hepatic or renal failure

● **Adverse reactions**
- Pulmonary fibrosis (with prolonged use), photosensitivity, corneal microdeposits, hypothyroidism, and peripheral neuropathy (amiodarone)
- AV block, bradycardia, ventricular arrhythmias, bronchospasm, and hypotension (sotalol)
- Severe hypotension (if I.V. amiodarone administered too quickly)

● **Interactions**
- Concurrent use with digoxin may increase digoxin levels and worsen arrhythmias
- Amiodarone increases quinidine, procainamide, and phenytoin levels
- Sotalol shouldn't be given with dolasetron or droperidol because of the increased risk of life-threatening arrhythmias

● **Nursing responsibilities**
- Assess lung, thyroid, and neurologic function in the patient receiving amiodarone to ensure prompt detection of adverse effects
- Don't administer sotalol unless the patient is unresponsive to other antiarrhythmics and has a life-threatening ventricular arrhythmia; monitor the patient's response carefully because the drug's proarrhythmic effects can be pronounced
- Teach the patient receiving amiodarone to use sunscreen and wear protective clothing to prevent photosensitivity reactions
- Teach the patient receiving amiodarone to use artificial tears to prevent corneal deposits
- Monitor the ECG continuously when starting treatment and periodically thereafter

CLASS IV ANTIARRHYTHMICS (CALCIUM CHANNEL BLOCKERS)

● **Mechanism of action**
- Block slow inward calcium channels, slowing conduction through the AV node

● **Pharmacokinetics**
- Absorption: Absorbed rapidly and completely from GI tract after oral administration

---

When NOT to use class III antiarrhythmics

- Breast-feeding
- Severe sinus node dysfunction
- Bradycardia-induced syncope
- Hypokalemia
- Heart block

Adverse reactions

- Hypotension, bradycardia
- Pulmonary fibrosis, corneal microdeposits

Key nursing actions

- Don't administer sotalol unless patient is unresponsive to other antiarrhythmics and has a life-threatening ventricular arrhythmia
- Assess lung, thyroid, and neurologic function in patient receiving amiodarone to ensure prompt detection of adverse effects.
- Teach patient to:
- use artificial tears and sunscreen and wear protective clothing if taking amiodarone.

Key facts about class IV antiarrhythmics

- Block the slow inward calcium channels, slowing conduction through the AV node
- Metabolized by the liver
- Excreted in the urine

When to use class IV antiarrhythmics

- Atrial fibrillation and flutter (except when associated with accessory bypass tracts)
- Supraventricular tachycardias
- Prinzmetal's or variant angina
- Unstable or chronic stable angina pectoris
- Hypertension

When NOT to use class IV antiarrhythmics

- Severe left ventricular dysfunction
- Cardiogenic shock
- Second- or third-degree heart block
- Sick sinus syndrome
- Severe heart failure
- Severe hypotension
- Atrial fibrillation and flutter associated with accessory bypass tracts
- In patients receiving I.V. beta-adrenergic blockers or with ventricular tachycardia (I.V. verapamil)

Adverse reactions

- Dizziness, hypotension, bradycardia, edema, constipation

Key nursing actions

- Advise patient to change position slowly.
- Encourage patient to increase fiber intake.
- If patient is receiving I.V. verapamil, monitor blood pressure and ECG continuously.

- **Distribution:** Highly protein-bound
- **Metabolism:** Metabolized by the liver; goes through first-pass metabolism
- **Excretion:** Excreted in urine

● **Drug examples**
- Diltiazem (Cardizem, Tiazac), verapamil (Calan, Covera-HS, Isoptin SR, Verelan)

● **Indications**
- Treat atrial fibrillation or flutter (except when associated with accessory bypass tracts) and supraventricular tachycardias
- Manage Prinzmetal's or variant angina and unstable or chronic stable angina pectoris
- Treat hypertension

● **Contraindications and precautions**
- Contraindicated in patients with severe left ventricular dysfunction, cardiogenic shock, second- or third-degree heart block, sick sinus syndrome (unless functioning pacemaker is present), atrial flutter or fibrillation associated with accessory bypass tracts, severe heart failure, or severe hypotension
- I.V. verapamil contraindicated in patients receiving I.V. beta-adrenergic blockers and in those with ventricular tachycardia
- Used cautiously in elderly patients and those with impaired hepatic or renal function or increased intracranial pressure (ICP)

● **Adverse reactions**
- Dizziness, hypotension, bradycardia, edema, constipation, heart failure, AV block, ventricular asystole, ventricular fibrillation, and nausea

● **Interactions**
- Use with digoxin increases risk of digoxin toxicity
- Use with beta-adrenergic blockers may increase risk of bradycardia and heart failure
- Use with antihypertensives or quinidine causes additive hypotension
- Furosemide I.V. forms precipitate if given with diltiazem I.V.
- Verapamil decreases lithium levels
- Grapefruit juice increases therapeutic effects and risk of toxicity

● **Nursing responsibilities**
- Advise the patient to change position slowly to minimize orthostatic hypotension
- Encourage the patient to increase fiber intake to prevent constipation
- Monitor blood pressure and ECG continuously if the patient is receiving I.V. verapamil
- Withhold the drug if the patient's heart rate is less than 60 beats/minute or systolic blood pressure is less than 90 mm Hg

MISCELLANEOUS ANTIARRHYTHMICS

● **Mechanism of action**
  - Adenosine: Interrupts reentrant pathways; slows conduction in the AV node
  - Atropine: Blocks muscarinic cholinergic receptors in the SA and AV nodes; blocks effects of vagus nerve on cardiac conduction

● **Pharmacokinetics**
  - Absorption: Administered I.V.
  - Distribution: Widely distributed; rapidly distributed (adenosine)
  - Metabolism: Metabolized in tissues (adenosine) and by the liver (atropine)
  - Excretion: Excreted in urine (atropine); excretion for adenosine unknown

● **Drug examples**
  - Adenosine (Adenocard), atropine sulfate

● **Indications**
  - Treat paroxysmal supraventricular tachycardia unresponsive to vagal maneuvers (adenosine)
  - Treat symptomatic sinus bradycardia and bradyarrhythmias (atropine)

● **Contraindications and precautions**
  - Adenosine contraindicated in patients with second- or third-degree AV block and sick sinus syndrome without a pacemaker, atrial fibrillation, atrial flutter, or ventricular tachycardia
  - Atropine contraindicated in patients with glaucoma, urine retention, or ileus
  - Used cautiously in patients with asthma

● **Adverse reactions**
  - Transient arrhythmias, dyspnea, facial flushing, and chest discomfort (adenosine)
  - Hallucinations (with high doses), tachycardia, dry mouth, and constipation (atropine)

● **Interactions**
  - Theophylline and caffeine decrease the effects of adenosine and atropine
  - Dipyridamole potentiates the effects of adenosine
  - Concurrent use of atropine with quinidine or tricyclic antidepressants causes additive anticholinergic effects

● **Nursing responsibilities**
  - Assess for paradoxical bradycardia when administering atropine in low doses or by slow infusion
  - Administer adenosine by rapid I.V. bolus under direct medical supervision to prevent complications; drug has a very short half-life
  - Monitor the patient's heart rate, respiratory rate, and blood pressure for signs of complications, such as heart failure and jugular vein distention
  - Monitor the ECG for new arrhythmias or exacerbation or resolution of an existing one

Key facts about adenosine and atropine

- Adenosine interrupts reentrant pathways and slows conduction in the AV node.
- Atropine blocks muscarinic cholinergic receptors in the SA and AV nodes and blocks the effects of the vagus nerve on cardiac conduction.
- Adenosine is metabolized in the tissues; atropine is metabolized by the liver.
- Atropine is excreted primarily in the urine.

When to use adenosine or atropine

- Paroxysmal supraventricular tachycardia unresponsive to vagal maneuvers (adenosine)
- Symptomatic sinus bradycardia and bradyarrhythmia (atropine)

When NOT to use adenosine or atropine

- Second- or third-degree AV block (adenosine)
- Sick sinus syndrome without a pacemaker (adenosine)
- Atrial fibrillation, atrial flutter, and ventricular tachycardia (adenosine)
- Glaucoma, urine retention, or ileus (atropine)

Adverse reactions

- Transient arrhythmias, dyspnea, facial flushing, tachycardia, dry mouth, and constipation

Key nursing actions

- Monitor heart rate, respiratory rate, blood pressure, and ECG.
- Give these drugs around the clock, as prescribed.
- Administer I.V. antiarrhythmics by infusion pump.
- Administer adenosine by rapid I.V. bolus

- Administer antiarrhythmics around the clock, as prescribed, to maintain therapeutic serum drug levels
- Know that I.V. antiarrhythmics must be administered by infusion pump for accuracy
- Teach the patient the purpose of the prescribed antiarrhythmic

ANTIHYPERTENSIVES

CENTRALLY ACTING ADRENERGIC INHIBITORS

- **Mechanism of action**
  - Stimulate alpha receptors in CNS to inhibit vasoconstriction and cardioacceleration, thus reducing peripheral resistance
  - Are commonly given with a diuretic

- **Pharmacokinetics**
  - Absorption: Well absorbed
  - Distribution: Widely distributed
  - Metabolism: Metabolized by the liver
  - Excretion: Excreted in urine and feces

- **Drug examples**
  - Clonidine (Catapres, Catapres-TTS), guanabenz (Wytensin), guanfacine (Tenex), methyldopa and methyldopate hydrochloride

- **Indications**
  - Treat moderate hypertension

- **Contraindications and precautions**
  - Contraindicated in patients with asthma, sinus bradycardia, cardiogenic shock, second- or third-degree heart block, or overt cardiac failure
  - Used cautiously in pregnant or breast-feeding patients and those with severe renal or hepatic impairment

- **Adverse reactions**
  - Depression, drowsiness, edema, dry mouth, and impotence (all centrally acting adrenergic inhibitors)
  - Dizziness and constipation (clonidine)
  - Headache, paresthesia, and sleep disturbances (methyldopa and methyldopate hydrochloride)

- **Interactions**
  - Clonidine may decrease the effectiveness of levodopa
  - Use of clonidine with beta-adrenergic-blocking agents, prazosin, or tricyclic antidepressants may block the antihypertensive effect of clonidine and cause life-threatening increases in blood pressure
  - Verapamil may cause severe hypotension when given with clonidine or methyldopate hydrochloride
  - Use of methyldopa with lithium increases risk of lithium toxicity
  - Use of methyldopa with monoamine oxidase inhibitors may lead to excessive sympathetic stimulation

---

Key facts about centrally acting adrenergic inhibitors

- Stimulate alpha receptors in the CNS to inhibit vasoconstriction and cardioacceleration, thus reducing peripheral resistance
- Metabolized by the liver
- Excreted in the urine and feces

When to use centrally acting adrenergic inhibitors

- Moderate hypertension

When NOT to use centrally acting adrenergic inhibitors

- Asthma
- Sinus bradycardia
- Cardiogenic shock
- Second- or third-degree heart block
- Overt cardiac failure

Adverse reactions

- Depression, drowsiness, edema, dry mouth, impotence

- Tricyclic antidepressants may reverse or attenuate the hypotensive effects of methyldopa
- Severe increases in blood pressure may occur if methyldopa is given with nonselective beta-adrenergic blockers, phenothiazines, sympathomimetics, or barbiturates

● **Nursing responsibilities**
- Monitor closely for worsening of depression when administering clonidine or methyldopa to a patient with a history of mental depression
- Instruct the patient to take clonidine at bedtime to minimize orthostatic hypotension
- Teach the patient how to use transdermal clonidine, if prescribed
- Warn the patient taking methyldopa that the drug may darken urine
- Monitor the patient for orthostatic hypotension, and help him change position slowly to minimize it

PERIPHERALLY ACTING ADRENERGIC INHIBITORS

● **Mechanism of action**
- Reduce effects of norepinephrine at peripheral nerve endings to decrease sympathetic vasoconstriction

● **Pharmacokinetics**
- Absorption: Readily absorbed from GI tract
- Distribution: Highly protein-bound
- Metabolism: Extensively metabolized by the liver
- Excretion: Excreted mostly in bile and feces; some in urine

● **Drug examples**
- Doxazosin (Cardura), guanadrel (Hylorel), guanethidine (Ismelin), prazosin (Minipress), reserpine, terazosin (Hytrin)

● **Indications**
- Treat moderate or essential hypertension

● **Contraindications and precautions**
- Contraindicated in patients with asthma, sinus bradycardia, cardiogenic shock, second- or third-degree heart block, or overt cardiac failure
- Used cautiously in pregnant or breast-feeding patients and those with impaired hepatic function

● **Adverse reactions**
- Drowsiness, edema, orthostatic hypotension, diarrhea, and nasal stuffiness (all peripherally acting adrenergic inhibitors)
- Weakness, bradycardia, and ejaculation failure (guanethidine)
- Depression, GI irritation, and impotence (reserpine)

● **Interactions**
- Use with antiarrhythmics may increase the risk of cardiac arrhythmias
- May decrease the antihypertensive effects of clonidine

Key nursing actions

- When administering clonidine or methyldopa to patient with history of mental depression, monitor closely for worsening depression.
- Know that methyldopa may darken urine.
- Teach patient to:
- take clonidine at bedtime
- use transdermal clonidine properly, if prescribed.

Key facts about peripherally acting adrenergic inhibitors

- Reduce the effects of norepinephrine at peripheral nerve endings to decrease sympathetic vasoconstriction
- Metabolized extensively by the liver
- Excreted mostly in the bile and feces; some is excreted in the urine

When to use peripherally acting adrenergic inhibitors

- Moderate or essential hypertension

When NOT to use peripherally acting adrenergic inhibitors

- Asthma
- Sinus bradycardia
- Cardiogenic shock
- Second- or third-degree heart block
- Overt cardiac failure

Adverse reactions

- Drowsiness, edema, orthostatic hypotension, diarrhea, nasal stuffiness

Key nursing actions

- If patient taking reserpine has history of mental depression, monitor closely for worsening of depression.
- Advise patient to take reserpine with food, milk, or water.

Key facts about peripheral vasodilating drugs

- Exert direct action on arteries alone or on arteries and veins to decrease peripheral vascular resistance
- Metabolized rapidly in the tissues and RBCs
- Excreted in the urine

When to use peripheral vasodilating drugs

- Moderate to severe hypertension
- Essential hypertension
- Hypertensive crisis

When NOT to use peripheral vasodilating drugs

- Asthma
- Sinus bradycardia
- Cardiogenic shock
- Second- or third-degree heart block
- Overt cardiac failure

Adverse reactions

- Fluid retention, tachycardia, orthostatic hypotension, severe hypotension (with I.V. doses)

- Verapamil and beta-adrenergic blockers may increase the acute postural hypotensive reaction when given with prazosin

● **Nursing responsibilities**
- Monitor closely for worsening of depression if the patient taking reserpine has a history of mental depression
- Advise the patient to take reserpine with food, milk, or water to minimize GI irritation

PERIPHERAL VASODILATING DRUGS

● **Mechanism of action**
- Exert direct action on arteries alone or on arteries and veins to decrease peripheral vascular resistance

● **Pharmacokinetics**
- Absorption: Usually administered I.V.
- Distribution: Unknown
- Metabolism: Metabolized rapidly in tissues and red blood cells (RBCs)
- Excretion: Excreted in urine

● **Drug examples**
- Diazoxide (Hyperstat I.V.), hydralazine (Apresoline), minoxidil, nitroprusside (Nitropress)

● **Indications**
- Treat moderate to severe hypertension
- Treat essential hypertension (hydralazine and minoxidil)
- Treat hypertensive crisis (diazoxide and nitroprusside)

● **Contraindications and precautions**
- Contraindicated in patients with asthma, sinus bradycardia, cardiogenic shock, second- or third-degree heart block, or overt cardiac failure
- Used cautiously in pregnant or breast-feeding patients and those with impaired hepatic function

● **Adverse reactions**
- Fluid retention, tachycardia, orthostatic hypotension, severe hypotension (with I.V. doses), angina, palpitations, headache, and severe pericardial effusion
- Excessive hair growth (minoxidil)

● **Interactions**
- Antihypertensives, general anesthetics, and sildenafil may potentiate antihypertensive effects of nitroprusside
- Concurrent use with pressor agents may increase blood pressure
- Drugs may produce an additive effect when given with nitrates

● **Nursing responsibilities**
- Closely monitor the patient for fluid volume excess
- Monitor the patient's blood pressure every 5 minutes at start of infusion and at least every 15 minutes throughout

- Weigh the patient daily; record daily intake and output
- Auscultate breath sounds for crackles
- Observe for jugular vein distention and peripheral edema
- Advise the patient taking minoxidil that excessive hair growth is likely to occur 3 to 6 months after therapy begins; reassure him that extra growth should disappear 1 to 6 months after therapy ends
- Monitor thiocyanate levels in the patient receiving nitroprusside

BETA-ADRENERGIC BLOCKERS

● **Mechanism of action**
  - Compete with epinephrine for beta-adrenergic receptor sites
  - Inhibit response to beta-adrenergic stimulation, thereby decreasing cardiac output

● **Pharmacokinetics**
  - Absorption: Partially absorbed
  - Distribution: Distributed in tissues
  - Metabolism: Minimally metabolized by the liver
  - Excretion: Excreted primarily in urine; partially in feces

● **Drug examples**
  - Acebutolol (Sectral), atenolol (Tenormin), betaxolol (Kerlone), carteolol (Cartrol), carvedilol (Coreg), labetalol (Normodyne, Trandate), metoprolol (Lopressor, Toprol), nadolol (Corgard), penbutolol (Levatol), pindolol (Visken), propranolol (Inderal), timolol (Blocadren)

● **Indications**
  - Treat mild hypertension

● **Contraindications and precautions**
  - Contraindicated in patients with asthma, chronic obstructive pulmonary disease (COPD), sinus bradycardia, cardiogenic shock, second- or third-degree heart block, or overt cardiac failure
  - Used cautiously in pregnant or breast-feeding patients and in those with impaired hepatic or renal function

● **Adverse reactions**
  - Bradycardia, nausea, vomiting, bronchospasm, diarrhea, hypotension, AV block, heart failure, and rash

● **Interactions**
  - Increased effect or toxicity if taken with digoxin, calcium channel blockers, or cimetidine
  - Decreased effect if taken with antacids, calcium salts, or anti-inflammatories
  - These drugs may alter the requirement for insulin and oral antidiabetic agents

Key nursing actions

- Closely monitor patient for fluid volume excess; monitor patient's blood pressure every 5 minutes at start of infusion and at least every 15 minutes during infusion.
- Weigh patient daily, and record daily intake and output.

Key facts about beta-adrenergic blockers

- Compete with epinephrine for beta-adrenergic receptor sites; inhibit the response to beta-adrenergic stimulation, thereby decreasing cardiac output
- Minimally metabolized by the liver
- Excreted primarily in the urine and partially in the feces

When to use beta-adrenergic blockers

- Mild hypertension

When NOT to use beta-adrenergic blockers

- Asthma
- Sinus bradycardia
- Cardiogenic shock
- Second- or third-degree heart block
- Overt cardiac failure
- COPD

Adverse reactions

- Bradycardia, hypotension, nausea, vomiting, bronchospasm, AV block

Key nursing actions

- Don't discontinue drug abruptly.
- Give propranolol with food.

Key facts about ACE inhibitors

- Block conversion of angiotensin I to angiotensin II, preventing peripheral vasoconstriction
- Metabolized by the liver
- Excreted in the urine and feces

When to use ACE inhibitors

- Mild hypertension
- Heart failure after MI
- Risk of MI, stroke, and death

When NOT to use ACE inhibitors

- Asthma
- Sinus bradycardia
- Cardiogenic shock
- Second- or third-degree heart block
- Overt cardiac failure

Adverse reactions

- Proteinuria (captopril)
- Nagging, nonproductive cough; angioedema; increased BUN and creatinine levels

● **Nursing responsibilities**
- Warn the patient not to stop taking the drug abruptly; doing so can exacerbate angina or precipitate an MI
- Administer propranolol consistently with meals; food may increase absorption
- Assess the patient's pulse rate; withhold drug and notify the practitioner if the rate is below 50 beats/minute (or according to facility policy)

ANGIOTENSIN-CONVERTING ENZYME (ACE) INHIBITORS

● **Mechanism of action**
- Block conversion of angiotensin I to angiotensin II, preventing peripheral vasoconstriction

● **Pharmacokinetics**
- Absorption: Absorbed from GI tract
- Distribution: Distributed in most body tissues
- Metabolism: Metabolized by the liver
- Excretion: Excreted in urine and feces

● **Drug examples**
- Benazepril (Lotensin), captopril (Capoten), enalapril (Vasotec), fosinopril (Monopril), lisinopril (Prinivil, Zestril), moexipril (Univasc), quinapril (Accupril), ramipril (Altace), trandolapril (Mavik)

● **Indications**
- Treat mild hypertension
- Treat heart failure after an MI and reduce the risk of MI, stroke, and death from cardiovascular causes (most drugs)

● **Contraindications and precautions**
- Contraindicated in patients with asthma, sinus bradycardia, cardiogenic shock, second- or third-degree heart block, or overt cardiac failure
- Used cautiously in pregnant or breast-feeding patients; patients with impaired hepatic function; and patients with renal impairment (dosage is reduced)

● **Adverse reactions**
- Nagging nonproductive cough, headache, fatigue, angioedema, GI reactions, hyperkalemia, and increased blood urea nitrogen (BUN) and creatinine levels
- Proteinuria (captopril)

● **Interactions**
- Antihypertensives, diuretics, and phenothiazines increase antihypertensive effects
- Aspirin and NSAIDs decrease the hypotensive effects
- Increased hypoglycemic effects if used with insulin and oral antidiabetic agents

- Concurrent use with potassium-sparing diuretics and potassium supplements should be avoided; may increase diuretic effects and the risk of hyperkalemia
- Increase serum lithium levels and the risk of toxicity

- **Nursing responsibilities**
  - Administer captopril on an empty stomach, preferably 1 hour before meals, for maximum effectiveness
  - Monitor the patient taking captopril for proteinuria every 2 to 4 weeks for the first 3 months of therapy to detect decreased renal function
  - Tell the patient to report light-headedness, especially in the first few days of starting therapy, so dosage may be adjusted
  - Advise the patient to avoid sudden position changes to minimize orthostatic hypotension
  - Encourage nonpharmacologic treatments for hypertension, such as sodium reduction, calorie reduction, stress management, and exercise

ANGIOTENSIN II RECEPTOR BLOCKING AGENTS (ARBs)

- **Mechanism of action**
  - Block the binding of angiotensin II to the angiotensin II receptor, preventing the vasoconstriction and aldosterone-secreting effects of angiotensin, thus lowering the blood pressure

- **Pharmacokinetics**
  - Absorption: Absorbed orally
  - Distribution: Highly bound to plasma proteins
  - Metabolism: Metabolized by the liver; olmesartan metabolized in the GI tract
  - Excretion: Excreted in feces and urine

- **Drug examples**
  - Candesartan (Atacand), eprosartan (Teveten), irbesartan (Avapro), losartan (Cozaar), olmesartan (Benicar), telmisartan (Micardis), valsartan (Diovan)

- **Indications**
  - Treat hypertension
  - Manage heart failure (valsartan)
  - Provide renal protective effect in type 2 diabetes (irbesartan and losartan)

- **Contraindications and precautions**
  - Contraindicated in patients with hypersensitivity to any ARB and during the second and third trimester of pregnancy
  - Used cautiously in patients with renal or hepatic dysfunction and those with hypovolemia
  - Telmisartan used cautiously in patients with biliary dysfunction

Adverse reactions

- Headache, fatigue, dizziness, cough, symptoms of upper respiratory tract infection

Key nursing facts

- Alert practitioner before surgery because of potential complications
- Monitor blood pressure carefully
- Instruct the patient to maintain fluid intake
- Stress the importance of continuing with nonpharmacologic therapies

Key facts about calcium channel blockers

- Dilate vessels by blocking the slow channel, preventing calcium from entering the cell
- Metabolized by the liver
- Excreted in the urine

When to use calcium channel blockers

- Mild hypertension

When NOT to use calcium channel blockers

- Cardiogenic shock
- Second- or third-degree heart block

● Adverse reactions

- Headache, fatigue, depression, dizziness, abdominal pain, nausea, cough, sinusitis, symptoms of upper respiratory tract infection
- Possible angioedema (olmesartan)

● Interactions

- Use with phenobarbital decreases drug effectiveness
- Effects of losartan may be decreased in patients also taking ketoconazole, fluconazole, or diltiazem
- Digoxin may increase serum levels of telmisartan
- Use with NSAIDs may reduce drug effectiveness
- Use with potassium supplements may result in hyperkalemia

● Nursing responsibilities

- Alert the practitioner that patient is taking an ARB before surgery because of potential complications from blocking the renin-angiotensin system
- Monitor the patient's blood pressure carefully; additive therapy may be required if drug doesn't achieve desired levels
- Instruct the patient to maintain fluid intake, especially when in a situation that can result in excessive fluid loss, such as diarrhea, vomiting, or excessive sweating
- Teach the patient ways to minimize orthostatic hypertension
- Stress the importance of continuing with nonpharmacologic therapies (diet modifications, exercise, and stress reduction)

CALCIUM CHANNEL BLOCKERS

● Mechanism of action

- Dilate vessels by blocking the slow channel, preventing calcium from entering the cell

● Pharmacokinetics

- Absorption: Absorbed rapidly and completely from GI tract
- Distribution: Highly protein-bound
- Metabolism: Metabolized by the liver; undergo first-pass metabolism
- Excretion: Excreted in urine

● Drug examples

- Amlodipine (Norvasc), diltiazem (Cardizem, Carizem LA), felodipine (Plendil), isradipine (DynaCirc), nicardipine (Cardene), nifedipine (Procardia), nisoldipine (Sular), verapamil (Calan, Isoptin SR)

● Indications

- Treat mild hypertension

● Contraindications and precautions

- Contraindicated in patients with severe left ventricular dysfunction, cardiogenic shock, second- or third-degree heart block, sick sinus syndrome (unless a functioning pacemaker is present), atrial flutter or fibrillation associated with accessory bypass tracts, severe heart failure, or severe hypotension

- I.V. verapamil contraindicated in patients receiving I.V. beta-adrenergic blockers and those with ventricular tachycardia
- Used cautiously in elderly patients and those with impaired hepatic or renal function or increased ICP

● **Adverse reactions**
- Dizziness, AV heart blocks, headache, edema, nausea, bradycardia, ventricular asystole, and ventricular fibrillation

● **Interactions**
- Increased risk of digoxin toxicity when used with digoxin
- Use with nifedipine may cause a reflex increase in heart rate and peripheral edema
- Use with beta-adrenergic blockers may increase the risk of bradycardia and heart failure
- Grapefruit juice increases the drug's therapeutic effects and the risk of toxicity

● **Nursing responsibilities**
- Know that nifedipine may be given S.L.
  - The patient can puncture the end of the capsule and squeeze the liquid under the tongue
  - Some institutions vary in this policy; the patient may be asked to swallow the capsule after S.L. dosing
- Withhold the dose and notify the practitioner if the patient's systolic pressure is less than 90 mm Hg or the heart rate is less than 60 beats/minute
- Monitor the patient for signs and symptoms of heart failure
- Warn the patient not to stop the drug abruptly; gradually reducing the dosage under practitioner's supervision helps prevent rebound hypertension

DIURETICS

● **Mechanism of action**
- Inhibit sodium and chloride reabsorption, thereby increasing urine output and decreasing edema, circulating blood volume, and cardiac output

● **Pharmacokinetics**
- See chapter 9 for the pharmacokinetics of specific types of diuretics

● **Drug examples**
- Chlorothiazide (Diuril), chlorthalidone (Hygroton), furosemide (Lasix), hydrochlorothiazide (Esidrix, HydroDIURIL, Oretic), indapamide (Lozol), metolazone (Mykrox, Zaroxolyn)

● **Indications**
- Treat mild hypertension

● **Contraindications and precautions**
- Contraindicated in patients with asthma, sinus bradycardia, cardiogenic shock, second- or third-degree heart block, or overt cardiac failure

Adverse reactions
- Dizziness, AV blocks, headache, edema, nausea, ventricular asystole

Key nursing actions
- Know that nifedipine may be given sublingually.
- Warn patient not to stop drug abruptly.
- Withhold dose and notify practitioner if systolic blood pressure is less than 90 mm Hg or heart rate is less than 60 beats/minute.

Key facts about diuretics
- Inhibit sodium and chloride reabsorption
- Increase urine output
- Decrease edema, circulating blood volume, and cardiac output
- Varied metabolism and excretion

When to use diuretics
- Mild hypertension

GO WITH THE FLOW

Managing antihypertensive therapy

The flowchart below is based on the approach to antihypertensive therapy endorsed by the Joint National Committee on the Detection, Evaluation, and Treatment of High Blood Pressure.

DIAGNOSIS OF HYPERTENSION SUSPECTED AND CONFIRMED

1
- Obtain baseline blood pressure readings
- Instruct patient in lifestyle modifications (weight reduction, moderate alcohol intake, regular physical activity, reduction of sodium intake, smoking cessation)

Adequate response? → **YES** → Continue therapy and monitoring

NO

2
- Continue instructions for lifestyle modifications; enlist aid of family members and support groups
- Prepare patient to begin drug therapy regimen
- Anticipate use of thiazide-type diuretics, angiotensin-converting enzyme (ACE) inhibitor, angiotensin receptor blocker (ARB), beta-adrenergic blocker (BB), calcium channel blocker (CCB), or a combination for stage 1 hypertension in the absence of compelling indications (see below)
- Instruct patient in drug therapy regimen
- Continue monitoring blood pressure
- Assess for signs and symptoms of adverse effects
- Anticipate use of a two-drug combination (usually a thiazide-type diuretic and an ACE inhibitor, ARB, BB, or CCB) for stage 2 hypertension in the absence of compelling indications (see below)
- Anticipate use of the following drugs if the patient has any of these compelling indications: heart failure—diuretic, BB, ACE inhibitor, ARB, or aldosterone antagonist; post-myocardial infarction—BB, ACE inhibitor, or aldosterone antagonist; high coronary disease risk—diuretic, BB, ACE inhibitor, or CCB; diabetes—diuretic, BB, ACE inhibitor, ARB, or CCB; chronic kidney disease—ACE inhibitor or ARB; recurrent stroke prevention—diuretic or ACE inhibitor

Adequate response? → **YES** → Continue therapy and monitoring

NO

3
- Anticipate change in drug therapy regimen (addition of second or third antihypertensive, addition of diuretic if not already prescribed)
- Instruct patient in new drug therapy regimen; reinforce previous instructions
- Continue monitoring blood pressure
- Assess for signs and symptoms of adverse effects

Source: U.S. Department of Health and Human Services, National Institutes of Health, National Heart, Lung, and Blood Institute (2003). The Seventh Report of the Joint National Committee on Detection, Evaluation, and Treatment of High Blood Pressure (JNC 7). Washington, D.C.: Government Printing Office.

TIME-OUT FOR TEACHING

Teaching about antihypertensives

Include these topics in your teaching plan for the patient receiving an antihypertensive:

- medication therapy regimen, including the drug's name, dose, frequency, duration, and possible adverse effects
- signs and symptoms of possible adverse effects and when to notify the practitioner
- continuation of drug even if the patient feels better
- need for adequate drug supply and instructions for missed doses
- dietary restrictions, including fluid and sodium restrictions as appropriate

- weight monitoring
- safety measures, including avoiding sudden position changes, driving, or hazardous activities until drug effects are known, and avoiding physical exertion, especially in hot weather
- avoidance of over-the-counter medications unless permitted by the practitioner
- lifestyle modifications
- measures to ensure compliance with therapy
- medical follow-up.

- Used cautiously in pregnant or breast-feeding patients and those with impaired hepatic function

● **Adverse reactions**

- Fatigue, dizziness, orthostatic hypotension, rash, hypokalemia, and hyperglycemia

● **Interactions**

- Concurrent use with similar-acting drugs and alcohol causes additive hypotension
- Concurrent use with antidepressants, antihistamines, appetite suppressants, decongestants, NSAIDs, and sympathomimetic bronchodilators may reduce drug's effects

● **Nursing responsibilities**

- Monitor the patient's vital signs, and assess for risk factors for hypertension
- Teach the patient about the importance of complying with therapy (see *Managing antihypertensive therapy*)
- Instruct the patient not to take a double dose after missing a dose
- Warn the patient not to stop the drug abruptly because this may cause rebound hypertension
- Instruct the patient to monitor blood pressure weekly (to help determine drug effectiveness) and to watch for weight gain and peripheral edema (to detect fluid retention)
- Advise the patient to change position slowly to minimize orthostatic hypotension
- Instruct the patient to avoid hot baths and showers; can lead to hypotension

Topics for patient discussion

- Therapy regimen
- Signs and symptoms of possible adverse effects and when to notify practitioner
- Continuation of drug even if the patient feels better
- Need for adequate drug supply
- Dietary restrictions
- Weight monitoring
- Safety measures
- Practitioner permission before taking over-the-counter drugs
- Lifestyle modifications
- Need for compliance with therapy
- Medical follow-up

When NOT to use diuretics

- Asthma
- Sinus bradycardia
- Cardiogenic shock
- Second- or third-degree heart block
- Overt cardiac failure

Adverse reactions

- Fatigue, dizziness, orthostatic hypotension, rash, hypokalemia, hyperglycemia

Key nursing actions

- Instruct patient not to take double dose after missing a dose.
- Warn patient not to stop drug abruptly.
- Teach patient to monitor blood pressure weekly and to watch for weight gain and peripheral edema.
- Instruct patient to avoid hot baths and showers.
- Caution patient not to consume excessive amounts of coffee, tea, or cola.

Key facts about nitrates

- Produce vasodilation, decrease preload and afterload, and reduce myocardial oxygen consumption
- Metabolized by liver
- Excreted in urine

When to use nitrates

- Acute angina
- Surgical hypertension

When NOT to use I.V. nitrates

- Hypersensitivity to these drugs
- Early MI
- Severe anemia
- Angle-closure glaucoma
- Orthostatic hypotension
- Cardiac tamponade

Adverse reactions

- Headache, dizziness, orthostatic hypotension, tachycardia, flushing, palpitations, nausea, vomiting

---

- Caution the patient not to consume excessive amounts of coffee, tea, or cola; may interfere with blood pressure control and drug effectiveness
- Encourage the patient to comply with additional antihypertensive interventions (weight reduction, low-sodium diet, smoking cessation, regular exercise, stress management, and alcohol restrictions)
- Instruct the patient to notify the practitioner if intolerable adverse effects occur (see *Teaching about antihypertensives*, page 161)

ANTIANGINALS

NITRATES

● Mechanism of action
- Produce vasodilation, decrease preload and afterload, and reduce myocardial oxygen consumption

● Pharmacokinetics
- Absorption: Well-absorbed in GI tract
  - Undergo first-pass metabolism, so they're incompletely absorbed systemically
  - Completely absorbed after S.L. administration
  - Well absorbed after topical administration
- Distribution: Widely distributed throughout body; about 60% protein-bound
- Metabolism: Metabolized by the liver
- Excretion: Excreted in urine

● Drug examples
- Isosorbide dinitrate (Isordil), isosorbide mononitrate (Imdur, ISMO), nitroglycerin (Nitro-Bid, Nitrodisc, Nitro-Dur, Nitrolingual, Nitrostat, TransdermNitro, Tridil)

● Indications
- Treatment and prophylactic management of acute angina
- Treat surgical hypertension (I.V. nitroglycerin)

● Contraindications and precautions
- I.V. form contraindicated in patients hypersensitive to nitrates and those with early MI, severe anemia, angle-closure glaucoma, orthostatic hypotension, hypertrophic cardiomyopathy, or cardiac tamponade
- Used cautiously in patients with hypotension or volume depletion, acute MI, heart failure, or constrictive pericarditis

● Adverse reactions
- Headache (most common), dizziness, orthostatic hypotension, tachycardia, flushing, palpitations, nausea, and vomiting

● Interactions
- Cause marked orthostatic hypotension when taken with calcium channel blockers

TIME-OUT FOR TEACHING

Teaching about nitrates

Include these topics in your teaching plan for the patient receiving a nitrate:
- medication therapy regimen, including the drug's name, dose, frequency, duration, and possible adverse effects
- forms of drug available and type prescribed
- signs and symptoms of possible adverse effects and when to notify the practitioner
- safety and emergency measures
- application and administration techniques
- measures to relieve common adverse effects, such as headache and orthostatic blood pressure
- skin-care measures if topical drugs are used
- cardiopulmonary resuscitation training
- storage guidelines
- dietary restrictions
- need for compliance with therapy, including taking drug as prescribed
- follow-up care.

- Erectile dysfunction drugs shouldn't be taken within 24 hours of nitrates because of increased hypotension
- Nitrates may cause severe hypotension if taken with alcohol

● **Nursing responsibilities**
- Know that nitroglycerin is available in several forms: I.V., S.L. tablet, sustained-release capsule, sustained-release buccal capsule, and transdermal ointment or patch
- Teach the patient about proper use and storage of nitroglycerin S.L. tablets
- Instruct the patient to sit down and take the drug at the first sign of an acute angina attack
- Teach the patient to repeat the dose if no relief occurs in 5 minutes and to seek emergency medical help if no relief occurs after taking 3 tablets in 15 minutes
- Advise the patient that S.L. tablets may be taken at the onset of activities known to cause angina such as sexual activity
- Advise the patient to discard unused tablets and replace them with fresh ones every 3 months
- Be aware that I.V. nitroglycerin must be mixed in either dextrose 5% in water or normal saline solution and hung in a glass bottle. Use the tubing specified by manufacturer; I.V. nitroglycerin will bind to plastic
- Inform the patient that headache is a common adverse effect of nitrates and typically subsides with continued therapy; advise him to take aspirin or acetaminophen for headache relief (see *Teaching about nitrates*)
- Teach the patient how to apply a transdermal patch or ointment, if prescribed; instruct him to remove the patch or ointment at bedtime to avoid tolerance
- Advise the patient to avoid alcoholic beverages; can increase hypotension

Key nursing actions

- Know that nitroglycerin is available in several forms.
- Teach patient about proper use of nitroglycerin S.L. tablets.
- Teach patient to repeat dose if no relief occurs in 5 minutes and to seek emergency medical help if no relief occurs after taking 3 tablets in 15 minutes.
- Inform patient that headache is common adverse effect of nitrates and typically subsides with continued therapy.
- Advise patient to avoid alcoholic beverages.
- Know that tolerance may develop.
- Know special procedures for I.V. nitroglycerin.

• Know that tolerance may develop and a nitrate-free period of 8 to 12 hours may be prescribed

CALCIUM CHANNEL BLOCKERS

● **Mechanism of action**
  • Prevent passage of calcium ions across the myocardial cell membrane and vascular smooth muscle, thereby dilating coronary and peripheral arteries and preventing coronary vasospasm

● **Pharmacokinetics**
  • Absorption: Absorbed rapidly and completely from GI tract
  • Distribution: Highly protein-bound
  • Metabolism: Metabolized by the liver; undergo first-pass metabolism
  • Excretion: Excreted in urine

● **Drug examples**
  • Amlodipine (Norvasc), diltiazem (Cardizem), nicardipine (Cardene), nifedipine (Procardia), verapamil (Calan, Isoptin SR)

● **Indications**
  • Long-term prevention of angina

● **Contraindications and precautions**
  • Contraindicated in patients with severe left ventricular dysfunction, sick sinus syndrome (unless a functioning pacemaker is present), atrial flutter or fibrillation associated with accessory bypass tracts, severe heart failure, cardiogenic shock, second- or third-degree heart block
  • Used cautiously in elderly patients and those with impaired hepatic or renal function
  • I.V. verapamil contraindicated in patients receiving I.V. beta-adrenergic blockers and those with ventricular tachycardia

● **Adverse reactions**
  • Constipation, dizziness, bradycardia, hypotension, edema, heart failure, and AV heart block
  • Reflex increase in heart rate and peripheral edema (nifedipine)

● **Interactions**
  • May increase the risk of digoxin toxicity when used with digoxin
  • Use with beta-adrenergic blockers increases the risk of bradycardia and heart failure

● **Nursing responsibilities**
  • Administer diltiazem before meals
  • Withhold the dose and notify the practitioner if the patient's systolic pressure is less than 90 mm Hg or heart rate is less than 60 beats/minute
  • Monitor the patient for signs and symptoms of heart failure, such as swelling of hands and feet and shortness of breath
  • Teach the patient about the need to continue concurrent nitrate therapy, if prescribed

---

Key facts about calcium channel blockers

• Dilate coronary and peripheral arteries and prevent coronary vasospasm
• Metabolized by the liver
• Excreted in the urine

When to use calcium channel blockers

• Prevention of angina

When NOT to use calcium channel blockers

• Cardiogenic shock
• Second- or third-degree heart block

Adverse reactions

• Reflex increase in heart rate, peripheral edema, constipation, dizziness, bradycardia

Key nursing actions

• If patient's systolic pressure is less than 90 mm Hg or heart rate is less than 60 beats/minute, withhold dose and notify practitioner.
• Monitor patient for signs and symptoms of heart failure.
• Teach patient about need to continue concurrent nitrate therapy, if prescribed.

BETA-ADRENERGIC BLOCKERS

● **Mechanism of action**
- Reduce myocardial oxygen demands by slowing the heart rate and decreasing the force of myocardial contractions

● **Pharmacokinetics**
- Absorption: Partially absorbed
- Distribution: Distributed in tissues
- Metabolism: Minimally metabolized by the liver
- Excretion: Excreted primarily in urine; partially in feces

● **Drug examples**
- Atenolol (Tenormin), carvedilol (Coreg), metoprolol (Lopressor, Toprol), nadolol (Corgard), propranolol (Inderal)

● **Indications**
- Treat angina pectoris

● **Contraindications and precautions**
- Contraindicated in patients with bradyarrhythmias, COPD, or asthma
- Used cautiously in patients with diabetes or hepatic or renal impairment

● **Adverse reactions**
- Bradycardia, bronchospasm, nausea, vomiting, diarrhea, hypotension, AV heart block, and rash

● **Interactions**
- These drugs cause additive hypotensive effects when used concurrently with alcohol, antihypertensives, other beta-adrenergic blockers, or calcium channel blockers
- Requirements for insulin and oral antidiabetic agents may need to be changed

● **Nursing responsibilities**
- Assess the location, duration, and intensity of anginal pain (signs and symptoms of angina resemble those of MI)
- Assess the patient's vital signs regularly; monitor ECG for changes in heart rate or rhythm
- Withdraw drug slowly; abrupt withdrawal may exacerbate symptoms of hyperthyroidism or cause thyroid storm
- Monitor blood pressure and the intensity and duration of the patient's response to drug
- Assess for factors that precipitate angina
- Instruct the patient to change position slowly to minimize orthostatic hypotension
- Caution the patient to avoid hot baths or showers; can lead to hypotension
- Warn the patient not to consume alcohol, which can lead to additive hypotension
- Observe for tolerance (tachyphylaxis)

Key facts about beta-adrenergic blockers

- Reduce myocardial oxygen demands
- Minimally metabolized by the liver
- Excreted mostly in the urine and partially in the feces

When to use beta-adrenergic blockers

- Angina pectoris

When NOT to use beta-adrenergic blockers

- Bradyarrhythmias
- COPD
- Asthma

Adverse reactions

- Hypotension, bronchospasm, bradycardia, AV heart block

Key nursing actions

- Assess location, duration, and intensity of anginal pain.
- Assess vital signs regularly and monitor ECG, blood pressure, and intensity and duration of patient's response to drug.
- Teach patient to change position slowly.
- Caution patient to avoid hot baths or showers.
- Warn patient to avoid alcohol.
- Observe for tolerance.
- Withdraw drug slowly.

- Assess the patient's pulse rate; withhold the drug and notify the practitioner if rate is less than 50 beats/minute
- Observe the patient with diabetes for sweating, hunger, and fatigue; signs of hypoglycemic shock may be masked
- Advise the patient receiving long-term therapy not to discontinue drug suddenly because this may precipitate an MI or arrhythmias

ANTILIPEMICS

BILE ACID SEQUESTRANTS

Key facts about bile acid sequestrants

- Bind bile acids in the GI tract to form an insoluble complex that is excreted, thereby increasing cholesterol clearance and lowering serum LDL levels
- Excreted unchanged 100% in the feces

When to use bile acid sequestrants

- Hyperlipoproteinemia
- Pruritus associated with partial biliary obstruction

When NOT to use bile acid sequestrants

- Hypersensitivity to these drugs
- Complete biliary obstruction

Adverse reactions

- Constipation with fecal impaction, flatulence, nausea, heartburn, increase in liver function test values

Key nursing actions

- Instruct patient to take drug before meals and at least 1 hour before or 4 to 6 hours after taking another drug.
- Monitor serum cholesterol, triglyceride, and liver enzyme levels during first 6 months.
- Instruct patient to follow recommended diet and exercise program, limit alcohol, and stop smoking.

● **Mechanism of action**
- Bind bile acids in GI tract to form an insoluble complex that's excreted, thereby increasing cholesterol clearance and lowering serum low-density lipoprotein (LDL) levels

● **Pharmacokinetics**
- Absorption: Bile adsorbed from GI tract
- Distribution: None
- Metabolism: None
- Excretion: Excreted unchanged 100% in feces

● **Drug examples**
- Cholestyramine (Questran), colesevelam (Welchol), colestipol (Colestid)

● **Indications**
- Treat hyperlipoproteinemia
- Relieve pruritus associated with partial biliary obstruction (cholestyramine)

● **Contraindications and precautions**
- Contraindicated in patients hypersensitive to bile acid–sequestering resins or drug components and those with complete biliary obstruction
- Treat diseases contributing to increased blood cholesterol level before starting drug therapy

● **Adverse reactions**
- Constipation (most common); may be accompanied by fecal impaction, flatulence, nausea, and heartburn
- Possible increase in liver function test values and malabsorption of fat-soluble vitamins (vitamins A, D, E, K, and folic acid)

● **Interactions**
- These drugs may bind orally administered drugs and vitamins and counteract their effectiveness
- These drugs may interfere with absorption of digoxin, oral phosphate supplements, and hydrocortisone

● **Nursing responsibilities**
- Instruct the patient to take drug before meals and at least 1 hour before or 4 to 6 hours after taking another drug
- Instruct the patient to mix powder form with beverages

- Advise the patient to swallow colestipol tablets whole and not to crush, chew, or cut them
- Monitor the patient's serum cholesterol, triglyceride, and liver enzyme levels periodically during the first 6 months of therapy
- As appropriate, instruct the patient to follow recommended diet and restrict intake of fats, cholesterol, carbohydrates, and alcohol; to stop smoking; and to follow a recommended exercise program
- Suggest a laxative, stool softener, or increased fluid and fiber intake to prevent constipation

FIBRIC ACID DERIVATIVES

- **Mechanism of action**
  - Decrease hepatic synthesis or accelerate breakdown of LDLs
  - Niacin: Increases serum high-density lipoprotein (HDL) levels and reduces the serum levels of LDLs, phospholipids, and very-low-density lipoproteins
- **Pharmacokinetics**
  - Absorption: Well absorbed in GI tract
  - Distribution: Peak plasma levels vary with each drug; fenofibrate 99% protein-bound
  - Metabolism: Varies with each drug
  - Excretion: Excreted in urine
- **Drug examples**
  - Fenofibrate (Tricor), gemfibrozil (Lopid), niacin (vitamin B_3 [Nicolar, Nicotinex])
- **Indications**
  - Adjunct therapy to diet in patients with hypertriglyceridemia and hypercholesterolemia
  - Reduce serum levels of LDL, cholesterol, and triglycerides and increase serum levels of HDL
  - Adjunct to diet therapy in reducing risk of coronary heart disease (gemfibrozil)
- **Contraindications and precautions**
  - Contraindicated in patients hypersensitive to drug or drug components and in those with hepatic or severe renal dysfunction (including primary biliary cirrhosis, unexplained and persistent liver function abnormalities, and preexisting gallbladder disease)
  - Treatment discontinued if gallstones develop during therapy
- **Adverse reactions**
  - Diarrhea, abdominal pain, epigastric pain, nausea, vomiting, dyspepsia, pancreatitis, cholelithiasis, and hypersensitivity reactions (including severe rashes and urticaria)
  - Possible increased liver enzyme levels

Key facts about fibric acid derivatives

- Decrease hepatic synthesis or accelerate breakdown of LDLs
- Increase serum HDL levels and reduce serum levels of LDLs, phospholipids, and very-low-density lipoproteins
- Metabolism varies with each drug
- Excreted in the urine

When to use fibric acid derivatives

- As adjunct in hypertriglyceridemia and hypercholesterolemia
- Reduction of LDL, cholesterol, and triglyceride levels
- Increase in HDL levels
- Reduction of coronary heart disease risk

When NOT to use fibric acid derivatives

- Hypersensitivity to these drugs
- Hepatic or severe renal dysfunction

Adverse reactions of fibric acid derivatives

- Diarrhea, abdominal pain, epigastric pain, nausea, vomiting, dyspepsia, pancreatitis, cholelithiasis, hyperglycemia, hypersensitivity reactions, increased liver enzyme levels

Key nursing actions

- Monitor patient's serum cholesterol, triglyceride, and liver enzyme levels during first 6 months.
- Instruct patient to take drug with evening meal.
- Instruct patient to follow his recommended diet and exercise program, avoid alcohol, and stop smoking.
- Inform patient that abdominal pain, diarrhea, nausea, and vomiting may occur; urge him to notify physician if these symptoms become pronounced or continue for prolonged period.

Key facts about HMG-CoA reductase inhibitors

- Block HMG-CoA reductase in the liver, preventing cholesterol synthesis
- Reduce serum cholesterol and LDL levels
- Metabolized extensively by the liver
- Excreted in bile

When to use HMG-CoA reductase inhibitors

- Hyperlipoproteinemia, hypercholesterolemia, hypertriglyceridemia
- Reduction of serum levels of LDL, cholesterol, and triglycerides
- Increase in serum levels of HDL
- Secondary prevention of cardiovascular events

● **Interactions**
- Use with oral anticoagulants may increase anticoagulant effect
- Use of clofibrate or gemfibrozil with sulfonylureas may increase hypoglycemic effects
- Use with 3-hydroxy-3-methylglutaryl (HMG) CoA reductase inhibitors may cause rhabdomyolysis and myopathy
- Cyclosporine levels may increase or decrease, depending on drug used

● **Nursing responsibilities**
- Monitor the patient's serum cholesterol, triglyceride, and liver enzyme levels periodically during the first 6 months of therapy
- Instruct the patient to take the drug with evening meal to enhance effectiveness
- Instruct the patient to follow recommended diet and restrict intake of fats, cholesterol, carbohydrates, and alcohol; to stop smoking; and to follow a recommended exercise program when appropriate
- Inform the patient that abdominal pain, diarrhea, nausea, and vomiting may occur; urge him to notify the practitioner if symptoms become pronounced or continue for a prolonged time

HMG-COA REDUCTASE INHIBITORS

● **Mechanism of action**
- Block HMG-CoA reductase in liver, preventing cholesterol synthesis
- Reduce serum cholesterol and LDL levels

● **Pharmacokinetics**
- Absorption: Rapidly absorbed
- Distribution: More than 90% protein-bound; 50% protein-bound (pravastatin)
- Metabolism: Extensively metabolized by the liver
- Excretion: Excreted in bile

● **Drug examples**
- Atorvastatin (Lipitor), ezetimibe and simvastatin (Vytorin), fluvastatin (Lescol), lovastatin (Mevacor), pravastatin (Pravachol), rosuvastatin (Crestor), simvastatin (Zocor)

● **Indications**
- Treat hyperlipoproteinemia, hypercholesterolemia, and hypertriglyceridemia
- Reduce serum levels of LDL, cholesterol, and triglycerides
- Increase serum levels of HDL
- Secondary prevention of cardiovascular events (all drugs but atorvastatin)

● **Contraindications and precautions**
- Contraindicated in patients hypersensitive to drug components, pregnant or breast-feeding patients, and those with active liver disease or unexplained and persistent elevated liver function test results

TIME-OUT FOR TEACHING

Teaching about HMG-CoA reductase inhibitors

Include these topics in your teaching plan for the patient receiving a 3-hydroxy-3-methylglutaryl (HMG) CoA reductase inhibitor:

- medication therapy regimen, including the drug's name, dose, frequency, duration, and possible adverse effects

- signs and symptoms of possible adverse effects and when to notify the practitioner
- dietary modifications
- need for compliance with therapy, including taking drug as prescribed
- follow-up care, including laboratory tests and practitioner visits.

- Secondary causes of hyperlipidemia should be ruled out before starting therapy

Adverse reactions
- Nausea, vomiting, diarrhea, abdominal cramps, constipation, flatulence, pancreatitis, hepatitis, and cirrhosis
- Possible rhabdomyolysis, myalgia, myopathy, and hypersensitivity reactions

Interactions
- Concurrent use of gemfibrozil and fibric acid derivatives with lovastatin may cause severe rhabdomyolysis and myopathy
- Use with cyclosporine, erythromycin, or nicotinic acid may increase the risk of rhabdomyolysis and myopathy
- Concurrent use of lovastatin and simvastatin with warfarin increases the effects of warfarin
- These drugs may increase digoxin levels

Nursing responsibilities
- Know that drug therapy is initiated only after diet therapy has proven ineffective; the patient should be on a standard cholesterol-lowering diet during therapy
- Give lovastatin with evening meal; absorption is enhanced and cholesterol biosynthesis is greater in evening
- Fluvastatin, pravastatin, and simvastatin are usually administered at bedtime, without regard to food
- Administer 1 hour before or 4 hours after bile sequestering drugs
- Monitor liver function tests frequently at the start of therapy and periodically thereafter
- Advise the patient to restrict alcohol intake
- Teach the patient about proper dietary management (restricting total fat and cholesterol intake), weight control, and exercise; explain their importance in controlling elevated serum lipid levels (see *Teaching about HMG-CoA reductase inhibitors*)

Topics for patient discussion

- Therapy regimen
- Signs and symptoms of possible adverse effects and when to notify the practitioner
- Dietary modifications
- Need for compliance with therapy
- Follow-up care

When NOT to use HMG-CoA reductase inhibitors

- Hypersensitivity to these drugs
- Active liver disease
- Elevated liver function test results
- Pregnancy
- Breast-feeding

Adverse reactions

- Nausea, vomiting, diarrhea, abdominal cramps, constipation, flatulence, rhabdomyolysis, myalgia, myopathy, hypersensitivity reactions

Key nursing actions

- Start these drugs only after diet therapy has proven ineffective.
- Give lovastatin with the evening meal; fluvastatin, pravastatin, and simvastatin are usually administered at bedtime.
- Advise patient to limit alcohol.
- Monitor liver function test results frequently at start of therapy and periodically thereafter.

Key facts about cholesterol absorption inhibitors

- Inhibit absorption from the small intestine, ultimately decreasing serum cholesterol levels
- Metabolized in the small intestine and by the liver
- Excreted in feces and urine

When to use cholesterol absorption inhibitors

- As adjunct in reducing cholesterol levels in primary hypercholesterolemia
- As adjunct to treat homozygous familial hypercholesterolemia

When NOT to use cholesterol absorption inhibitors

- Hypersensitivity to drug
- Patients with active liver disease (if used with atorvastatin or simvastatin)

Adverse reactions

- Headache, dizziness, fatigue, abdominal pain, diarrhea, cough, back pain, myalgia

Key nursing actions

- Teach about diet and exercise as adjuncts to medication.
- Tell the patient to take drug at least 2 hours before or 4 hours after bile sequestering drugs.
- Inform the patient of the need for liver function and cholesterol tests.

CHOLESTEROL ABSORPTION INHIBITORS

- **Mechanism of action**
  - Inhibit absorption of cholesterol from the small intestine, leading to a decrease in the delivery of dietary cholesterol to the liver, which increases the clearance of cholesterol from the bloodstream, thereby decreasing serum cholesterol levels

- **Pharmacokinetics**
  - Absorption: Absorbed orally
  - Distribution: Highly bound to plasma proteins
  - Metabolism: Metabolized in the small intestine and by the liver
  - Excretion: Excreted in feces and urine

- **Drug examples**
  - Ezetimibe (Zetia)

- **Indications**
  - Adjunctive therapy with diet modification to reduce cholesterol and LDL levels in primary hypercholesterolemia
  - Adjunctive therapy with atorvastatin or simvastatin to treat homozygous familial hypercholesterolemia

- **Contraindications and precautions**
  - Contraindicated in patients hypersensitive to drug
  - If used concurrently with atorvastatin or simvastatin, contraindicated in patients with active liver disease
  - Used cautiously in elderly patients and those with liver dysfunction

- **Adverse reactions**
  - Headache, dizziness, fatigue, abdominal pain, diarrhea, cough, back pain, and myalgia

- **Interactions**
  - Cholestyramine may decrease serum levels of ezetimibe
  - Fenofibrate and gemfibrozil increase serum levels of ezetimibe
  - Concurrent use of cyclosporine increases serum levels and the risk of ezetimibe toxicity

- **Nursing responsibilities**
  - Know that the patient should begin a low-cholesterol diet at least 2 weeks before starting ezetimibe
  - Teach the patient about a low-cholesterol diet and exercise program as adjunctive therapy with medication
  - Instruct the patient to take drug at least 2 hours before or 4 hours after any bile sequestering drugs
  - Inform the patient of the need for periodic liver function and cholesterol blood tests

NCLEX CHECKS

It's never too soon to begin your NCLEX® preparation. Now that you've reviewed this chapter, carefully read each of the following questions and choose the best answer. Then compare your responses with the correct answers.

1. A 78-year-old client is hospitalized and receives I.V. digoxin (Lanoxin). The nurse should withhold the drug and notify the physician if the client's:

☐ **1.** pulse rate is 54 beats/minute.

☐ **2.** history reveals liver failure.

☐ **3.** blood pressure is 72/40 mm Hg.

☐ **4.** respiratory rate is less than 14 breaths/minute.

2. A client is receiving digoxin (Lanoxin) for treatment of atrial flutter. Upon entering the room to give the medication, the nurse finds the client irritable, complaining of nausea and blurred vision, and disoriented to place and time. The most appropriate action at this time is to:

☐ **1.** try to reorient the client while helping him take the digoxin.

☐ **2.** return to the room later and see if the client will take the digoxin.

☐ **3.** withhold the digoxin and notify the physician about the assessment findings.

☐ **4.** check the medication profile for possible drug interactions after giving the digoxin to the client.

3. Which statement about antiarrhythmics is most accurate?

☐ **1.** Antiarrhythmics act by decreasing myocardial contractility and oxygen demand.

☐ **2.** Most antiarrhythmics are commonly prescribed across the life span.

☐ **3.** Most antiarrhythmics cause new arrhythmias.

☐ **4.** Electrolyte imbalance is the most common cause of arrhythmias that require drug therapy.

4. A client has tachycardia that hasn't responded well to propranolol (Inderal). The physician orders amiodarone (Cordarone). Before giving this class III antiarrhythmic, the nurse reviews the client's drug history. Which drug is most likely to interact with amiodarone?

☐ **1.** Digoxin (Lanoxin)

☐ **2.** Morphine

☐ **3.** Theophylline (Theo-Dur)

☐ **4.** Verapamil (Calan)

5. A client with hypertension requires a selective beta-adrenergic blocker for blood pressure control. Which drug is a selective beta-adrenergic blocker?

☐ **1.** Atenolol (Tenormin)

☐ **2.** Benazepril (Lotensin)

☐ **3.** Captopril (Capoten)

☐ **4.** Clonidine (Catapres)

TOP 5

Items to study for your next test on drugs and the cardiovascular system

1. Indications for inotropic drugs, antiarrhythmics, antihypertensives, antianginals, and antilipemics

2. Mechanisms of action of cardiac drugs and antilipemics

3. Common adverse effects of cardiac drugs and antilipemics

4. Nursing responsibilities when administering a cardiac drug or antilipemic

5. Appropriate teaching for the patient receiving a cardiac drug or an antilipemic

6. Which adverse reaction associated with ACE inhibitors is the most common and typically leads to disruption of therapy?

☐ **1.** Constipation
☐ **2.** Cough
☐ **3.** Sexual dysfunction
☐ **4.** Tachycardia

7. A client develops hypotension while receiving I.V. nitroglycerin (Tridil). The nurse should:

☐ **1.** monitor the client closely for signs of alcohol intoxication.
☐ **2.** have the client sit up slowly to minimize hypotensive effects.
☐ **3.** monitor the client for headache, and then give a prescribed analgesic.
☐ **4.** elevate the client's legs, and then retake the blood pressure before slowing the I.V. rate.

8. A client comes to the emergency department complaining of chest pains, which started 1 hour ago while he was playing golf. Nitroglycerin (Nitrostat), 0.4 mg, was given sublingually as ordered. Which adverse reaction is most likely to occur?

☐ **1.** Hypotension
☐ **2.** Dizziness
☐ **3.** Headache
☐ **4.** GI distress

9. Cholestyramine (Questran) is ordered for a client diagnosed with hypercholesterolemia. What information should the nurse include in the teaching plan?

☐ **1.** Vitamin C excretion will increase.
☐ **2.** Absorption of fat-soluble vitamins will be affected.
☐ **3.** Unlimited fats in the diet are allowed while taking this drug.
☐ **4.** The drug should be taken on an empty stomach.

10. A cardiologist orders diltiazem (Cardizem), 20 mg, as an I.V. bolus over 2 minutes for a client diagnosed with atrial fibrillation. The pharmacy dispenses a 5 mg/ml vial. How many milliliters should the nurse administer?

_____ milliliters

ANSWERS AND RATIONALES

1. CORRECT ANSWER: 1
The usual parameter for withholding digoxin is a heart rate less than 60 beats/minute. Liver failure isn't a contraindication for its use, and the drug has no effect on respirations or blood pressure.

2. CORRECT ANSWER: 3

Irritability, nausea, blurred vision, and confusion are signs and symptoms of digoxin toxicity. The digoxin dose should be withheld and the physician notified while the digoxin level is checked. The nurse should also try to reorient the client and prepare for possible emergency treatment pending the laboratory results. Even if the digoxin level is normal (0.5 to 2 ng/ml), clients vary greatly in response, and the dose should be withheld if the client shows signs of toxicity. Also, the client's medication profile should be reviewed for possible drug interactions before giving further doses of digoxin.

3. CORRECT ANSWER: 3

Most antiarrhythmics can cause new arrhythmias or worsen existing ones, so the benefits need to be weighed against the risks. Only class IV antiarrhythmics decrease myocardial contractility and oxygen demand; the other classes of antiarrhythmics have different mechanisms of action. Antiarrhythmics mainly are prescribed for adults and not across the life span. Ischemia, not electrolyte imbalance, is the most common cause of arrhythmias.

4. CORRECT ANSWER: 1

Amiodarone can interact with digoxin, increasing the serum digoxin level, thereby increasing the risk of digoxin toxicity and worsening arrhythmias. Amiodarone may also interact with other drugs, such as warfarin, procainamide, quinidine, and phenytoin. Amiodarone doesn't interact with verapamil, morphine, or theophylline.

5. CORRECT ANSWER: 1

Atenolol is a selective beta-adrenergic blocker. In addition to treating hypertension, atenolol is used to treat chronic stable angina and reduce cardiovascular mortality in clients with acute myocardial infarction. Benazepril is an ACE inhibitor that blocks the conversion of angiotensin I to angiotensin II. Captopril is also an ACE inhibitor. Clonidine is a centrally acting alpha-adrenergic inhibitor that inhibits the central vasomotor centers, decreasing sympathetic outflow to the heart, kidneys, and peripheral vasculature.

6. CORRECT ANSWER: 2

Cough leads to the discontinuation of ACE inhibitor therapy in more than 10% of clients taking this class of antihypertensive because it disrupts the client's sleep patterns. Constipation is a common adverse reaction to calcium channel blockers and doesn't usually cause discontinuation of therapy. Sexual dysfunction is a common cause of therapy disruption when treating hypertension with antihypertensives, but it isn't an adverse reaction of ACE inhibitors. Tachycardia is usually a reflex response that ends shortly after the start of therapy.

7. CORRECT ANSWER: 4

The best course of action would be to position the hypotensive client to promote venous return to the heart, such as elevating his legs. If the client's blood pressure is still hypotensive, the nurse should slow the I.V. rate, call the physician, and continue monitoring the heart rate and blood pressure every 5 to 15 minutes. I.V. nitroglycerin therapy doesn't cause alcohol intoxication. Sitting the client upright will worsen the hypotension and is contraindicated. Headaches are the most common adverse reaction to I.V. nitroglycerin and can be treated with analgesics, but treating the headache won't resolve the client's hypotension.

8. CORRECT ANSWER: 3

The most common reaction to nitrates is headache because nitrates dilate the blood vessels in the meningeal layers between the brain and the cranium. Hypotension, GI distress, and dizziness may occur, but the likelihood varies with each client.

9. CORRECT ANSWER: 2

Cholestyramine reduces the absorption of cholesterol and fat by binding with bile acids. Decreased fat absorption may lead to decreased absorption of fat-soluble vitamins, such as A, D, E, and K. Vitamin C is a water-soluble vitamin, so its excretion isn't affected by cholestyramine therapy. Cholestyramine should be mixed with fluids or pulpy fruits, not taken on an empty stomach. Cholestyramine is given with dietary restrictions.

10. CORRECT ANSWER: 4

The nurse should use the following formula to calculate drug dosages:

Dose on hand/Quantity on hand = Dose desired/X

In this example, the equation is as follows:

$$\frac{5 \text{ mg}}{\text{ml}} = \frac{20 \text{ mg}}{X}$$

$$5X = 20 \text{ ml}$$

$$X = 4 \text{ ml}$$

9

Drugs and the urinary system

PRETEST

1. Which medication is commonly used to treat edema associated with heart failure?

☐ 1. Trospium (Sanctura)
☐ 2. Carvedilol (Coreg)
☐ 3. Furosemide (Lasix)
☐ 4. Dopamine (Inocor)

CORRECT ANSWER: 3

2. Which group of diuretics works by increasing the osmotic pressure of the glomerular filtrate, inhibiting reabsorption of water and electrolytes?

☐ 1. Osmotic diuretics
☐ 2. Loop diuretics
☐ 3. Carbonic anhydrase inhibitors
☐ 4. Thiazide diuretics

CORRECT ANSWER: 1

3. A major adverse effect that's unique to potassium-sparing diuretics is:

☐ 1. hyperglycemia.
☐ 2. hyperkalemia.
☐ 3. dizziness.
☐ 4. orthostatic hypotension.

CORRECT ANSWER: 2

4. Before administering torsemide (Demadex), the nurse should check which laboratory value?

- ☐ 1. Hematocrit
- ☐ 2. Calcium
- ☐ 3. Magnesium
- ☐ 4. Potassium

CORRECT ANSWER: 4

5. A nurse should instruct a client to take oxybutynin (Oxytrol):

- ☐ 1. with meals.
- ☐ 2. 1 hour before meals.
- ☐ 3. 12 hours after meals.
- ☐ 4. at bedtime.

CORRECT ANSWER: 1

LEARNING OBJECTIVES

After studying this chapter, you should be able to:

- Identify medications commonly used as diuretics.
- Describe the mechanisms of action and rationales for using thiazide and thiazide-like diuretics, loop diuretics, potassium-sparing diuretics, osmotic diuretics, and carbonic anhydrase inhibitors.
- Name the major adverse effects of each type of diuretic.
- Identify nursing responsibilities when administering each type of diuretic.
- Discuss patient teaching related to each type of diuretic.

CHAPTER OVERVIEW

Diuretics increase urine formation and promote fluid loss. They're used to treat edema caused by heart failure or other drugs, to treat hypertension and glaucoma, and to prevent acute tubular necrosis. Knowing a diuretic's mechanism of action helps the nurse understand why specific drugs are selected.

ANATOMY AND PHYSIOLOGY

● **Anatomy**
- Kidneys
  - Are bean-shaped organs embedded in dorsal part of abdomen retroperitoneally
  - Consist of three regions
    - Outer region (renal cortex), containing blood-filtering mechanisms
    - Middle region (renal medulla)
    - Inner region (renal pelvis)
- Nephron
  - Is the structural and functional unit of the kidney; over 1 million in each kidney
  - Contains a glomerular capsule, or *Bowman's capsule*
    - Appears as a long tubule with a closed end
    - Is divided into three portions
      - Proximal convoluted tubule
      - Loop of Henle
      - Distal convoluted tubule

● **Physiology**
- Kidneys
  - Receive and filter a large volume of blood from the renal artery
  - Use tubular absorption and secretion to convert glomerular filtrate into urine
- Nephrons
  - Use glomeruli to filter blood
  - Flow filtrate through the renal tubules
- Tubules
  - Reabsorb and secrete various substances from the filtrate
  - Change filtrate composition and concentration, ultimately producing urine
- Glomerular filtration rate (GFR)—depends on glomerular capillary permeability, blood pressure, and effective filtration rate
- Kidney cells—secrete renin in response to decreased blood pressure, blood volume, or plasma sodium concentration

● **Function**
- Dispose wastes and excess ions in the form of urine
- Filter blood, regulating its volume and chemical makeup

A&P highlights
- The kidneys are two bean-shaped organs embedded in the dorsal part of the abdomen retroperitoneally.
- Nephrons are the structural and functional units of the kidney.
- Each kidney contains over 1 million nephrons.
- The kidneys receive and filter a large volume of blood from the renal artery; tubular absorption and secretion convert glomerular filtrate into urine.
- Within the nephrons, glomeruli filter the blood; then the filtrate flows through the renal tubules.
- The glomerular filtration rate depends on glomerular capillary permeability, blood pressure, and effective filtration rate.
- The kidneys dispose of wastes and excess ions in the form of urine; filter blood; maintain fluid, electrolyte, and acid-base balances; produce several hormones and enzymes; convert vitamin D to a more active form; and regulate blood pressure and blood volume.

- Maintain fluid, electrolyte, and acid-base balances
- Produce several hormones and enzymes
- Convert vitamin D to a more active form
- Regulate blood pressure and blood volume by secreting renin

THIAZIDE AND THIAZIDE-LIKE DIURETICS

● **Mechanism of action**
- Increase water excretion by either increasing the GFR or decreasing or inhibiting sodium reabsorption from the tubules

● **Pharmacokinetics**
- Absorption: Absorbed rapidly but incompletely from GI tract after oral administration
- Distribution: 65% to 95% protein-bound
- Metabolism: Unknown
- Excretion: Excreted primarily in urine

● **Drug examples**
- Chlorothiazide (Diuril), chlorthalidone (Hygroton), hydrochlorothiazide (Esidrix, HydroDIURIL, Oretic), indapamide (Lozol), metolazone (Mykrox, Zaroxolyn)

● **Indications**
- Treat hypertension, edema, and heart failure
- Prevent recurrence of renal calculi

● **Contraindications and precautions**
- Metolazone contraindicated in patients sensitive to sulfonamides and those with anuria, hepatic coma, or precoma
- Used cautiously in pregnant patients and those with systemic lupus erythematosus, hypercholesterolemia, or diabetes mellitus
- Chlorothiazide shouldn't be given with whole blood or blood derivatives; given only in emergency or to adults who can't take oral medication

● **Adverse reactions**
- Orthostatic hypotension, dizziness, light-headedness, headache, weakness, restlessness, insomnia, anorexia, nausea, vomiting, abdominal pain, diarrhea, constipation, impotence or reduced libido, rash, necrotizing angiitis, and photosensitivity
- Possible hypokalemia, hyperglycemia, hyponatremia, hypomagnesemia, and other fluid and electrolyte imbalances
- Possible life-threatening reactions include uremia, aplastic anemia, hemolytic anemia, leukopenia, agranulocytosis, thrombocytopenia, and neutropenia

● **Interactions**
- These drugs may decrease excretion of lithium, causing lithium toxicity
- Use with other potassium-depleting drugs and digoxin may cause additive hypokalemia, increasing the risk of digoxin toxicity

---

Key facts about thiazide and thiazide-like diuretics

- Increase water excretion by increasing the GFR or decreasing or inhibiting sodium reabsorption from the tubules
- Excreted primarily in the urine

When to use thiazide and thiazide-like diuretics

- Hypertension
- Edema
- Heart failure

When NOT to use thiazide and thiazide-like diuretics

- Hypersensitivity to sulfonamides
- Anuria
- Hepatic coma
- Precoma
- With whole blood or blood derivatives

Adverse reactions

- Orthostatic hypotension, dizziness, light-headedness, headache, weakness, restlessness, insomnia, anorexia, nausea, vomiting, abdominal pain, diarrhea, constipation, impotence or reduced libido, rash, necrotizing angiitis, photosensitivity, hypokalemia, electrolyte imbalances

- Nonsteroidal anti-inflammatory drugs (NSAIDs) may reduce the antihypertensive effect of thiazide diuretics
- These drugs may produce additive hypotension when used with antihypertensives
- Blood glucose levels may increase, requiring higher doses of insulin or oral antidiabetic drugs

● **Nursing responsibilities**
- Monitor digoxin levels in the patient receiving digoxin concurrently with a thiazide or thiazide-like diuretic
- Instruct the patient to use a sunscreen and wear protective clothing to prevent photosensitivity reactions
- Carefully monitor the patient for signs and symptoms of hypokalemia (drowsiness, paresthesia, muscle cramps, and hyporeflexia)
  - Administer prescribed potassium supplements
  - Advise the patient to eat foods high in potassium
- Give the drug in morning or early afternoon, if possible, to prevent nocturia from disrupting the patient's sleep at night
- Keep a urinal or bedpan within the patient's reach or ensure that bathroom is easily accessible

LOOP DIURETICS

● **Mechanism of action**
- Inhibit sodium and chloride reabsorption from the loop of Henle and distal tubule
- Increase sodium and water excretion by inhibiting sodium and chloride reabsorption in the proximal tubule

● **Pharmacokinetics**
- Absorption: Well absorbed from GI tract
- Distribution: Rapidly distributed; extensively protein-bound
- Metabolism: Metabolized partially or completely by the liver; furosemide excreted primarily unchanged
- Excretion: Excreted in urine

● **Drug examples**
- Bumetanide (Bumex), ethacrynic acid (Edecrin), furosemide, torsemide (Demadex)

● **Indications**
- Treat edema associated with heart failure, hepatic cirrhosis, and renal disease, including nephrotic syndrome
- Treat hypertension
- Short-term management of ascites due to malignancy, idiopathic edema, or lymphedema (ethacrynic acid)
- Adjunct to other diuretics for additive diuretic effects (ethacrynic acid)
- Adjunct to mannitol to treat cerebral edema (furosemide)

Key nursing actions

- Monitor digoxin levels in patients taking digoxin concurrently with these drugs.
- Monitor patient for signs and symptoms of hypokalemia.
- Give diuretic in morning or early afternoon, if possible.

Key facts about loop diuretics

- Inhibit sodium and chloride reabsorption from the loop of Henle and the distal tubule
- Increase sodium and water excretion by inhibiting sodium reabsorption in the proximal tubule
- Metabolized partially or completely by the liver, except for furosemide, which is excreted primarily unchanged
- Excreted in the urine

When to use loop diuretics

- Edema associated with heart failure
- Hepatic cirrhosis
- Renal disease
- Hypertension
- Short-term management of ascites due to malignancy, idiopathic edema, or lymphedema
- Additive diuretic effects
- Cerebral edema

When NOT to use loop diuretics

- When less potent diuretics are sufficient
- Hypersensitivity to these drugs
- Anuria
- Hepatic coma
- Severe, uncorrected electrolyte depletion
- Sulfa allergy

Adverse reactions

- Metabolic alkalosis, hypovolemia, hypochloremia, hypochloremic alkalosis, hyperuricemia, dehydration, hyponatremia, hypokalemia, hypomagnesemia, transient deafness, tinnitus, diarrhea, nausea, vomiting, abdominal pain, impaired glucose tolerance, dermatitis, paresthesia, hepatic dysfunction, photosensitivity, orthostatic hypotension

Key nursing actions

- Monitor serum digoxin levels in patients receiving digoxin and these drugs concurrently.
- Monitor patient for signs and symptoms of hypokalemia.
- Administer I.V. doses slowly over 1 to 2 minutes.
- Know that bumetanide is 40 times more potent than furosemide.
- Be especially alert for changes in patient's sodium and potassium levels.
- Give diuretic in morning or early afternoon, if possible.
- Monitor patient for signs of dehydration.
- Check vital signs to detect signs of hypovolemia; if signs are present, notify practitioner.
- Accurately record fluid intake and output.
- Give diuretic with food or milk if GI upset occurs.

● Contraindications and precautions

- Most potent diuretics available, producing greatest volume of diuresis but also having highest potential for severe adverse reactions and electrolyte depletion
- Contraindicated in patients hypersensitive to drug or drug components; patients with anuria or hepatic coma; and those with severe, uncorrected electrolyte depletion
- Used cautiously in elderly patients, pregnant or breast-feeding patients, and those with hepatic cirrhosis, ascites, or systemic lupus erythematosus
- Furosemide and torsemide contraindicated in patients with sulfa allergy

● Adverse reactions

- Fluid and electrolyte imbalances (most common), including metabolic alkalosis, hypovolemia, hypochloremia, hypochloremic alkalosis, hyperuricemia, dehydration, hyponatremia, hypokalemia, hypomagnesemia, and hyperglycemia
- Possible transient deafness, tinnitus, diarrhea, nausea, vomiting, abdominal pain, impaired glucose tolerance, dermatitis, paresthesia, hepatic dysfunction, photosensitivity, and orthostatic hypotension

● Interactions

- Excretion of lithium may decrease, causing lithium toxicity
- Use with digoxin may cause additive hypokalemia, increasing the risk of digoxin toxicity and arrhythmias
- Use with aminoglycosides and cisplatin increases the risk of ototoxicity
- Use with anticoagulants may increase anticoagulant effects
- Use with NSAIDs and probenecid may decrease diuretic effects
- Use with thiazide diuretics causes synergistic effect that may result in profound diuresis and serious electrolyte abnormalities

● Nursing responsibilities

- Monitor serum digoxin levels in patients receiving digoxin and loop diuretics concurrently
- Instruct the patient to use a sunscreen and wear protective clothing to prevent photosensitivity reactions
- Monitor the patient for signs and symptoms of hypokalemia (drowsiness, paresthesia, muscle cramps, and hyporeflexia)
  - Administer prescribed potassium supplements
  - Advise the patient to eat foods high in potassium
- Administer I.V. doses slowly over 1 to 2 minutes to prevent hypotension and tinnitus
- Know that bumetanide is 40 times more potent than furosemide; check the dosage with extreme care
- Be especially alert for changes in the patient's sodium and potassium levels
- Use the Z-track method to minimize skin irritation when giving furosemide I.M.

- Give the drug in morning or early afternoon, if possible, to prevent nocturia from disrupting the patient's sleep at night
- Keep a urinal or bedpan within the patient's reach or ensure that the bathroom is easily accessible
- Monitor the patient for signs of dehydration (poor skin turgor and dry mucous membranes)
- Check the patient's vital signs to detect signs of hypovolemia (tachycardia, hypotension, and dyspnea); if signs are present, notify the practitioner
- Record the patient's fluid intake and output accurately; if a large discrepancy occurs, notify the practitioner and expect to decrease the diuretic dosage
- Give the drug with food or milk if GI upset occurs

POTASSIUM-SPARING DIURETICS

- **Mechanism of action**
  - Act at the distal tubule to cause excretion of sodium, bicarbonate, and calcium, but conserve potassium excretion
  - Spironolactone: Acts by competing with aldosterone for receptor sites and blocks the action of aldosterone on distal tubules
- **Pharmacokinetics**
  - Absorption: Absorbed in GI tract
  - Distribution: Unknown
  - Metabolism: Metabolized by the liver; amiloride isn't metabolized
  - Excretion: Excreted primarily in urine
- **Drug examples**
  - Amiloride (Midamor), spironolactone, triamterene (Dyrenium)
- **Indications**
  - Conserve potassium or enhance effects of loop or thiazide diuretics
  - Treat hyperaldosteronism, cirrhosis of the liver accompanied by edema or ascites, nephrotic syndrome, and hypokalemia (spironolactone)
  - Treat idiopathic edema or edema associated with heart failure, hepatic cirrhosis, nephrotic syndrome, steroid use, or hyperaldosteronism (triamterene)
- **Contraindications and precautions**
  - Contraindicated in patients hypersensitive to drug; patients with a serum potassium level greater than 5.5 mEq/L; patients receiving antikaliuretic therapy, potassium supplementation, or another potassium-sparing diuretic; and those with impaired renal function or anuria
  - Used with extreme caution in pregnant or breast-feeding patients, diabetic patients, and those with (or at risk for) metabolic or respiratory acidosis or renal or hepatic impairment
- **Adverse reactions**
  - Possible hyperkalemia, increased blood urea nitrogen level, nausea, vomiting, diarrhea, anorexia, abdominal pain, muscle cramping, headache, and dizziness

Topics for patient discussion

- Therapy regimen
- Signs and symptoms of possible adverse effects and when to notify the practitioner
- Signs and symptoms of hyperkalemia
- Dietary restrictions
- Weight monitoring
- Intake and output
- Safety measures
- Measures to relieve minor adverse effects
- Need for compliance with therapy
- Follow-up care

Key nursing actions

- Monitor patient for signs and symptoms of hyperkalemia; notify practitioner immediately if symptoms occur.
- Instruct patient to avoid salt substitutes and potassium-rich foods, except with practitioner approval.
- Advise patient to avoid driving or performing activities requiring mental alertness or physical dexterity.

 TIME-OUT FOR TEACHING

Teaching about potassium-sparing diuretics

Include these topics in your teaching plan for the patient receiving a potassium-sparing diuretic:

- medication therapy regimen, including the drug's name, dose, frequency, duration, and possible adverse effects
- signs and symptoms of possible adverse effects and when to notify the practitioner
- signs and symptoms of hyperkalemia
- dietary restrictions such as alcohol
- weight monitoring
- intake and output
- safety measures
- measures to relieve minor adverse effects
- need for compliance with therapy, including taking the drug as prescribed
- follow-up care, including laboratory tests and practitioner visits.

● Interactions

- Giving drug with potassium supplements, other potassium-sparing diuretics, or angiotensin-converting enzyme inhibitors increases the risk of hyperkalemia
- Concurrent use of spironolactone and digoxin increases the risk of digoxin toxicity
- Salicylates decrease effects of spironolactone

● Nursing responsibilities

- Monitor the patient for signs and symptoms of hyperkalemia (confusion, hyperexcitability, muscle weakness, flaccid paralysis, arrhythmias, abdominal distention, and diarrhea); notify the practitioner immediately if any of these symptoms occurs
- Instruct the patient to avoid salt substitutes and potassium-rich foods, except with practitioner's approval (see *Teaching about potassium-sparing diuretics*)
- Administer amiloride with food for maximum effectiveness; triamterene, after meals
- Give the drug in morning or early afternoon, if possible, to prevent nocturia from disrupting the patient's sleep at night.
- Advise the patient to avoid driving or performing activities requiring mental alertness or physical dexterity because potassium-sparing diuretics may cause dizziness, headache, or vision disturbances

OSMOTIC DIURETICS

● **Mechanism of action**
- Increase osmotic pressure of glomerular filtrate, inhibiting reabsorption of water and electrolytes
- Create osmotic gradient in the glomerular filtrate and blood
  - In glomerular filtrate, gradient prevents sodium and water reabsorption
  - In blood, gradient allows fluid to be drawn from intracellular spaces into intravascular spaces
  - Resulting increase in intravascular volume may cause fluid overload in patients with impaired kidney function

● **Pharmacokinetics**
- Absorption: Administered I.V.
- Distribution: Distributed rapidly
- Metabolism: slightly metabolized (mannitol); freely filtered by glomeruli
- Excretion: Excreted primarily in urine

● **Drug examples**
- Glycerin (Osmoglyn), isosorbide (Ismotic), mannitol (Osmitrol), urea (Ureaphil)

● **Indications**
- Treat cerebral edema and reduce intracranial and intraocular pressure
- Promote diuresis in acute renal failure and urinary excretion of toxic substances (mannitol)
- Interrupt acute attacks of glaucoma (glycerin and isosorbide)

● **Contraindications and precautions**
- Contraindicated in patients with well-established anuria, severe dehydration, frank or impending acute pulmonary edema, severe cardiac decompensation, or hypersensitivity to drug
- Mannitol contraindicated in patients with anuria due to severe renal disease, severe pulmonary congestion, frank pulmonary edema, active intracranial bleeding (unless during a craniotomy), or severe dehydration and in patients who develop progressive renal damage or dysfunction, heart failure, or pulmonary congestion after starting mannitol therapy

● **Adverse reactions**
- Nausea, vomiting, confusion, headache, disorientation, dizziness, light-headedness, syncope, vertigo, gastric disturbances, hyponatremia, dehydration, circulatory overload (from osmotic effects), and thrombophlebitis or local irritation at infusion site
- Possible rebound increased intracranial pressure (ICP) (8 to 12 hours after diuresis), chest pains, blurred vision, rhinitis, thirst, and urine retention (mannitol)

● **Interactions**
- Urea may increase renal excretion of lithium, decreasing lithium's effects

Key facts about osmotic diuretics

- Increase osmotic pressure of the glomerular filtrate, inhibiting reabsorption of water and electrolytes
- Create an osmotic gradient in the glomerular filtrate and the blood
- Mannitol is only slightly metabolized; the other drugs are freely filtered by the glomeruli
- Excreted primarily in the urine

When to use osmotic diuretics

- Cerebral edema
- Reduction of intracranial and intraocular pressure
- Promotion of diuresis in acute renal failure
- Promotion of urinary excretion of toxic substances
- Interruption of acute attacks of glaucoma

When NOT to use osmotic diuretics

- Well-established anuria, severe dehydration, frank or impending acute pulmonary edema, severe cardiac decompensation, or hypersensitivity to these drugs

Adverse reactions

- Nausea, vomiting, confusion, headache, disorientation, dizziness, light-headedness, syncope, vertigo, gastric disturbances, hyponatremia, dehydration, circulatory overload, thrombophlebitis or local irritation at the infusion site

Key nursing actions

- Monitor vital signs, urine output, and central venous pressure for signs of circulatory overload and fluid volume depletion.
- Assess neurologic status and intracranial pressure.

Key facts about carbonic anhydrase inhibitors

- Inhibit the action of the enzyme carbonic anhydrase
- In the kidney, carbonic anhydrase inhibition decreases the availability of hydrogen ions, blocking sodium-hydrogen exchange mechanisms, thus increasing urinary excretion of sodium, potassium, bicarbonate, and water
- In the eye, carbonic anhydrase inhibition reduces aqueous humor production, thereby reducing intraocular pressure
- Excreted in the urine

When to use carbonic anhydrase inhibitors

- Glaucoma
- Epilepsy
- Acute mountain sickness

When NOT to use carbonic anhydrase inhibitors

- Pregnancy
- Decreased sodium or potassium levels
- Marked kidney or liver disease
- Adrenocortical insufficiency
- Severe pulmonary obstruction
- Chronic noncongestive angle-closure glaucoma (long-term use)

● **Nursing responsibilities**
- Monitor the patient's vital signs, urine output, and central venous pressure for signs of circulatory overload and fluid volume depletion; assess for circulatory overload when urine output is less than 30 ml/hour
- Assess the patient's neurologic status and ICP for signs of increased ICP

CARBONIC ANHYDRASE INHIBITORS

● **Mechanism of action**
- Inhibit action of the enzyme carbonic anhydrase
- Decrease availability of hydrogen ions in kidney, blocking sodium-hydrogen exchange mechanisms, thus increasing urinary excretion of sodium, potassium, bicarbonate, and water
- Reduce aqueous humor production in eye, thereby reducing intraocular pressure

● **Pharmacokinetics**
- Absorption: Absorbed from GI tract; some systemic absorption occurs after ophthalmic administration
- Distribution: Distributed in tissues with high carbonic anhydrase content (erythrocytes, plasma, kidneys, eyes, liver, and muscles)
- Metabolism: Unknown
- Excretion: Excreted in urine

● **Drug examples**
- Acetazolamide (Diamox), methazolamide (GlaucTabs)

● **Indications**
- Promote diuresis
- Treat glaucoma
- Treat epilepsy and acute mountain sickness (acetazolamide)

● **Contraindications and precautions**
- Contraindicated in pregnant patients and those with decreased sodium or potassium levels, marked kidney or liver disease, adrenocortical insufficiency, or severe pulmonary obstruction; also for long-term use in chronic noncongestive angle-closure glaucoma
- Rarely used for diuresis in patients with drug-induced edema or heart failure because they may cause metabolic acidosis
- Used with extreme caution in patients with hepatic impairment; methazolamide may cause hepatic coma
- Used cautiously in patients allergic to sulfonamides; cross-sensitivity reaction may occur

● **Adverse reactions**
- Fatigue, malaise, drowsiness, headache, paresthesia, urticaria, pruritus, Stevens-Johnson syndrome, and photosensitivity; also hypokalemia, metabolic acidosis, and other electrolyte imbalances

Interactions
- Salicylates may cause carbonic anhydrase inhibitor toxicity (central nervous system depression and metabolic acidosis)
- Use with diflunisal (Dolobid) may increase intraocular pressure
- Concurrent use of acetazolamide and cyclosporine (Sandimmune) may increase cyclosporine levels and the risk of neurotoxicity
- Concurrent use of acetazolamide and primidone (Mysoline) may decrease serum and urine levels of primidone

Nursing responsibilities
- Give the drug with food if GI upset occurs
- Advise the patient to avoid prolonged or unprotected exposure to sunlight during therapy; risk of photosensitivity reactions

ANTIMUSCARINICS

Mechanism of action
- Decrease bladder contractions by blocking muscarinic receptors

Pharmacokinetics
- Absorption: Absorbed orally
- Distribution: Widely distributed
- Metabolism: Metabolized by the liver
- Excretion: Excreted in urine and feces

Drug examples
- Darifenacin (Enablex), dicyclomine (Antispas, Bentyl, Dibent, Di-Spaz), oxybutynin (Oxytrol, Oxytrol Transdermal System), solifenacin (Vesicare), tolterodine (Detrol, Detrol LA), trospium (Sanctura)

Indications
- Treat overactive bladder in patients with symptoms of urinary frequency, urgency, or incontinence

Contraindications and precautions
- Contraindicated in patients with urine retention, narrow-angle glaucoma, or gastric retention
- Used cautiously in patients with renal or hepatic impairment
- Darifenacin used cautiously in patients with severe constipation, ulcerative colitis, and myasthenia gravis

Adverse reactions
- Blurred vision, headache, somnolence, rash, nausea, vomiting, constipation, dyspepsia, dry mouth, urine retention, weight gain, pain, acute myopia, and secondary angle-closure glaucoma

Interactions
- Use with other anticholinergic agents may increase dry mouth, constipation, and other anticholinergic effects
- Dose may need to be decreased if patient is also taking fluoxetine, ketoconazole, flecainide, or tricyclic antidepressants

Adverse reactions
- Hypokalemia, metabolic acidosis, other electrolyte imbalances, fatigue, malaise, drowsiness, headache, paresthesia, urticaria, pruritus, Stevens-Johnson syndrome, photosensitivity

Key nursing actions
- Give drug with food if GI upset occurs.
- Advise patient to avoid prolonged or unprotected exposure to sunlight during therapy.

Key facts about antimuscarinics
- Block muscarinic receptors, thereby decreasing bladder contractions
- Metabolized in the liver
- Excreted in urine and feces

When to use antimuscarinics
- Overactive bladder

When NOT to use antimuscarinics
- Urine retention
- Narrow angle glaucoma

Adverse reactions
- Blurred vision, dry mouth, secondary angle-closure glaucoma, constipation, urine retention

● **Nursing responsibilities**
- Administer the drug as prescribed
- Provide small, frequent meals, if necessary, to prevent GI upset
- Teach the patient about safety precautions if blurred vision occurs

TOP 5

Items to study for your next test on drugs and the urinary system

1. Medications commonly used as diuretics
2. Mechanisms of action and rationales for using thiazide diuretics, loop diuretics, potassiumsparing diuretics, osmotic diuretics, and carbonic anhydrase inhibitors
3. Major adverse effects of each type of diuretic
4. Nursing responsibilities when administering each type of diuretic
5. Patient teaching related to each type of diuretic

NCLEX CHECKS

It's never too soon to begin your NCLEX® preparation. Now that you've reviewed this chapter, carefully read each of the following questions and choose the best answer. Then compare your responses with the correct answers.

1. A nurse should observe for which electrolyte imbalance in a client receiving furosemide (Lasix)?
- ☐ **1.** Hypercalcemia
- ☐ **2.** Hypernatremia
- ☐ **3.** Hypokalemia
- ☐ **4.** Hypophosphatemia

2. During the course of treatment for heart failure, a client begins to complain of tinnitus. The nurse suspects that this symptom may be a result of:
- ☐ **1.** hypokalemia.
- ☐ **2.** hypovolemia.
- ☐ **3.** insufficient diuretic use.
- ☐ **4.** excessive diuretic use.

3. A client is taking a potassium-sparing diuretic, which has weaker antihypertensive and diuretic effects than other diuretics but preserves potassium levels in the body. Serum potassium levels should be closely monitored if the client is also taking:
- ☐ **1.** cetirizine (Zyrtec).
- ☐ **2.** epoprostenol (Flolan).
- ☐ **3.** ibutilide (Corvert).
- ☐ **4.** trandolapril (Mavik).

4. A client with a history of heart failure has sustained a head injury. He's receiving mannitol (Osmitrol) because he has developed cerebral edema. The nurse should monitor the client for:
- ☐ **1.** rashes.
- ☐ **2.** bradycardia.
- ☐ **3.** disorientation.
- ☐ **4.** circulatory overload.

5. A nurse is instructing a client about taking acetazolamide (Diamox) at home. Which element is most important to include in the teaching plan?
- ☐ **1.** The drug is safe to use and should cause few adverse reactions.
- ☐ **2.** Instill 2 drops into each eye every morning and before bedtime.
- ☐ **3.** If weakness, heart palpitations, or paresthesia occur, notify the physician.
- ☐ **4.** The drug may cause dim vision in low light, so night driving could be dangerous.

6. A client is being treated for heart failure. One of the diuretics the client will receive is furosemide (Lasix). The nurse checks the other drugs the client is taking before giving the furosemide. Which drug is likely to interact with this diuretic?

- ☐ **1.** Aspirin
- ☐ **2.** Captopril (Capoten)
- ☐ **3.** Lithium (Lithonate)
- ☐ **4.** Penicillin G (Pfizerpen)

7. A client is ordered furosemide (Lasix), 40 mg daily. The nurse knows the best time to administer this medication is:

- ☐ **1.** with breakfast.
- ☐ **2.** at noon.
- ☐ **3.** with dinner.
- ☐ **4.** at bedtime.

8. A client is being treated with hydrochlorothiazide (HydroDIURIL) for edema associated with mild heart failure and minimal urine output. Which drugs should the nurse expect the physician to order to potentiate the diuretic effect of hydrochlorothiazide?

- ☐ **1.** Bumetanide (Bumex)
- ☐ **2.** Ethacrynic acid (Edecrin)
- ☐ **3.** Furosemide (Lasix)
- ☐ **4.** Metolazone (Zaroxolyn)

9. A nurse is preparing discharge instructions for a client taking tolterodine (Detrol) for urinary frequency. The nurse should teach the client about which adverse effect?

- ☐ **1.** Tachycardia
- ☐ **2.** Diarrhea
- ☐ **3.** Blurred vision
- ☐ **4.** Anxiety

10. A client comes to the facility with acute pulmonary edema. The physician orders furosemide (Lasix), 80 mg, I.V. b.i.d. with a 40-mg I.V. bolus. What signs and symptoms should the nurse look for when administering the bolus? Select all that apply.

- ☐ **1.** Tinnitus
- ☐ **2.** Dizziness
- ☐ **3.** Headache
- ☐ **4.** Abdominal pain
- ☐ **5.** Increased urination
- ☐ **6.** Fever

ANSWERS AND RATIONALES

1. CORRECT ANSWER: 3

The client's potassium level should be monitored carefully for hypokalemia. Furosemide, a loop diuretic that promotes sodium and potassium excretion, may also cause hypocalcemia and hyponatremia (not hypercalcemia or hypernatremia) because of the increased excretion of calcium and sodium in the urine. Furosemide only minimally affects phosphorus levels.

2. CORRECT ANSWER: 4

Excessive diuretic use or too-rapid administration can cause tinnitus, transient deafness and, in extreme cases, varying degrees of permanent hearing loss. The symptoms of hypokalemia typically include muscle cramps and paresthesia, not tinnitus. Hypovolemia can cause light-headedness and dizziness, orthostasis, and increased thirst, not tinnitus.

3. CORRECT ANSWER: 4

Trandolapril is an angiotensin-converting enzyme inhibitor, which may increase potassium levels. Trandolapril given with a potassium-sparing diuretic increases the risk of hyperkalemia. Cetirizine, epoprostenol, and ibutilide don't increase potassium levels or cause hyperkalemia.

4. CORRECT ANSWER: 4

Mannitol is an osmotic diuretic that draws fluid from the tissues into the vascular system. Because of the additional fluid in the vascular system from the cerebral edema, a client with heart failure may develop fluid, or circulatory, overload. Rashes and bradycardia aren't common with this drug. Mannitol may increase orientation because it decreases intracranial pressure.

5. CORRECT ANSWER: 3

Acetazolamide increases urine output and can cause significant electrolyte imbalances, which may be indicated by weakness, palpitations, and paresthesia. If these symptoms occur, the client should notify the physician because the dosage may need adjustment. Acetazolamide is safe to use, but it has many adverse reactions. This drug is given by mouth, I.V., or I.M.; it isn't available in eyedrop form. Acetazolamide doesn't cause miotic effects.

6. CORRECT ANSWER: 3

Loop diuretics such as furosemide can alter renal function and enhance certain effects of drugs, such as lithium, by increasing reabsorption of the drug by the kidneys. Potassium-sparing (not loop) diuretics can interact with salicylates such as aspirin, reducing the effects of the diuretic; they also can interact with captopril, causing a reduction in potassium excretion and a subsequent higher incidence of hyperkalemia. Loop diuretics don't interact with penicillin.

7. CORRECT ANSWER: 1

Furosemide should be given in the morning to prevent sleep disruption from the frequent need to urinate.

8. CORRECT ANSWER: 4

Metolazone, a thiazide-like diuretic, is given 30 minutes before a thiazide or loop diuretic to potentiate the diuretic effect. Bumetanide, furosemide, and ethacrynic acid are loop diuretics and don't potentiate the effect of hydrochlorothiazide.

9. CORRECT ANSWER: 3

Blurred vision is a common adverse effect of antimuscarinics. Other common adverse effects include headache, rash, nausea, vomiting, constipation, and urine retention. Tachycardia, diarrhea, and anxiety aren't adverse effects of tolterodine.

10. CORRECT ANSWER: 1, 2, 4, 6

Furosemide must be administered slowly over 1 to 2 minutes. Administering the drug too quickly causes furosemide toxicity. Symptoms of toxicity include tinnitus (ringing in the ears), severe abdominal pain, dizziness, sore throat, and fever. Increased urination is the desired effect of furosemide administration. Headache isn't a sign of furosemide toxicity.

10

Drugs and the hematologic system

PRETEST

1. Which drug helps replace depleted iron stores in the body?
- [ ] 1. Ferrous gluconate (Fergon)
- [ ] 2. Folic acid (Folvite)
- [ ] 3. Epoetin alfa (Procrit)
- [ ] 4. Enoxaparin (Lovenox)

CORRECT ANSWER: 1

2. Which test is used to monitor the effectiveness of heparin?
- [ ] 1. Complete blood count
- [ ] 2. Platelet count
- [ ] 3. Partial thromboplastin time
- [ ] 4. Prothrombin time

CORRECT ANSWER: 3

3. A common adverse reaction of clopidogrel (Plavix) is:
- [ ] 1. hepatic dysfunction.
- [ ] 2. bleeding.
- [ ] 3. fever.
- [ ] 4. anorexia.

CORRECT ANSWER: 2

4. What should a nurse have available when administering a thrombolytic drug?

- ☐ 1. Indwelling urinary catheter
- ☐ 2. Endotracheal intubation supplies
- ☐ 3. Suction catheter
- ☐ 4. Typed and crossmatched blood

CORRECT ANSWER: 4

5. How much fluid should a client taking an iron preparation drink daily?

- ☐ 1. No more than 64 ounces
- ☐ 2. At least 64 ounces
- ☐ 3. At least 128 ounces
- ☐ 4. There's no recommendation

CORRECT ANSWER: 2

LEARNING OBJECTIVES

After studying this chapter, you should be able to:

- Explain the rationale for using hematopoietics, anticoagulants, and thrombolytics.
- Describe the mechanism of action and adverse effects of drugs used to treat the hematologic system.
- Identify laboratory tests used to monitor patients receiving hematopoietics, anticoagulants, and thrombolytics.
- Identify the nurse's responsibilities when administering hematopoietics, anticoagulants, and thrombolytics.

CHAPTER OVERVIEW

Hematopoietic factors help form cellular elements of blood. These drugs contribute to the production and formation of red blood cells (RBCs) in iron deficiency anemia and megaloblastic anemia. They also contribute to the production and formation of RBCs and white blood cells (WBCs) in anemia of bone marrow failure or suppression. Anemia may result from vitamin or mineral deficiencies that impair the manufacture of RBCs; treatment focuses on replacing the deficient vitamins or minerals.

Anticoagulants and thrombolytics are used in the prophylaxis and treatment of thromboembolic disorders, such as myocardial infarction (MI), pulmonary embolism, stroke, and deep vein thrombosis (DVT). Anticoagulants prevent clots from forming or existing clots from enlarging; thrombolytics cause clot dissolution. When used within 2 to 4 hours of the onset of MI, thrombolytics may minimize myocardial damage.

ANATOMY AND PHYSIOLOGY

Anatomy

- Blood
  - Made up of RBCs (erythrocytes), WBCs, and platelets (thrombocytes) in a viscous fluid called plasma
  - RBCs: most numerous elements in blood
  - WBCs
    - Are less numerous than RBCs
    - Have two classifications
      - Granulocytes (neutrophils, eosinophils, and basophils)
      - Agranulocytes (lymphocytes and monocytes)
  - Platelets
    - Are anucleated cells resembling small plates
    - Are about one-third the size of RBCs
    - Are formed from large multinucleated cells called megakaryocytes in bone marrow
- Plasma
  - Accounts for about 55% of total blood volume
  - Consists of albumin, globulins, and fibrinogen

Physiology

- RBCs
  - Produced in marrow of certain bones (erythropoiesis); regulated by oxygen content of arterial blood
  - Require hemoglobin to mature and function
    - Iron
      - Is an essential part of hemoglobin
      - Circulates in small amounts in plasma with the iron-binding transport protein transferrin
    - Transferrin

Anatomy highlights

- Blood consists of RBCs, WBCs, and platelets that are in a viscous fluid called plasma.
- RBCs are the most numerous elements in the blood.
- WBCs are classified as granulocytes (neutrophils, eosinophils, and basophils) and agranulocytes (lymphocytes and monocytes).
- Platelets resemble small plates and are anucleated cells about one-third the size of RBCs.
- Plasma accounts for about 55% of the total blood volume and consists of albumin, globulins, and fibrinogen.

- Transports iron from the GI tract (where iron is absorbed) and mononuclear phagocytes (where iron is recovered from RBC breakdown) to bone marrow, the liver, and the spleen (where extra iron is stored as ferritin and hemosiderin)
- WBCs
  - Mature in bone marrow
  - Circulate in blood and enter tissues
  - Participate in inflammatory and immune responses
    - Ingest and digest solid substances (other cells, bacteria, necrotic tissues, and foreign particles) through phagocytosis
    - Release chemicals in response to foreign antigens or bacteria that enter the body
- Clotting and coagulation
  - Involves various substances that help blood to clot, thus stopping the bleeding
    - Platelets
    - Coagulation factors (clotting activators and fibrin)
    - RBCs
  - Involves coagulation inhibitors and anticoagulants, which counterbalance coagulation factors and mechanisms to prevent excessive (disseminated) intravascular coagulation
    - Antithrombin—found in plasma; inhibits thrombin formation
    - Heparin—found in basophils and mast cells; has anticoagulant properties
    - Prostaglandin derivatives—inhibit platelet aggregation and phospholipid release that initiate coagulation
  - Leads to *fibrinolysis,* a process in which the clot dissolves after the bleeding blood vessel heals
    - Is activated simultaneously with the coagulation mechanism
    - Restricts clotting to a limited area, thereby preventing excessive intravascular coagulation
    - Activates plasmin, a proteolytic (protein-digesting) enzyme, which breaks down clot's fibrin strands

● Function
- Blood
  - Delivers oxygen to body cells from lungs and delivers nutrients to body cells from GI tract
  - Transports carbon dioxide to lungs and nitrogenous wastes to kidneys for elimination
  - Transports hormones from endocrine glands to target tissues
  - Maintains body temperature by absorbing and distributing body heat
  - Maintains acid-base balance
    - Contains blood proteins and other solutes that act as buffers to prevent sudden changes in blood pH
    - Stores bicarbonate atoms (important component of blood-buffer system needed to maintain normal blood pH)

Physiology highlights

- RBC production is called erythropoiesis.
- WBCs mature in the bone marrow, circulate in the blood, and enter the tissues.
- WBCs participate in the inflammatory and immune responses.
- Platelets, coagulation factors, RBCs, and other blood components help blood to clot.
- After a bleeding blood vessel has healed and the clot is no longer needed, it must be lysed.
- Coagulation inhibitors and anticoagulants that retard clotting counterbalance coagulation factors and mechanisms and prevent excessive intravascular coagulation.
- Fibrinolysis is a clot-dissolving system that's activated simultaneously with the coagulation mechanism.

Function highlights

- Blood
- Delivers oxygen and nutrients to body cells
- Transports carbon dioxide to lungs and nitrogenous wastes to kidneys for elimination
- Transports hormones from endocrine glands to target tissues
- Maintains body temperature
- Maintains acid-base balance
- Stores bicarbonate atoms
- Maintains adequate fluid volume
- Helps prevent blood loss through hemostasis
- Plasma
- Helps maintain colloid osmotic pressure of blood
- Transports enzymes, hormones, vitamins, and other substances
- Plays a major role in blood coagulation

– Maintains adequate fluid volume
  - Contains salts (such as sodium chloride) and proteins (such as albumin) to prevent excessive fluid loss
  - Prevents loss of blood from body through hemostasis, which involves vascular spasm, platelet formation, and coagulation
– Helps prevent infection through the action of antibodies, complement proteins, and WBCs
- Plasma
  – Albumin: helps maintain colloid osmotic pressure of blood, thus regulating fluid flow between capillaries and interstitial tissues
  – Globulins: transport enzymes, hormones, vitamins and other substances
  – Gamma globulins: act as antibodies, defending body against infection
  – Fibrinogen: converts to fibrin (protein that forms a meshlike network across wound) when blood coagulates

HEMATOPOIETICS

IRON PRODUCTS

● **Mechanism of action**
- Supplement and replace depleted iron stores in bone marrow to assist in erythropoiesis (RBC production)

● **Pharmacokinetics**
- Absorption: Absorbed primarily in duodenum and upper jejunum
  – Depends partially on body stores of iron
  – Increases when body stores are low
  – Decreases when body stores are high
- Distribution: Transported by blood and bound to transferrin, its carrier plasma-protein
- Metabolism: Occurs in closed system where most of iron that's broken down is reused by body
- Excretion: Excreted in urine, feces, and sweat and through intestinal cell sloughing

● **Drug examples**
- Ferrous fumarate (Femiron, Feostat, Ircon, Hemocyte), ferrous gluconate (Fergon), ferrous sulfate (Feosol, Fer-In-Sol, Fer-gen-Sol, Feratab, Ferralyn), iron dextran (INFeD, DexFerrum), iron sucrose (Venofer), sodium ferric gluconate (Ferrlecit)

● **Indications**
- Prevent and treat iron deficiency and iron deficiency anemia
- Dietary supplement for iron

Key facts about iron products

- Supplement and replace depleted iron stores in the bone marrow to assist in erythropoiesis
- Metabolism occurs in a closed system where most of the iron that's broken down is reused by the body
- Excreted in the urine, feces, and sweat and through intestinal cell sloughing

When to use iron products

- Iron deficiency
- Iron deficiency anemia
- As dietary iron supplement

Contraindications and precautions
- Contraindicated in patients with hemochromatosis, hemosiderosis, hemolytic anemias, peptic ulcer disease, inflammatory bowel disorders, or hypersensitivity to drug, tartrazine, or sulfites
- Not intended for long-term use in patients with normal iron stores

Adverse reactions
- Oral iron preparations: Nausea, vomiting, constipation, dark stools, diarrhea, and GI distress
- Parenteral iron preparations: Nausea, vomiting, headache, staining at the I.M. injection site, localized phlebitis at the I.V. injection site, and anaphylaxis
- Liquid iron preparations: May temporarily stain teeth
- Iron sucrose injection: Heart failure, sepsis, and mild to moderate hypersensitivity reactions (wheezing, dyspnea, hypotension, rash, pruritus)

Interactions
- Cimetidine, and histamine-2 (H_2) receptor agonists decrease absorption of oral iron preparations
- Oral iron products decrease absorption of tetracycline, methyldopa, quinolones, levofloxacin, ciprofloxacin, levothyroxine, and penicillamine

Nursing responsibilities
- Administer drug according to the prescribed route
  - For oral administration
    - Give drug between meals
    - If GI distress occurs, give drug with meals
    - Give tablets with juice or water, not with milk or antacids; orange juice or ascorbic acid promotes iron absorption
    - Dilute liquid iron preparations, and give with straw to avoid staining teeth
  - For I.M. administration
    - Use Z-track technique to prevent leakage and staining into subcutaneous tissues
  - For I.V. administration
    - Check facility policy before giving I.V.; some facilities don't permit infusions because safety is controversial
    - Use I.V. route in these situations
      - Insufficient muscle mass for deep I.M. injection
      - Impaired absorption from muscle caused by stasis or edema
      - Possibility of uncontrolled I.M. bleeding from trauma (may occur in hemophilia)
      - Massive, prolonged parenteral therapy (may be necessary with chronic substantial blood loss)
    - Give initial test dose to rule out hypersensitivity before administering drug I.V.

When NOT to use iron products
- Hypersensitivity to tartrazine or sulfites
- Hemochromatosis
- Hemosiderosis
- Hemolytic anemias

Adverse reactions
- Nausea, vomiting, constipation, dark stools, diarrhea, GI distress, headache, staining at I.M. injection site, localized phlebitis at I.V. injection site, anaphylaxis, temporary staining of teeth

Key nursing actions
- Administer drugs according to prescribed route.
- Monitor patient's CBC, hemoglobin, and plasma iron level.
- Check for constipation.
- Caution parents to be alert for iron poisoning in children.
- Know that signs and symptoms of iron poisoning include nausea, vomiting, diarrhea, and GI bleeding, which can lead to shock, coma, and death.
- Teach patient to:
  - continue regular dosing schedule after missing dose; caution against doubling dose
  - drink at least 2 L of fluid daily (unless contraindicated) and to exercise regularly
  - avoid antacids, coffee, tea, dairy products, eggs, and whole grain breads for 1 hour before and 2 hours after taking oral iron preparations
  - be aware that iron preparations may turn stools dark green or black.

Topics for patient discussion

- Therapy regimen
- Available forms and proper administration method
- Signs and symptoms of possible adverse effects and when to notify the practitioner
- Dietary allowances
- Changes in stool color
- Measures to relieve minor adverse effects
- Need for compliance with therapy
- Follow-up care

TIME-OUT FOR TEACHING

Teaching about iron products

Include these topics in your teaching plan for the patient receiving an iron product:

- medication therapy regimen, including the drug's name, dose, frequency, duration, and possible adverse effects
- available forms and proper administration method
- signs and symptoms of possible adverse effects and when to notify the practitioner
- dietary allowances, including the need for high-iron foods
- changes in stool color
- measures to relieve minor adverse effects such as constipation
- need for compliance with therapy, including taking the drug as prescribed
- follow-up care, including laboratory tests and practitioner visits.

- Flush vein with 10 ml of 0.9% sodium chloride solution on completion of I.V. iron dextran infusion
- Instruct the patient to rest for 15 to 30 minutes after infusion
- Monitor the patient's laboratory test results
  - Complete blood count (CBC)
  - Hemoglobin levels
  - Plasma iron level
- Check for constipation
  - Record color, amount, and consistency of stools
  - Teach dietary measures for preventing constipation (see *Teaching about iron products*)
- Instruct the patient to continue the regular dosing schedule after missing a dose; caution against doubling doses
- Caution parents to be aware of iron poisoning in children and to contact their pediatrician or local poison control center immediately if signs and symptoms occur
  - Signs and symptoms include nausea, vomiting, diarrhea, and GI bleeding; can lead to shock, coma, and death
  - Poisoning can occur within minutes to hours after swallowing tablets
- Instruct the patient to drink at least 2 qt (2 L) of fluid daily (unless contraindicated), to increase fiber intake, and to exercise regularly to prevent constipation
- Advise the patient to avoid antacids, coffee, tea, dairy products, eggs, and whole grain breads for 1 hour before and 2 hours after taking oral iron preparations; may interfere with absorption
- Inform the patient that iron preparations may turn stools dark green or black

VITAMINS

● **Mechanism of action**
  • Replace depleted vitamin stores

● **Pharmacokinetics**
  • Absorption
    – Vitamin B_{12}: Absorbed by simple diffusion, but depends on intrinsic factor (secreted by parietal cells of gastric mucosa; regulates amount of vitamin B_{12} absorbed); therefore, parenteral form is usually used
    – Hydroxocobalamin (vitamin B_{12}; crystalline): Absorbed more slowly from injection site than cyanocobalamin
    – Folic acid and leucovorin: Undergo hydrolysis in GI tract before being completely absorbed
  • Distribution
    – Vitamin B_{12}: Protein-bound and distributed in tissues
    – Folic acid and leucovorin: Distributed rapidly to all body tissues
  • Metabolism: Vitamin B_{12}, folic acid, leucovorin, and cyanocobalamin are metabolized and stored in liver
  • Excretion
    – Vitamin B_{12}: Excreted in urine; some excreted in bile, then reabsorbed in ileum; also excreted in breast milk
    – Folic acid and leucovorin: Excreted in urine and feces; some excreted in breast milk

● **Drug examples**
  • Cyanocobalamin (Nascobal), hydroxocobalamin, vitamin B_{12} (Big Shot B-12); folic acid or vitamin B_9 (Folvite); leucovorin (folinic acid, citrovorum factor)

● **Indications**
  • Treat megaloblastic anemia (vitamin B_{12} deficiency) (cyanocobalamin)
  • Treat vitamin B_{12} deficiency resulting from pernicious anemia (nasal form and parenteral form [hydroxocobalamin])
  • Treat megaloblastic anemia caused by folic acid deficiency (folic acid and parenteral leucovorin)
  • Treat toxicity associated with methotrexate therapy (oral and parenteral forms of leucovorin)

● **Contraindications and precautions**
  • Cyanocobalamin contraindicated in patients hypersensitive to these vitamins or cobalt
  • Folic acid and leucovorin contraindicated in patients with pernicious anemia and other megaloblastic anemias caused by vitamin B_{12} deficiency

● **Adverse reactions**
  • Headache, infection, nausea, mild diarrhea, asthenia, paresthesia, itching, and rash (cyanocobalamin)
  • Allergic reaction, itching, nausea, irritability, and allergic bronchospasm (folic acid)

Key facts about vitamins

● Replace depleted vitamin stores
● Vitamin B_{12}, folic acid, and leucovorin metabolized and stored in the liver
● Vitamin B_{12} excreted in the urine but some excreted in the bile and then reabsorbed in the ileum; also excreted in breast milk
● Folic acid and leucovorin excreted in the urine and feces; some excreted in breast milk

When to use vitamins

● Vitamin B_{12} deficiency
● Megaloblastic anemia due to folic acid deficiency
● Toxicity associated with methotrexate therapy

When NOT to use vitamins

● Hypersensitivity to these vitamins or cobalt
● Pernicious anemia, other megaloblastic anemias caused by vitamin B_{12} deficiency

Adverse reactions

● Headache, infection, nausea, mild diarrhea, asthenia, paresthesia, itching, rash, allergic reaction or allergic bronchospasm

- Heart failure, hypokalemia, pulmonary edema, and polycythemia vera (parenteral B$_{12}$)

● **Interactions**
- Folic acid may increase metabolism or counteract effects of anticonvulsants, causing subtherapeutic phenytoin level and increasing the risk of seizures
- Alcohol, aspirin, neomycin, chloramphenicol, and colchicine may reduce absorption of cyanocobalamin, impairing vitamin's effectiveness
- Aspirin, hormonal contraceptives, methotrexate, triamterene, pentamidine, trimethoprim, and sulfasalazine may decrease folate levels
- Large doses of folic acid may counteract effect of anticonvulsants

● **Nursing responsibilities**
- Inform the patient with pernicious anemia of the need for lifelong monthly injections of vitamin B$_{12}$
  – Failure to do so will result in return of anemia and development of incapacitating and irreversible damage to spinal cord nerves
- Take seizure precautions in a patient receiving large doses of folic acid while on anticonvulsant therapy
- Encourage the patient to eat foods rich in vitamin B$_{12}$ (meat, seafood, eggs, legumes, and liver)
- Monitor laboratory test results, such as hematocrit and reticulocyte counts, to determine therapy's effectiveness
- Check folate levels in the patient receiving more than 10 mcg of vitamin B$_{12}$ daily; hematologic results may seem normal but may mask folate deficiency, possible cause of megaloblastic anemia
- Monitor potassium level during first 48 hours of treatment, particularly if the patient has addisonian pernicious anemia or megaloblastic anemia

BIOLOGIC RESPONSE MODIFIERS

● **Mechanism of action**
- Stimulate RBC production in bone marrow by boosting erythropoietin production

● **Pharmacokinetics**
- Absorption: Slow and rate limiting with subcutaneous (subQ) administration
- Distribution: Distribution of darbepoetin alfa confined to vascular space; distribution of epoetin alfa is unknown
- Metabolism: Unknown
- Excretion: Unknown

● **Drug examples**
- Darbepoetin alfa (Aranesp), epoetin alfa (Epogen, Procrit)

● Indications

- Treat anemia associated with chronic renal failure, whether or not the patient is on dialysis (darbepoetin alfa)
- Treat anemia associated with end-stage renal disease, chemotherapy, or zidovudine therapy (epoetin alfa)
- Decrease need for perioperative blood transfusions in surgery patients (epoetin alfa)

● Contraindications and precautions

- Contraindicated in patients with uncontrolled hypertension or hypersensitivity to drug or drug components (such as mammalian-derived products or human albumin)
- Epoetin alfa not intended for patients with chronic renal disease and severe anemia or for patients infected with human immunodeficiency virus or cancer patients with anemia that's caused by other factors, such as iron or folate deficiencies, hemolysis, or GI bleeding that should be managed appropriately
- Used with extreme caution in pregnant and breast-feeding patients
- Darbepoetin alfa used with extreme caution in patients with underlying hematologic disease (such as hemolytic anemia, sickle cell anemia, thalassemia, or porphyria); safety not established

● Adverse reactions

- Hypertension, seizures, iron deficiency, increased risk of thrombotic events (including MI, stroke, or transient ischemic attack), hypersensitivity, and allergic reactions
- Vascular access thrombosis, heart failure, sepsis, cardiac arrhythmias, infection, hypertension, hypotension, myalgia, headache, vomiting, chest pain, and diarrhea (darbepoetin alfa)

● Interactions

- None reported

● Nursing responsibilities

- Monitor hemoglobin levels and hematocrit frequently, especially early in therapy, to evaluate drug effectiveness
  - Rapid rise in hematocrit associated with seizures and hypertension
  - Adequate iron, folic acid, and vitamin B_{12} stores required for erythropoiesis
- Institute seizure precautions, and closely monitor neurologic status
- Monitor blood pressure for signs of hypertension frequently
- Teach the patient or family the proper technique for subQ injection

COLONY-STIMULATING FACTOR

● Mechanism of action

- Stimulates production of granulocytes and macrophages in bone marrow by binding to specific cell surface receptors or stimulating leukopoiesis

---

When to use biologic response modifiers

- Anemia associated with chronic renal failure, end-stage renal disease, chemotherapy, or zidovudine therapy
- Decrease in need for perioperative blood transfusions

When NOT to use biologic response modifiers

- Hypersensitivity to these drugs
- Uncontrolled hypertension

Adverse reactions

- Hypertension, seizures, iron deficiency, increased risk of thrombotic events, hypersensitivity, allergic reactions

Key nursing actions

- Monitor hemoglobin and hematocrit frequently, especially early in therapy.
- Institute seizure precautions and closely monitor patient's neurologic status.
- Frequently monitor patient's blood pressure for signs of hypertension.
- Teach proper technique for subQ injection.

Key facts about colony-stimulating factor

- Stimulates production of granulocytes and macrophages in bone marrow by binding to specific cell surface receptors

When to use colony-stimulating factor

- Aplastic anemia secondary to chemotherapy
- Acceleration of bone marrow recovery in malignant lymphoma and Hodgkin's disease
- Failed bone marrow transplant
- Increase of WBCs during zidovudine therapy

When NOT to use colony-stimulating factor

- Hypersensitivity to these drugs
- Excessive leukemic myeloid blasts in the bone marrow or peripheral blood
- Simultaneous administration of cytotoxic chemotherapy or radiotherapy
- Within 24 hours before or after chemotherapy or radiotherapy

Adverse reactions

- Respiratory symptoms, supraventricular arrhythmias, bone pain, arthralgia, myalgia, anorexia, nausea, vomiting, diarrhea, stomatitis, fluid retention, hypersensitivity reactions

Key nursing actions

- Monitor WBC count.
- Discontinue drug when absolute neutrophil count is 10,000 for filgrastim and 20,000 for sargramostim.
- Teach proper technique for subQ injection.
- Teach importance of maintaining nutritionally balanced diet and complying with therapy.

● Pharmacokinetics
- Unknown

● Drug examples
- Aldesleukin (interleukin-2), filgrastim (Neupogen), pegfilgrastim (Neulasta), sargramostim (Leukine)

● Indications
- Treat aplastic anemia secondary to chemotherapy
- Accelerate bone marrow recovery in malignant lymphoma and Hodgkin's disease
- Treat delayed or failed bone marrow transplant
- Increase WBCs in patients taking zidovudine

● Contraindications and precautions
- Filgrastim and pegfilgrastim contraindicated in patients with hypersensitivity to *Escherichia coli*–derived proteins or other drug components
- Sargramostim contraindicated in patients with excessive leukemic myeloid blasts in bone marrow or peripheral blood (10% or more) or hypersensitivity to drug or its components; in patients receiving simultaneous administration of cytotoxic chemotherapy or radiotherapy; and within 24 hours before or after chemotherapy or radiotherapy
- Aldesleukin contraindicated in patients with serious cardiovascular disease

● Adverse reactions
- Respiratory symptoms, supraventricular arrhythmias, bone pain, arthralgia, myalgia, anorexia, nausea, vomiting, diarrhea, stomatitis, fluid retention, and hypersensitivity reactions

● Interactions
- Concurrent use with lithium may potentiate release of neutrophils
- Lithium, corticosteroids, and other drugs may potentiate myeloproliferative effects of sargramostim

● Nursing responsibilities
- Monitor WBC count
- Monitor for signs and symptoms of infection
- Discontinue drug when absolute neutrophil count is 10,000 for filgrastim and 20,000 for sargramostim
- Know that pegfilgrastim is longer-acting than filgrastim
- Don't administer filgrastim within 24 hours of antineoplastic drugs
- Instruct the patient or family in proper technique for subQ injection
- Teach the patient the importance of maintaining nutritionally balanced diet and complying with therapeutic regimen

ANTICOAGULANTS

HEPARIN AND HEPARIN DERIVATIVES

- **Mechanism of action**
  - Prevent extension and formation of clots by inhibiting factors in clotting cascade

- **Pharmacokinetics**
  - Absorption: Varies based on administration
  - Distribution: Varies after subQ administration
  - Metabolism: Metabolized by liver
  - Excretion: Excreted in urine

- **Drug examples**
  - I.V. forms: bivalirudin (Angiomax), heparin, lepirudin (Refludan), tinzaparin (Innohep)
  - SubQ forms: dalteparin (Fragmin), enoxaparin (Lovenox)
  - Oral forms: warfarin (Coumadin, Jantoven)

- **Indications**
  - Treat or prevent thromboembolic disorders (such as DVT, pulmonary embolus, and atrial fibrillation with embolization) and ischemic complications
  - Adjunct to aspirin in patients with unstable angina undergoing percutaneous transluminal coronary angioplasty (bivalirudin)
  - Treat or prevent heparin-induced thrombocytopenia (lepirudin)

- **Contraindications and precautions**
  - Contraindicated in patients with underlying coagulation disorders, ulcer disease, recent surgery, cancer, or active bleeding; patients with severe thrombocytopenia or uncontrolled bleeding; and those with hypersensitivity to drug or drug components
  - Enoxaparin sodium not recommended for patients with prosthetic heart valves; higher risk for thromboembolism

- **Adverse reactions**
  - Fever, pain at injection site, nausea, constipation, and insomnia
  - Hyperlipidemia, thrombocytopenia (with heparin), hemorrhages, and spinal or epidural hematoma (with indwelling catheters)

- **Interactions**
  - Androgens, chloral hydrate, chloramphenicol, metronidazole, acetaminophen, allopurinol, tricyclic antidepressants, quinidine, sulfonamides, thrombolytics, and valproic acid increase the risk of bleeding and enhance effects of warfarin
  - Alcohol, barbiturates, estrogen-containing hormonal contraceptives, and foods high in vitamin K increase the risk of clotting and may decrease effects of warfarin

Key facts about anticoagulants

- Prevent extension and formation of clots by inhibiting factors in the clotting cascade
- Heparin metabolized by the liver
- Excreted in urine

When to use anticoagulants

- Thromboembolic disorders
- Ischemic complications
- Unstable angina in percutaneous transluminal coronary angioplasty

When NOT to use anticoagulants

- Hypersensitivity to these drugs
- Underlying coagulation disorders
- Ulcer disease
- Recent surgery
- Cancer
- Active bleeding
- Severe thrombocytopenia
- Uncontrolled bleeding

Adverse reactions

- Hyperlipidemia, thrombocytopenia, hemorrhages, spinal or epidural hematoma, fever, pain at injection site, nausea, constipation, insomnia

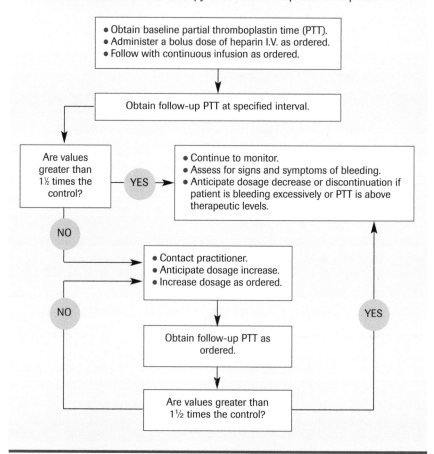

GO WITH THE FLOW

Monitoring heparin therapy

When monitoring a patient who's receiving heparin, the nurse plays a key role in ensuring maximum effectiveness while minimizing possible adverse effects. Use the flowchart below to initiate therapy and monitor the patient's response.

- Obtain baseline partial thromboplastin time (PTT).
- Administer a bolus dose of heparin I.V. as ordered.
- Follow with continuous infusion as ordered.

Obtain follow-up PTT at specified interval.

Are values greater than 1½ times the control?

YES
- Continue to monitor.
- Assess for signs and symptoms of bleeding.
- Anticipate dosage decrease or discontinuation if patient is bleeding excessively or PTT is above therapeutic levels.

NO

- Contact practitioner.
- Anticipate dosage increase.
- Increase dosage as ordered.

NO

Obtain follow-up PTT as ordered.

Are values greater than 1½ times the control?

YES

Key nursing actions

- Don't give heparin by I.M. route.
- Minimize venipunctures and injections; apply pressure to all puncture sites.
- Inject subQ heparin and enoxaparin into abdomen; don't aspirate or rub injection site and rotate injection sites.
- Assess for signs and symptoms of bleeding; instruct patient to report bleeding immediately.
- Monitor hemoglobin and clotting factor and platelet levels.
- Caution patients not to increase dietary vitamin K or drastically and suddenly change diet.
- Teach patient to:
– inform physician and dentist of therapy regimen before undergoing any medical treatments
– be aware of importance of routine laboratory tests to monitor coagulation times
– carry identification describing disease and drug regimen
– not take drugs or vitamins, including over-the-counter or herbal products, without medical approval.

- Concurrent use with other drugs that affect platelet function (such as aspirin, dextran, dipyridamole, and nonsteroidal anti-inflammatory drugs [NSAIDs]) increases the risk of bleeding

● **Nursing responsibilities**
- Don't give heparin by I.M. route
- Minimize venipunctures and injections; apply pressure to all puncture sites to prevent bleeding
- Know that heparin is given initially because of its rapid action
  – The patient may then be started on warfarin, which takes several days to reach therapeutic levels
  – Once therapeutic levels are reached, heparin will be discontinued and the patient maintained on warfarin

TIME-OUT FOR TEACHING
Teaching about anticoagulants

Include these topics in your teaching plan for the patient receiving an anticoagulant:
- medication therapy regimen, including the drug's name, dose, frequency, duration, and possible adverse effects
- signs and symptoms of possible adverse effects and when to notify the practitioner
- subcutaneous administration technique, if indicated
- safety measures and bleeding precautions
- avoidance of over-the-counter products unless permitted by the practitioner
- need for compliance with therapy, including taking the drug as prescribed
- follow-up care, including laboratory tests and practitioner visits.

Topics for patient discussion
- Therapy regimen
- Signs and symptoms of possible adverse effects and when to notify the practitioner
- Subcutaneous administration technique, if indicated
- Safety measures and bleeding precautions
- Avoidance of over-the-counter products unless permitted by the practitioner
- Need for compliance with therapy
- Follow-up care

- Be aware that heparin directly affects partial thromboplastin time (PTT) and warfarin directly affects prothrombin time (PT) and international normalized ratio (INR)
- Monitor PTT in the patient taking argatroban
- Know that enoxaparin usually doesn't significantly affect INR, PT, PTT, or platelet function (see *Monitoring heparin therapy*)
- Inject subQ heparin and enoxaparin into abdomen
    - Don't aspirate or rub injection site
    - Rotate injection sites
- Know that protamine sulfate is an antidote for heparin and that phytonadione (vitamin K) is an antidote for warfarin
- Assess for bleeding; instruct the patient to report signs and symptoms of bleeding immediately
- Monitor hemoglobin and clotting factor and platelet levels
- Instruct the patient to use a soft toothbrush and an electric razor to prevent trauma and bleeding (see *Teaching about anticoagulants*)
- Instruct the patient to inform the practitioner and dentist of the medication regimen before undergoing any medical treatments
- Caution the patient not to increase dietary vitamin K or drastically and suddenly change diet; doing either of these can impair warfarin's effectiveness
- Teach the patient the importance of routine laboratory tests to monitor coagulation times
- Instruct the patient to carry identification describing disease and drug regimen
- Instruct the patient not to take any drugs or vitamins, including over-the-counter or herbal preparations, unless directed by the practitioner

Key facts about antiplatelet drugs

- Interfere with platelet aggregation in different drug-specific and dose-specific ways, preventing thromboembolic events
- Metabolized in liver
- Depending on the form, may be excreted in bile, urine, or feces

When to use antiplatelet drugs

- As prophylaxis for thromboembolic events and intermittent claudication

When NOT to use antiplatelet drugs

- Active bleeding
- Thrombocytopenia
- Severe liver impairment
- Underlying coagulation disorders
- Ulcer disease
- Recent surgery
- Cancer

Adverse reactions

- Bleeding, pancytopenia, neutropenia or agranulocytosis, hemorrhage, thrombotic thrombocytopenic purpura, dizziness, diarrhea, abnormal stools, headache, infection, rash, nausea, pain at injection site

ANTIPLATELET DRUGS

- ● **Mechanism of action**
  - Interfere with platelet aggregation in different drug-specific and dose-specific ways, preventing thromboembolic events

- ● **Pharmacokinetics**
  - Absorption: Varies with each drug
  - Distribution: Usually distributed quickly and widely throughout body; highly protein-bound
  - Metabolism: Metabolized in liver
  - Excretion: Depending on form, may be excreted in bile, urine, or feces

- ● **Drug examples**
  - Aspirin, cilostazol (Pletal), clopidogrel (Plavix), dipyridamole (Persantine), ticlopidine (Ticlid)

- ● **Indications**
  - Prophylaxis for thromboembolic events and intermittent claudication
  - Reduce risk of death in patients with previous MI or unstable angina and risk of transient ischemic attacks in men (aspirin)
  - Reduce symptoms of intermittent claudication (cilostazol)
  - Reduce risk of cardiovascular event and death in patients with recent MI or stroke, established peripheral arterial disease, or acute coronary syndrome (clopidogrel)
  - Second-line drug in prevention of stroke in high-risk individuals (ticlopidine)

- ● **Contraindications and precautions**
  - Contraindicated in patients with active bleeding, thrombocytopenia, history of hemorrhagic stroke, severe liver impairment, underlying coagulation disorders, ulcer disease, recent surgery, or cancer

- ● **Adverse reactions**
  - Dizziness, diarrhea, abnormal stools, headache, infection, rash, nausea, and pain at injection site
  - Possible bleeding, pancytopenia, neutropenia or agranulocytosis (ticlopidine), hemorrhage, or thrombotic thrombocytopenic purpura

- ● **Interactions**
  - Use with other drugs that affect platelet function (such as aspirin, dextran, dipyridamole, or NSAIDs) may increase risk of bleeding
  - Antacids decrease plasma level of ticlopidine
  - Use with sulfinpyrazone increases risk of bleeding

- ● **Nursing responsibilities**
  - Monitor for bruising and evidence of bleeding
  - Instruct the patient to report signs and symptoms of bleeding immediately

- Monitor hemoglobin and clotting factor and platelet levels
- Minimize venipunctures and injections; apply pressure to all puncture sites to prevent bleeding
- Stop drug 5 to 7 days before surgery, or as ordered by the practitioner
- Withhold dose and notify the practitioner if the patient develops bleeding, salicylism, or adverse GI reactions

FACTOR Xa INHIBITORS

Mechanism of action
- Block factor Xa, altering the clot formation process

Pharmacokinetics
- Absorption: Absorbed rapidly and completely with 100% bioavailability
- Distribution: Widely distributed
- Metabolism: Unknown
- Excretion: Excreted in urine

Drug examples
- Fondaparinux (Arixtra)

Indications
- Prevention of DVT in patients undergoing abdominal surgery or surgery for hip fracture, hip replacement, or knee replacement
- Adjunct to warfarin for treatment of acute DVT and pulmonary embolism

Contraindications and precautions
- Contradicted in patients with active bleeding, thrombocytopenia, severe renal impairment, or bacterial endocarditis and in those weighing less than 110 lb (50 kg)
- Used cautiously in patients with bleeding disorders, renal impairment, uncontrolled hypertension, GI ulcer, or diabetic retinopathy and in those who had a recent spinal puncture

Adverse reactions
- Fever, spinal and epidural hematoma, nausea, hemorrhage, thrombocytopenia, injection site irritation, rash, and anemia

Interactions
- Use with drugs that increase risk of bleeding (NSAIDs, aspirin, and anticoagulants) increases risk of hemorrhage

Nursing responsibilities
- Monitor for signs and symptoms of bleeding
- Monitor the patient who had epidural or spinal anesthesia for formations of spinal or epidural hematoma
- Monitor laboratory results, including CBC, platelet count, and renal function tests

---

Key nursing actions

- Monitor and assess patient for bruising or bleeding.
- Tell patient to report signs and symptoms of bleeding immediately.
- Monitor hemoglobin and clotting factor and platelet levels.
- Minimize venipunctures and injections; apply pressure to all puncture sites to prevent bleeding.

Key facts about Factor Xa inhibitors

- Alter the clot formation process by blocking factor Xa
- Excreted in urine

When to use Factor Xa inhibitors

- Prevention of DVT
- Acute DVT
- Pulmonary embolism

When NOT to use Factor Xa inhibitors

- Active bleeding
- Thrombocytopenia
- Renal impairment
- Bacterial endocarditis

Adverse reactions

- Fever, spinal and epidural hematoma, nausea, hemorrhage, thrombocytopenia

Key nursing actions

- Monitor for signs and symptoms of bleeding.
- Monitor laboratory results.
- Keep in mind that factor Xa inhibitors aren't interchangeable with heparin or heparin derivatives.

- Know that PT and PTT tests are ineffective in monitoring drug levels
- Be aware that factor Xa inhibitors aren't interchangeable with heparin or heparin derivatives
- Don't massage the injection site after administration

THROMBOLYTICS

Mechanism of action
- Activate plasminogen, leading to its conversion to plasmin (clot-degrading substance)

Pharmacokinetics
- Absorption: Administered I.V.
- Distribution: Distributed immediately
- Metabolism: Varies with each drug
- Excretion: Varies with each drug

Drug examples
- Alteplase (tissue plasminogen activator [Activase]), drotrecogin alfa (activated) (Xigris), reteplase (Retavase), streptokinase (Streptase), tenecteplase (TNKase), urokinase (Abbokinase)

Indications
- Lysis of thrombi and treatment of massive pulmonary emboli, acute ischemic stroke, and acute MI
- Treat DVT and clear arterial catheters and arteriovenous cannulas
- Reduce risk of death in patients with severe sepsis associated with acute organ dysfunction (drotrecogin alfa)

Contraindications and precautions
- Contraindicated in patients with recent streptococcal infection (streptokinase), active internal bleeding, recent stroke, underlying coagulation disorders, ulcer disease, recent surgery, cancer, or uncontrolled hypertension
- Streptokinase not indicated for arterial embolism originating from left side of heart because of increased risk of new embolic phenomena (such as cerebral embolism)

Adverse reactions
- Bleeding and arrhythmias (most common), hypersensitivity reactions, urticaria, fever, and hemorrhage

Interactions
- Use with other drugs that affect platelet function (such as aspirin, dextran, dipyridamole, and NSAIDs) may increase risk of bleeding
- Aminocaproic acid (Amicar) inhibits streptokinase and can be used to reverse its fibrinolytic effects

Nursing responsibilities
- Know that thrombolytics should be given only when patient's hematologic function and clinical response can be monitored

---

Key facts about thrombolytics

- Activate plasminogen, leading to its conversion to plasmin
- Metabolism varies with each drug
- Excretion varies with each drug

When to use thrombolytics

- Lysis of thrombi
- Massive pulmonary emboli, DVT, acute ischemic stroke, and acute MI
- Clearing of arterial catheters and arteriovenous cannuli
- Reduction of mortality in severe sepsis associated with acute organ dysfunction and a high risk of death

When NOT to use thrombolytics

- Recent streptococcal infection
- Active internal bleeding
- Recent stroke
- Underlying coagulation disorders
- Ulcer disease
- Recent surgery
- Cancer
- Uncontrolled hypertension

Adverse reactions

- Bleeding, arrhythmias, hypersensitivity reactions, urticaria, fever, hemorrhage

- Assess the patient for signs and symptoms of bleeding, monitor coagulation values, and implement appropriate safety measures to prevent bleeding
- Ensure that antidote for thrombolytic overdose (aminocaproic acid) is readily available
- Minimize venipunctures, injections, and other invasive procedures to decrease risk of bleeding; apply pressure to all puncture sites
- Monitor hemoglobin and clotting factor and platelet levels
- Assess for signs and symptoms of bleeding; instruct the patient to report signs and symptoms of bleeding immediately
- Monitor vital signs for indications of bleeding or hypotension frequently; check peripheral pulses to ensure adequate circulation to extremities
- Keep typed and crossmatched blood on hand in case of hemorrhage

NCLEX CHECKS

It's never too soon to begin your NCLEX® preparation. Now that you've reviewed this chapter, carefully read each of the following questions and choose the best answer. Then compare your responses with the correct answers.

1. A client on a weight-reduction diet is diagnosed with iron deficiency anemia. What drug information should the nurse give this client?

- ☐ **1.** Iron products are absorbed through the liver and kidneys.
- ☐ **2.** Peak drug levels occur at the same time no matter which administration route is used.
- ☐ **3.** Iron deficiency anemia is correctable with an oral iron preparation.
- ☐ **4.** Normal hemoglobin levels and body iron stores are restored after 1 month of iron therapy.

2. Which agent would a nurse use to treat anemia related to renal disease?

- ☐ **1.** Cyanocobalamin (Nascobal)
- ☐ **2.** Epoetin alfa (Procrit)
- ☐ **3.** Ferrous sulfate (Feosal)
- ☐ **4.** Folic acid (Folvite)

3. A 21-year-old client takes hormonal contraceptives and is a heavy smoker. She develops a thrombus in her leg, is admitted to the hospital, and is started on heparin. Which action by the nurse is most important?

- ☐ **1.** Keeping the client on strict bed rest
- ☐ **2.** Limiting the client's smoking to one pack per day
- ☐ **3.** Giving the client aspirin for headaches and joint stiffness
- ☐ **4.** Having the client walk after 4 hours to prevent joint stiffness

4. A client receiving heparin is also ordered warfarin (Coumadin) therapy. Which rationale explains why these two drugs are given together?

- ☐ **1.** Heparin activates warfarin.
- ☐ **2.** Heparin hastens warfarin's onset of action.
- ☐ **3.** Warfarin and heparin have an antagonistic effect.
- ☐ **4.** Warfarin's therapeutic effects don't start until clotting factors are depleted.

Key nursing actions

- Assess for signs and symptoms of bleeding; tell patient to report bleeding immediately.
- Ensure that aminocaproic acid is readily available.
- Minimize venipunctures, injections, and other invasive procedures; apply pressure to puncture sites to prevent bleeding.
- Keep typed and crossmatched blood on hand to administer in case of hemorrhage.

TOP 6

Items to study for your next test on drugs and the hematologic system

1. Rationale for using hematopoietics, anticoagulants, thrombolytics, and antiplatelets
2. Mechanisms of action of hematopoietics, anticoagulants, thrombolytics, and antiplatelets
3. Laboratory tests used to monitor the patient who is receiving a hematopoietic, anticoagulant, thrombolytic, or antiplatelet drug
4. Common adverse effects of hematopoietics, anticoagulants, thrombolytics, and antiplatelet drugs
5. Nursing responsibilities when administering hematopoietics, anticoagulants, thrombolytics, and antiplatelet drugs
6. Appropriate teaching for the patient who is receiving a hematopoietic, anticoagulant, thrombolytic, or antiplatelet drug

5. A client who's allergic to salicylates is ordered an antiplatelet drug to help prevent stroke. What drug would the nurse expect to administer?
- ☐ **1.** Dipyridamole (Persantine)
- ☐ **2.** Folic acid (Folvite)
- ☐ **3.** Ticlopidine (Ticlid)
- ☐ **4.** Warfarin (Coumadin)

6. A client is admitted to the emergency department with an acute inferior wall MI. After receiving oxygen, I.V. nitroglycerin, and I.V. morphine, he still feels pain. The physician orders streptokinase (Streptase), 140,000 International Units by intracoronary infusion. Which condition contraindicates the use of streptokinase?
- ☐ **1.** Age 60 or older
- ☐ **2.** History of MI
- ☐ **3.** Acute pulmonary thromboembolism
- ☐ **4.** Stroke in the past 2 months

7. A client undergoing chemotherapy has been receiving filgrastim (Neupogen) subQ daily for 5 days. Which finding indicates filgrastim therapy is effective?
- ☐ **1.** Increased platelet count
- ☐ **2.** Decreased tumor cell level
- ☐ **3.** Decreased immunoglobulin level
- ☐ **4.** Increased WBC count

8. A nurse is instructing a client on foods that affect the absorption of ferrous sulfate (Feosol). Because the client likes to take the pills with breakfast, the nurse instructs the client to avoid taking the ferrous sulfate with:
- ☐ **1.** bacon.
- ☐ **2.** eggs.
- ☐ **3.** oatmeal.
- ☐ **4.** toast.

9. A nurse is teaching a client with pernicious anemia about vitamin B_{12} injections. Which statement by the client indicates teaching has been successful?
- ☐ **1.** "The injections must be done every 6 months."
- ☐ **2.** "The injections must be continued for the rest of my life."
- ☐ **3.** "The injections can be stopped when my symptoms go away."
- ☐ **4.** "I can switch to an oral form when a therapeutic blood level of vitamin B_{12} is achieved."

10. A nurse is caring for a client receiving heparin. Place the steps for monitoring the client's heparin therapy in the correct order. Use all the options.

| **1.** Obtain a follow-up PTT at a specified interval. |
| **2.** Obtain a baseline PTT. |
| **3.** Change the dosage as indicated by the physician. |
| **4.** Start heparin therapy as ordered. |
| **5.** Monitor for signs and symptoms of bleeding. |
| **6.** Contact the physician with PTT results. |

| |
| |
| |
| |
| |
| |

ANSWERS AND RATIONALES

1. CORRECT ANSWER: 3

Iron deficiency anemia, which is commonly caused by inadequate dietary intake of iron, is correctable with oral iron preparations. Iron products are absorbed primarily in the duodenum and upper jejunum. It usually takes 6 months of iron therapy to restore normal hemoglobin levels and create iron stores in the body. Peak levels differ according to the route of administration and absorption factors. For example, drug levels may peak in 4 weeks with oral administration and within 4 to 8 weeks with I.V. and I.M. administration.

2. CORRECT ANSWER: 2

Epoetin alfa imitates erythropoietin, which is necessary for the stimulation of RBC production. It may be used to correct normocytic anemia related to renal disease. Cyanocobalamin is used to treat pernicious anemia. Ferrous sulfate is used to prevent and treat iron deficiency anemia. Folic acid is used to treat megaloblastic anemia related to folic acid deficiency.

3. CORRECT ANSWER: 1

A client with a thrombus needs to be on strict bed rest to prevent dislodgment of the clot, which could migrate to the pulmonary system and cause a pulmonary embolus. Smoking constricts blood vessels and may contribute to clot formation, so it should be avoided entirely. Aspirin potentiates the effects of anticoagulants and should be avoided while the client is receiving heparin. The client shouldn't walk because bed rest is needed to prevent dislodgment of the clot.

4. CORRECT ANSWER: 4

Therapeutic anticoagulation with warfarin or other oral anticoagulants may not be achieved until 3 to 5 days after initiation of therapy, when clotting factors are depleted. Heparin administration provides continued anticoagulation during this transition to oral anticoagulation therapy. Heparin accelerates the interaction between thrombin and antithrombin III, but it doesn't activate or hasten the onset of the effects of warfarin. Heparin doesn't antagonize the effects of warfarin.

5. CORRECT ANSWER: 3

For clients with salicylate (aspirin) sensitivity, ticlopidine is typically used as a prophylactic against stroke. Dipyridamole's status as an antiplatelet drug is questionable because research has shown mixed results. Folic acid and warfarin aren't antiplatelet drugs.

6. CORRECT ANSWER: 4

Streptokinase is contraindicated when a client has had a stroke within the past 2 months, is undergoing intracranial or intraspinal surgery, or has active internal bleeding, intracranial neoplasm, severe uncontrolled hypertension, or drug hypersensitivity because bleeding is an adverse reaction of this drug. Acute pulmonary thromboembolism and a history of MI aren't contraindications to streptokinase therapy. Streptokinase should be used with caution in clients older than age 75. There's no age-related caution for clients age 75 and younger.

7. CORRECT ANSWER: 4

Chemotherapy typically decreases the number of neutrophils. Filgrastim accelerates the maturation and growth of neutrophils, thereby increasing WBC count. Filgrastim has no effect on platelet production, tumor cells, or immunoglobulin levels.

8. CORRECT ANSWER: 2

Because eggs, milk, coffee, and tea interfere with the absorption of iron, the nurse should advise the client to take the ferrous sulfate 2 hours after any breakfast that includes these foods—not with the meal. Bacon, toast, and oatmeal aren't known to change iron's absorption.

9. CORRECT ANSWER: 2

Vitamin B_{12} doesn't cure the underlying pathologic cause of pernicious anemia, so it must be taken for life. The usual interval for administration is every 3 to 4 weeks after initial treatment. Symptoms will return if the injections are stopped. It's unlikely that the oral form will be effective if the client lacks intrinsic factor.

10. CORRECT ANSWER:

2. Obtain a baseline PTT.

4. Start heparin therapy as ordered.

5. Monitor for signs and symptoms of bleeding.

1. Obtain a follow-up PTT at a specified interval

6. Contact the physician with PTT results.

3. Change the dosage as indicated by the physician.

When monitoring a client's heparin therapy, the nurse begins by obtaining a baseline PTT, then initiating the heparin therapy, as ordered. Once therapy is started, the nurse monitors for signs and symptoms of bleeding. The nurse obtains a follow-up PTT at a specified interval and informs the physician of the PTT result. Dosage changes are made based on the physician's orders.

Drugs and the endocrine system

11

PRETEST

1. Antidiuretic hormones work by:

- ☐ 1. enhancing water reabsorption in the kidneys.
- ☐ 2. accelerating heat production and oxygen consumption.
- ☐ 3. increasing glucose transport into cells.
- ☐ 4. simulating the action of endogenous growth hormones.

CORRECT ANSWER: 1

2. During the first few months of taking a thyroid hormone, a child may experience:

- ☐ 1. bradycardia.
- ☐ 2. lethargy.
- ☐ 3. hair loss.
- ☐ 4. weight gain.

CORRECT ANSWER: 3

3. Which insulin can be administered I.V. or subcutaneously?

- ☐ 1. Ultralente
- ☐ 2. NPH
- ☐ 3. Lantus
- ☐ 4. Regular

CORRECT ANSWER: 4

4. When teaching a client about insulin injections, the nurse should instruct him to inject the insulin:

- ☐ 1. in the same place each time.
- ☐ 2. in a different injection site each time.
- ☐ 3. in his arms only.
- ☐ 4. in his abdomen only.

CORRECT ANSWER: 2

5. When administering an antihypercalcemic drug, a nurse should monitor which laboratory value?

- ☐ 1. Sodium
- ☐ 2. Potassium
- ☐ 3. Phosphate
- ☐ 4. Chloride

CORRECT ANSWER: 3

LEARNING OBJECTIVES

After studying this chapter, you should be able to:

- Identify and describe the rationale for using different types of drugs to treat endocrine disorders.
- Describe the mechanism of action and major adverse effects of growth hormones, antidiuretic hormones, thyroid hormones, antithyroid drugs; parathyroid and antihypercalcemic drugs.
- Discuss the nursing responsibilities and patient teaching required for administration of endocrine system drugs.

CHAPTER OVERVIEW

Endocrine drugs include growth hormones, antidiuretic hormones, thyroid hormones, antithyroid drugs, parathyroid and antihypercalcemic drugs and antidiabetics such as insulin. Growth hormones replace hormones in states of deficiency. Antidiuretic hormones enhance reabsorption of water in kidneys and smooth-muscle contraction (vasoconstriction), thereby promoting an antidiuretic effect and regulating fluid balance. Thyroid hormones replace endogenous thyroid hormone in deficiency states, and antithyroid drugs treat hypersecretion and decrease the size and vascularity of the thyroid gland before surgery. Parathyroid and antihypercalcemic drugs regulate calcium imbalances, which usually result from underlying disorders. Antidiabetics are used to control hyperglycemia secondary to diabetes mellitus, stress responses, total parenteral nutrition, hyperkalemia, medications, and other disorders.

A&P highlights

- The endocrine system includes the pituitary gland, thyroid gland, parathyroid glands, adrenal glands, and the islets of Langerhans (in the pancreas).
- These endocrine glands release various hormones:
- Anterior pituitary gland secretes GH, TSH, ACTH, FSH, LH, and prolactin.
- Posterior pituitary gland secretes oxytocin and ADH.
- Thyroid gland secretes T_3, T_4, and thyrocalcitonin.
- Parathyroid glands secrete PTH.
- Adrenal cortex secretes glucocorticoids, mineralocorticoids, and sex hormones.
- Adrenal medulla secretes epinephrine and norepinephrine.
- Islets of Langerhans secrete glucagon, insulin, and somatostatin.

ANATOMY AND PHYSIOLOGY

- **Anatomy of the endocrine system**
  - Includes endocrine glands (ductless glands located throughout body) and other structures
  - Major glands
    - Pituitary gland (master gland)
      - Is located at the base of brain
      - Has two main lobes—anterior and posterior
    - Thyroid gland
      - Is one of largest endocrine glands
      - Is located in lower anterior portion of neck
    - Parathyroid glands
      - Are four pea-size glands (smallest of endocrine glands)
      - Are located on thyroid gland's posterior surface
    - Adrenal glands
      - Are located on top of each kidney
      - Consist of the adrenal cortex (bulk of the gland) and adrenal medulla (inner part), which function as separate endocrine glands
    - Islets of Langerhans
      - Are clusters of six different hormone-secreting cells
      - Millions are scattered throughout pancreas
    - Ovaries and testes (discussed in chapter 15)
  - Minor glands: pineal and thymus glands

- **Physiology**
  - Endocrine glands—release hormones (chemical substances that regulate activities of specific organs) directly into blood or lymph
  - Hormones—secreted into bloodstream and travel to target tissues, where they alter the metabolism of specific cells
  - Pituitary gland—receives chemical and nervous stimulation from hypothalamus
  - Hypothalamus

- Activates, controls, and integrates various endocrine functions
- Releases hormones stored in the anterior and posterior pituitary glands
- Controls hormone release with negative feedback mechanism, whereby further hormone output is suppressed when there's an elevated level of hormone or hormone-regulated substance in body
- Anterior pituitary gland—secretes growth hormone (GH), thyroid-stimulating hormone (TSH), adrenocorticotropic hormone (ACTH), follicle-stimulating hormone (FSH), luteinizing hormone (LH), and prolactin
- Posterior pituitary gland—secretes oxytocin and antidiuretic hormone (ADH)
- Thyroid gland
  - Secretes triiodothyronine (T_3) and thyroxine (T_4), which regulate metabolic rate
  - Secretes thyrocalcitonin, which helps control calcium metabolism
- Parathyroid glands—secrete parathyroid hormone (PTH), the principal regulator of calcium metabolism
- Adrenal cortex—secretes glucocorticoids, mineralocorticoids, and sex hormones
- Adrenal medulla—secretes epinephrine and norepinephrine
- Islets of Langerhans—contain alpha cells (secrete glucagon), beta cells (secrete insulin), and delta cells (secrete somatostatin)

● **Function**
- Controls body functions through glandular release of hormones
- Anterior pituitary hormones
  - GH: stimulates bone and muscle growth
  - TSH: stimulates thyroid gland to release thyroid hormone
  - ACTH: stimulates adrenal cortex to release glucocorticoid
  - FSH: stimulates ovarian follicle maturation and production in females and sperm production in males
  - LH: stimulates ovulation and ovarian production of progesterone and testicular production of male testosterone
  - Prolactin: stimulates milk production in breasts
- Posterior pituitary hormones
  - Oxytocin: stimulates contraction of pregnant uterus
  - ADH: causes cells of renal and collecting tubules to be more permeable to water, thus altering urine concentration
- Thyroid hormones
  - T_3 and T_4: control rate of metabolism, which is necessary for normal growth and development and for development and maturation of nervous system
  - Thyrocalcitonin: maintains blood calcium level by inhibiting calcium release from bone (thereby lowering blood calcium level)
- PTH
  - Helps regulate calcium metabolism by adjusting rate at which kidneys remove calcium and magnesium ions from urine

Functions of the anterior pituitary gland

- GH: stimulates bone and muscle growth
- TSH: causes the release of thyroid hormone
- ACTH: causes the release of glucocorticoid
- FSH: stimulates ovarian follicle production and sperm production
- LH: stimulates ovulation
- Prolactin: stimulates the breasts to produce milk

Functions of the posterior pituitary gland

- Oxytocin: stimulates uterine contraction
- ADH: causes cells to be more permeable to water

Functions of the thyroid gland

- T_3 and T_4: control the rate of metabolism
- Thyrocalcitonin: maintains blood calcium level

Functions of PTH in the parathyroid glands

- Helps regulate calcium metabolism
- Raises the blood calcium level

Functions of the adrenal cortex

- Glucocorticoids: raise the blood glucose level
- Mineralocorticoids: regulate electrolyte and water balance
- Sex hormones: responsible for the sex drive

Functions of norepinephrine and epinephrine in the adrenal medulla

- Cause physiologic effects in response to stress
- Increase heart rate, cardiac output
- Cause vasoconstriction
- Increase blood glucose level

Functions of the islets of Langerhans

- Glucagon: increases blood glucose level
- Insulin: controls carbohydrate metabolism and increases glucose use
- Somatostatin: inhibits insulin and glucagon secretion; suppresses growth hormone

Key facts about growth hormones

- Therapeutically equivalent to and simulate the action of endogenous growth hormones
- Stimulate linear growth and increase the number and size of muscle cells
- Decrease carbohydrate metabolism; increase protein metabolism
- Reduce body fat stores, increase lipid mobilization, and decrease mean cholesterol levels
- Metabolized by liver and kidneys
- Excreted in urine and feces

– Raises blood calcium level
- Adrenal cortex hormones
  - Glucocorticoids: raise the blood glucose level by decreasing glucose metabolism and promoting glucose formation from protein and fat (also known as *gluconeogenesis*)
  - Mineralocorticoids: regulate electrolyte and water balance by promoting sodium absorption and potassium excretion by the renal tubules
  - Sex hormones: are responsible for the sex drive in men and women
- Adrenal medulla hormones (norepinephrine and epinephrine)
  - Cause widespread physiologic effects in response to stress, also known as *fight-or-flight response*
  - Increase heart rate and cardiac output; cause vasoconstriction
  - Increase blood glucose level and nervous system response
- Islets of Langerhans hormones
  - Glucagon (secreted by alpha cells): increases blood glucose level in response to hypoglycemia
  - Insulin (secreted by beta cells in response to blood glucose elevation): controls carbohydrate metabolism and increases use of glucose as source of energy, thereby decreasing blood glucose levels
  - Somatostatin (secreted by delta cells): inhibits insulin and glucagon secretion and suppresses growth hormone, resulting in decreased blood glucose levels; also inhibits glucose absorption from GI tract

GROWTH HORMONES

- **Mechanism of action**
  - Therapeutically equivalent to and simulate action of endogenous growth hormones; interact with specific plasma membrane receptors to stimulate linear growth and increase number and size of muscle cells to stimulate skeletal growth
  - Decrease carbohydrate metabolism by decreasing insulin sensitivity in children with hypopituitarism
  - Increase protein metabolism by retaining nitrogen and increasing cellular protein synthesis
  - Reduce body fat stores, increase lipid mobilization, and increase plasma fatty acids to increase lipid metabolism and decrease mean cholesterol levels
  - Stimulate synthesis of chondroitin and collagen and urine excretion of hydroxyproline to cause connective tissue metabolism

- **Pharmacokinetics**
  - Absorption: I.M. or subcutaneously (subQ)
  - Distribution: Distributed to highly perfused organs, particularly liver and kidneys
  - Metabolism: Metabolized by liver and kidneys
  - Excretion: Excreted in urine and feces

● **Drug examples**
  - Somatrem, somatropin (Genotropin, Humatrope, Norditropin, Nutropin, Nutropin AQ, Nutropin Depot, Saizen, Serostim)

● **Indications**
  - Treat growth failure caused by lack of adequate endogenous growth hormones (all drugs except Serostim)
  - Treat growth failure in children with chronic renal failure (Nutropin and Nutropin AQ)
  - Treat cachexia or wasting caused by acquired immunodeficiency syndrome (Serostim)
  - Long-term treatment of short stature associated with Turner's syndrome (Humatrope, Nutropin, and Nutropin AQ)
  - Treat somatropin deficiency syndrome (Humatrope)
  - Treat growth failure in patients with Prader-Willi syndrome and those born small for gestational age who don't achieve catch-up growth by age 2 (Genotropin)

● **Contraindications and precautions**
  - Contraindicated in patients with closed epiphyses or evidence of intracranial tumors or active neoplasia
  - Some drugs contain benzyl alcohol, which is contraindicated in neonates and patients hypersensitive to it
  - Humatrope contraindicated in patients allergic to glycerin
  - Used cautiously in breast-feeding patients and those with diabetes or glucose tolerance

● **Adverse reactions**
  - Malignant transformation of skin lesions, clipped capital femoral epiphysis or avascular necrosis of femoral head, gynecomastia, and intracranial hypertension (accompanied by vision changes, headache, nausea, or vomiting)
  - Possible leukemia in children
  - Swelling, musculoskeletal discomfort, and carpal tunnel syndrome (Serostim)
  - Pain at injection site, mild and transient edema, glucose intolerance, headache, weakness, localized muscle pain, and antibodies to growth hormones
  - Mild and transient peripheral edema, increased growth of preexisting nevi, and pancreatitis (Nutropin AQ)

● **Interactions**
  - Use with androgens, estrogens, or thyroid hormones may cause epiphyseal closure
  - Use with glucocorticoids diminishes growth rate

● **Nursing responsibilities**
  - Monitor serum and urine glucose levels regularly to prevent glucose intolerance
  - Monitor thyroid function tests regularly

When to use growth hormones

- Growth failure; short stature
- Cachexia or wasting
- Somatropin deficiency syndrome

When NOT to use growth hormones

- Closed epiphyses, intracranial tumors, or active neoplasia
- Drug allergies
- Neonates

Adverse reactions

- Malignant transformation of skin lesions, clipped capital femoral epiphysis or avascular necrosis of femoral head, gynecomastia, intracranial hypertension, leukemia, swelling, musculoskeletal discomfort, carpal tunnel syndrome, pain at injection site, mild and transient edema, glucose intolerance, headache, weakness, localized muscle pain, antibodies to growth hormones, increased growth of preexisting nevi, pancreatitis

- Know that injection of growth hormones may cause pain and swelling; rotate injection sites to decrease these effects
- Teach the patient self-injection techniques if appropriate
- Stress importance of regular blood and urine glucose monitoring to detect adverse effects
- Recommend annual bone age determinations for children receiving growth hormone
- Monitor for intracranial hypertension by performing periodic funduscopic examinations

ANTIDIURETIC HORMONES

Mechanism of action

- Enhance reabsorption of water in kidneys and smooth-muscle contraction (vasoconstriction), thereby promoting an antidiuretic effect and regulating fluid balance
- Promotes vasoconstriction and decreases hepatic blood flow (vasopressin)

Pharmacokinetics

- Absorption
  - Intranasal desmopressin: Absorbed in nasal mucosa
  - Oral desmopressin: Absorbed minimally in GI tract; bioavailability is 5% compared with that of intranasal administration and 0.16% compared with that of I.V. administration
  - Vasopressin: Unknown
- Distribution
  - Desmopressin: Unknown but appears in breast milk
  - Vasopressin: Widely distributed
- Metabolism
  - Desmopressin: Unknown
  - Vasopressin: Metabolized in liver and kidneys
- Excretion
  - Desmopressin: Unknown
  - Vasopressin: Excreted unchanged in urine

Drug examples

- Desmopressin (DDAVP, Stimate), vasopressin (Pitressin)

Indications

- Treat diabetes insipidus
- Treat nocturnal enuresis (nighttime bedwetting) (desmopressin)
- Control bleeding in hemophilia A and mild to moderate von Willebrand's disease (type I) with factor VIII levels greater than 5% (desmopressin)
- Prevent and treat postoperative abdominal distention and dispel interfering gas shadows in abdominal roentgenography (vasopressin)

Contraindications and precautions

- Desmopressin contraindicated in patients with type IIB or pseudo (platelet-type) von Willebrand's disease

- Vasopressin contraindicated in patients with anaphylaxis or hypersensitivity to drug or its components and those with chronic nephritis with nitrogen retention
- Vasopressin used with extreme caution in pregnant or breast-feeding patients and those with vascular disease (especially coronary artery disease), epilepsy, migraines, asthma, heart failure, or states in which a rapid increase in extracellular water may result in further compromise

● **Adverse reactions**
- Water intoxication, hyponatremia, abdominal cramps, nausea, nasal congestion or changes (with nasal administration), facial flushing, hypertension, chest pain, headache, epistaxis, sore throat, cough, and injection site redness, swelling, or burning

● **Interactions**
- Use with alcohol, demeclocycline, epinephrine, heparin, or lithium reduces antidiuretic hormone activity
- Use with carbamazepine, chlorpropamide, fludrocortisone, tricyclic antidepressants, or urea increases antidiuretic hormone activity

● **Nursing responsibilities**
- Monitor fluid intake and output and urine osmolality frequently
- Teach the patient how to use intranasal drug form if prescribed
- Instruct the patient to consult the practitioner if rhinitis or nasal congestion occurs; may decrease effects of intranasal therapy
- Caution the patient to abstain from alcohol to prevent adverse drug interactions and dehydration
- Teach the patient to self-administer and alternate injection sites to prevent tissue damage if appropriate
- Warn the patient, especially if the patient is a child or elderly person, to ingest only enough fluid to satisfy thirst to decrease the risk of water intoxication and hyponatremia
- Teach that early signs of water intoxication include drowsiness and listlessness and that headaches precede coma and seizures
- Know that desmopressin has greater antidiuretic response than vasopressin; response time following I.V. administration is about 10 times greater than that following intranasal administration

THYROID HORMONES

● **Mechanism of action**
- Control metabolic rate of tissues and accelerate heat production and oxygen consumption
- Produce T_3 activity and replace hormonal deficits or suppress excessive hormone production (synthetic thyroid hormones)

● **Pharmacokinetics**
- Absorption: Absorbed from GI tract; fasting increases absorption
- Distribution: More than 99% protein-bound

Adverse reactions
- Water intoxication, hyponatremia, abdominal cramps, nausea, nasal congestion, facial flushing, hypertension, chest pain, headache, epistaxis, sore throat, cough, injection site redness, swelling, or burning

Key nursing actions
- Monitor fluid intake and output and urine osmolality frequently.
- Warn patients to ingest only enough fluid to satisfy thirst to decrease risk or water intoxication and hyponatremia.

Key facts about thyroid hormones
- Control metabolic rate of tissues
- Accelerate heat production and oxygen consumption
- Result in T_3 activity
- Used to replace hormonal deficits or suppress excessive hormone production
- Metabolized in liver
- Excreted in feces

When to use thyroid hormones

- Primary or secondary hypothy-roidism
- Goiters
- Thyrotoxicosis

When NOT to use thyroid hormones

- Acute MI or thyrotoxicosis
- Coexistence of hypothyroidism and hypoadrenalism, unless treatment of hypoadrenalism with adrenocortical steroids precedes initiation of thyroid therapy

Adverse reactions

- Hyperthyroidism, tachycardia, arrhythmias, palpitations, ner-vousness, sweating, heat intol-erance, insomnia, weight loss, headache, decreased bone den-sity, partial hair loss

- Metabolism: Metabolized in liver
- Excretion: Excreted in feces

● **Drug examples**
- Levothyroxine (T_4 [Levothroid, Levoxine, Levoxyl, Synthroid, Thyro-Tabs, Unithroid]), liothyronine (T_3 [Cytomel], Triostat), liotrix (Thyrolar)

● **Indications**
- Thyroid hormone replacement in primary or secondary hypothyroidism (including cretinism, myxedema, and nontoxic goiter) and hypothyroidism caused by functional deficiency, primary atrophy, partial or total absence of thyroid gland, or effects of surgery, radiation, or drugs
- Treat or prevent goiters by suppressing secretion of TSH from pituitary gland
- Adjunct to antithyroid drugs to treat thyrotoxicosis, prevent goitrogenesis and hypothyroidism, and prevent thyrotoxicosis during pregnancy

● **Contraindications and precautions**
- Contraindicated in patients with acute myocardial infarction (MI) or thy-rotoxicosis uncomplicated by hypothyroidism; if hypothyroidism is a com-plication, thyroid hormones may be used judiciously
- Contraindicated when hypothyroidism and hypoadrenalism (Addison's disease) coexist, unless treatment of hypoadrenalism with adrenocortical steroids precedes initiation of thyroid therapy
- Used cautiously in patients with heart disease, hypertension, diabetes mellitus or insipidus, myxedema, or adrenal insufficiency
- Not intended for use as primary or adjunctive therapy in weight control programs

● **Adverse reactions**
- Signs and symptoms of hyperthyroidism or aggravated existing hyperthy-roidism (after prolonged or excessive use)
- Signs of overdose (tachycardia, arrhythmias, palpitations, nervousness, hypertension, angina, diarrhea, tremors, sweating, heat intolerance, in-somnia, weight loss, and headache)
- Possible decreased bone density with long-term use in women
- Possible partial hair loss in children in first few months of therapy (usually temporary)

● **Interactions**
- Thyroid hormones increase effects of oral anticoagulants
- Colestipol and cholestyramine decrease effects of thyroid hormones and may cause hypothyroidism
- Thyroid hormones may decrease serum digoxin levels
- Thyroid hormones may increase theophylline levels
- Antacids containing aluminum, sucralfate, cholestyramine, iron products, and insulin may decrease amount of levothyroxine available in body

● **Nursing responsibilities**
- Administer drug in morning to prevent insomnia

- Teach the patient to take drug 1 hour before meals or 2 hours after meals to improve drug absorption
- Give drugs at least 4 hours apart because colestipol and cholestyramine decrease effects of thyroid hormones
- Monitor pulse rate, and evaluate results of thyroid function studies
- Caution the patient not to change medication brands; potency differs among brands
- Teach the patient importance of complying with therapy
- Instruct the patient to notify the practitioner if headache, nervousness, diarrhea, excessive sweating, heat intolerance, chest pain, increased pulse rate, and palpitations (symptoms of hyperthyroidism) or other unusual events occur

ANTITHYROID DRUGS

- ### Mechanism of action
  - Iodine: Circulates into thyroid gland as iodide, which when oxidized helps yield thyroid hormones; large doses of iodide can inhibit T_3 and T_4 synthesis
  - Propylthiouracil (PTU) and methimazole: Inhibit synthesis of thyroid hormones; PTU partially inhibits conversion of T_4 to T_3
  - Sodium iodide I 131 (^{131}I): Limits thyroid hormone secretion by destroying thyroid tissue

- ### Pharmacokinetics
  - Absorption: Absorbed in GI tract
  - Distribution: Varies by drug
  - Metabolism: Unknown
  - Excretion: Excreted in urine

- ### Drug examples
  - Iodine (Strong Iodine Solution, USP [Lugol's solution], Thyro-Block), methimazole (Tapazole), PTU, sodium iodide ^{131}I (Iodotope, Sodium iodide ^{131}I Therapeutic)

- ### Indications
  - Treat hyperthyroidism (Graves' disease)
  - Treat hyperthyroidism when thyroidectomy is contraindicated or inadvisable (PTU)
  - Adjunctive therapy to treat hyperthyroidism and reduce thyroid friability before surgery and to treat thyrotoxic crisis or neonatal thyrotoxicosis (iodine)
  - Thyroid blocking during radiation emergency (iodine)
  - Palliative treatment in selected cases of thyroid carcinoma (sodium iodine ^{131}I)

Topics for patient discussion

- Therapy regimen
- Signs and symptoms
- Dietary restrictions

When NOT to use antithyroid drugs

- Pregnancy and breast-feeding
- Hypersensitivity to iodides

Adverse reactions

- Hypothyroidism, diarrhea, hypersensitivity, iodism, nausea, vomiting, agranulocytosis, rash, bone marrow depression, acute leukemia, anemia, radiation sickness, chest pains, tachycardia, itching, neck tenderness or swelling, sore throat, cough, and temporary thinning of the hair

Key nursing actions

- Administer drug at a consistent time 1 hour before or 2 hours after meals.
- Assess for signs and symptoms of overdose or underdose.

TIME-OUT FOR TEACHING

Teaching about thyroid hormones

Include these topics in your teaching plan for the patient receiving a thyroid hormone:

- medication regimen, including the drug's name, dosage, frequency, duration, and possible adverse effects
- signs and symptoms to discuss with the practitioner, including those relating to adverse effects and thyroid hormone deficiency or excess (including toxicity)
- consistency regarding time of administration and brand used
- possible dietary restrictions, such as foods containing iodine
- avoidance of other products containing iodine
- compliance with therapy, including taking the drug as prescribed
- follow-up care, including laboratory tests and practitioner visits.

Contraindications and precautions

- Iodine contraindicated in pregnant patients and those hypersensitive to iodides
- Methimazole contraindicated in pregnant and breast-feeding patients
- Sodium iodide ^{131}I contraindicated in patients who are pregnant, breast-feeding, or contemplating pregnancy; patients younger than age 30; and those with preexisting vomiting and diarrhea
- PTU and methimazole used cautiously in breast-feeding patients

Adverse reactions

- Hypothyroidism, diarrhea, hypersensitivity, and iodism (vomiting, abdominal pain, metallic taste, rash, and sore salivary glands) (iodine)
- Nausea, vomiting, agranulocytosis, and rash (methimazole and PTU)
- Bone marrow depression, acute leukemia, anemia, radiation sickness, chest pains, tachycardia, itching, neck tenderness or swelling, sore throat, cough, and temporary hair thinning (sodium iodide ^{131}I)

Interactions

- Iodine used with lithium may cause hypothyroidism

Nursing responsibilities

- Give drug at regular intervals (usually every 8 hours, unless directed otherwise by the practitioner) and at a consistent time (1 hour before or 2 hours after meals) because food may affect drug absorption
- Dilute strong iodine solution with water or fruit juice to improve taste
- Monitor serum thyroid levels and thyroid function test results
- Assess for signs and symptoms of overdose (hypothyroidism) or underdose (thyrotoxicosis)
- Advise the patient to consult the practitioner before eating iodized salt and iodine-rich foods (see *Teaching about thyroid hormones*)
- Instruct the patient to avoid aspirin and drugs containing iodine

- Explain importance of complying with therapy and undergoing routine follow-up evaluation

PARATHYROID AND ANTIHYPERCALCEMIC DRUGS

● **Mechanism of action**
- Parathyroid drugs: Increase serum calcium level, causing a corresponding decrease in the serum phosphate level
- Antihypercalcemic drugs: Reduce serum calcium level by reducing bone resorption, increasing GI absorption of calcium, and interfering with renal calcium clearance

● **Pharmacokinetics**
- Absorption
  - Parathyroid drugs: Readily absorbed in GI tract after oral administration
  - Antihypercalcemic drugs: Rapid absorption by bone; food reduces bioavailability of drug
- Distribution
  - Parathyroid drugs: Widely distributed; protein-bound
  - Antihypercalcemic drugs: Varies
- Metabolism
  - Parathyroid drugs: Metabolized in liver and kidneys
  - Antihypercalcemic drugs: Not metabolized
- Excretion
  - Parathyroid drugs: Excreted primarily in feces
  - Antihypercalcemic drugs: Excreted in urine

● **Drug examples**
- Parathyroid drugs: calcitriol (Calcijex, Rocaltrol), calcium carbonate (Os-Cal), calcium citrate, calcium chloride, calcium gluconate, calcium lactate
- Antihypercalcemic drugs: alendronate (Fosamax), calcitonin (salmon [Calcimar]), etidronate (Didronel), gallium (Ganite), ibandronate (Boniva), pamidronate (Aredia), risedronate (Actonel), teriparatide (Forteo), tiludronate (Skelid), zoledronic (Zometa)

● **Indications**
- Treat hypocalcemia, hypoparathyroidism, and pseudohypoparathyroidism (parathyroid drugs)
- Prevent and treat osteoporosis (parathyroid drugs)
- Treat hypercalcemia, Paget's disease, osteoporosis, heterotopic ossification following total hip replacement or spinal cord injury, hypercalcemia of malignancy, metastasis of breast cancer, and osteolytic lesions of multiple myeloma (antihypercalcemic drugs)

Key facts about parathyroid and antihypercalcemic drugs

- Parathyroid drugs: increase serum calcium level; metabolized in liver and kidneys; excreted in feces
- Antihypercalcemic drugs: reduce serum calcium level; not metabolized; excreted in urine

When to use parathyroid and antihypercalcemic drugs

- Parathyroid drugs: hypocalcemia, hypoparathyroidism, pseudohypoparathyroidism, osteoporosis
- Antihypercalcemic drugs: hypercalcemia, Paget's disease, osteoporosis, heterotopic ossification following total hip replacement or spinal cord injury, hypercalcemia of malignancy, metastases of breast cancer, osteolytic lesions of multiple myeloma

● Contraindications and precautions

- Parathyroid drugs contraindicated in patients with hypercalcemia or vitamin D toxicity
- Antihypercalcemic drugs contraindicated in patients with hypersensitivity to bisphosphonates or other drug components, hypocalcemia, abnormalities of the esophagus that delay gastric emptying, inability to stand or sit upright for at least 30 minutes, clinically overt osteomalacia, or severe renal impairment
- Parathyroid drugs used cautiously in patients with renal failure
- Antihypercalcemic drugs used cautiously in pregnant or breast-feeding patients (except zoledronic, which is contraindicated) and those with asthma or upper GI problems

● Adverse reactions

- Parathyroid drugs: Hypercalcemia (nausea, vomiting, anorexia, polyuria, polydipsia, constipation, arrhythmias, calculi, and lethargy)
- Antihypercalcemic drugs: Hypocalcemia (nausea, vomiting, facial flushing, tetany, positive Trousseau's sign, and positive Chvostek's sign)

● Interactions

- Use with magnesium-containing antacids may cause hypermagnesemia
- Use of calcium salts with cardiac glycosides increases the risk of digoxin toxicity
- Oral calcium salts reduce absorption of tetracyclines
- Aminoglycosides may potentiate antihypercalcemic effects

● Nursing responsibilities

- Instruct the patient to take antihypercalcemic drugs on an empty stomach with 6 to 8 ounces of water either 2 hours before or after meals or 30 minutes before first food of day
- Monitor serum electrolyte levels to prevent imbalances
- Assess for hypocalcemia and hypercalcemia
- Instruct the patient receiving an oral antihypercalcemic drug to avoid excessive consumption of spinach, whole grains, and rhubarb and to maintain adequate intake of calcium and vitamin D

ANTIDIABETICS

INSULIN

● Mechanism of action

- Reduces serum glucose level by increasing glucose transport into cells and promoting glucose conversion to glycogen

● Pharmacokinetics

- Absorption: Administered parenterally; destroyed in GI tract
- Distribution: Widely distributed throughout body
- Metabolism: Metabolized in liver and kidneys
- Excretion: Excreted in urine and feces

Comparing types of insulin

This chart compares rapid-acting, intermediate-acting, and long-acting insulins. Onset of action, peak concentration levels, and duration of action are based on subcutaneous administration. Only regular insulin can be administered intravenously.

	GENERIC NAME	TRADE NAME	ONSET (HOURS)	PEAK (HOURS)	DURATION (HOURS)
Rapid-acting	Insulin injection (regular)	Humulin R Novolin R Regular Iletin II Velosulin BR	½ to 1	Unknown	8 to 12
	Lispro insulin solution	Humalog	¼	½ to 1½	6 to 8
	Insulin aspart solution	NovoLog	¼	1 to 3	3 to 5
Intermediate-acting	Isophane insulin suspension (NPH)	Novolin N Humulin N NPH Iletin II	1 to 1½	4 to 12	24
	Insulin zinc suspension (lente)	Humulin L Lente Iletin II	1 to 2½	7 to 15	24
Long-acting	Insulin glargine solution	Lantus	1.1	5	24
	Extended insulin zinc suspension (Ultralente)		4 to 8	10 to 30	36

Duration of insulin

- Insulin injection: 8 to 12 hours
- Lispro insulin solution: 6 to 8 hours
- Insulin aspart solution: 3 to 5 hours
- Isophane insulin suspension: 24 hours
- Insulin zinc suspension: 24 hours
- Insulin glargine solution: 24 hours
- Extended insulin zinc suspension: 36 hours

Drug examples

- Rapid-acting insulins: insulin aspart (NovoLog), insulin lispro (Humalog), regular insulin (Humulin R, Novolin R, Regular Iletin II, Velosulin BR)
- Intermediate-acting insulins: isophane insulin suspension (NPH [Humulin N, Novolin N, NPH Iletin II]), insulin zinc suspension (lente [Humulin L, Lente Iletin II])
- Long-acting insulins: extended insulin zinc suspension (Ultralente), insulin glargine (Lantus) (see *Comparing types of insulin*)
- Mixed insulins: 30% regular insulin and 70% NPH insulin (Humulin 70/30, Novolin 70/30), 50% lispro protamine and 50% insulin lispro (Humalog Mix 50/50, Humalog Mix 75/25), 50% regular insulin and 50% NPH insulin (Humulin 50/50)

When to use insulin

- Type 1 and type 2 diabetes mellitus

When NOT to use insulin

- Hypersensitivity

Adverse reactions

- Hypoglycemia, rebound hyperglycemia, lipodystrophy, skin reactions at injection site

Key nursing actions

- Know that only regular insulin can be administered I.V., if needed in an emergency.
- When administering mixed insulin, draw regular insulin into the syringe first to avoid contaminating the clear regular insulin vial with the cloudy, longer-acting insulin mixture.
- Don't shake the insulin vial; instead, roll it between hands.
- Schedule snacks to coincide with insulin's peak action.

● **Indications**
- Treat type 1 (insulin-dependent) and type 2 (non-insulin-dependent) diabetes mellitus that's unresponsive to dietary measures and oral hypoglycemics
- Treat diabetic ketoacidosis and hyperosmolar hyperglycemic nonketotic syndrome
- Treat hyperkalemia by forcing potassium ions to shift from bloodstream into cells (regular insulin)

● **Contraindications and precautions**
- Contraindicated in patients with known hypersensitivity to pork products

● **Adverse reactions**
- Hypoglycemia, rebound hyperglycemia (Somogyi effect), lipodystrophy, skin reactions at injection site (warmth, stinging, swelling), and insulin resistance

● **Interactions**
- Use with beta-adrenergic blockers may mask signs and symptoms of hypoglycemia
- Use with corticosteroids, sympathomimetics, or thiazide diuretics may cause hyperglycemia, necessitating increased insulin dosage
- Alcohol, anabolic steroids, monoamine oxidase (MAO) inhibitors, salicylates, or sulfonamides may cause hypoglycemia, possibly requiring decreased insulin dosage

● **Nursing responsibilities**
- Know that only regular insulin can be administered I.V., if needed in an emergency
- Draw regular insulin into syringe first when administering mixed insulin to avoid contaminating the clear regular insulin vial with the cloudy, longer-acting insulin mixture
- Don't shake the insulin vial; instead, roll it between hands
- Teach the patient how to inject insulin, rotate injection sites, and dispose of used syringes
- Be aware that some patients may be allergic to certain types of insulin
- Schedule snacks to coincide with insulin's peak action, when hypoglycemia is most likely to occur; know that the patient receiving more than one type of insulin may be at risk for hypoglycemia several times daily
- Monitor blood glucose levels
- Assess for and teach patient to recognize signs and symptoms of hypoglycemia or hyperglycemia and what to do if they occur
- Monitor the glycosylated hemoglobin level periodically because it reflects degree of glycemic control for previous 2 to 3 months
- Be aware that stress, fever, trauma, infection, and surgery may increase insulin requirements

- Know that I.V. glucose or glucagon may be necessary in severe hypoglycemia
- Inform the patient that antidiabetics control but don't cure diabetes; emphasize the need for lifelong therapy
- Teach the patient to follow recommended diabetic diet and to use the exchange system when planning meals
- Emphasize importance of regular exercise, daily foot inspection, sick-day rules, and alcohol restriction
- Instruct the patient to contact the practitioner if he can't eat, such as from illness; inadequate intake increases the risk of hypoglycemia
- Instruct the patient to carry sugar or a glucose-raising substance (hard candy, glucose tablets) and identification describing the disease and drug regimen in case of a hypoglycemic reaction
- Refrigerate insulin

ORAL HYPOGLYCEMICS

● **Mechanism of action**
- Stimulate the pancreas to produce more insulin and increase the sensitivity of peripheral receptors to insulin, ultimately decreasing the serum glucose level

● **Pharmacokinetics**
- Absorption: Well absorbed in GI tract
- Distribution: Widely distributed
- Metabolism: Metabolized in liver
- Excretion: Excreted in urine

● **Drug examples**
- Alpha-glucoside inhibitors: acarbose (Precose), miglitol (Glyset)
- Biguanides: metformin (Glucophage, Glucophage XR, Glumetza)
- Combination: glyburide and metformin (Glucovance), rosiglitazone maleate and metformin (Avandamet), glipizide and metformin (Metaglip)
- Meglitinides: repaglinide (Prandin), nateglinide (Starlix)
- Sulfonylureas: acetohexamide (Dymelor), chlorpropamide (Diabinese), glimepiride (Amaryl), glipizide (Glucotrol, Glucotrol XL), glyburide (Dia-Beta, Micronase), tolazamide, tolbutamide (Orinase)
- Thiazolidinediones: rosiglitazone maleate (Avandia), pioglitazone hydrochloride (Actos)

● **Indications**
- Treat type 2 diabetes mellitus unresponsive to dietary measures and exercise

● **Contraindications and precautions**
- Sulfonylureas contraindicated in patients allergic to sulfa drugs
- Thiazolidinediones contraindicated in patients with liver cirrhosis or heart failure; used cautiously in patients with liver impairment or edema

---

Key facts about oral hypoglycemics

- Stimulate the pancreas to produce more insulin and decrease the serum glucose level
- Metabolized in liver
- Excreted in urine

When to use oral hypoglycemics

- Type 2 diabetes mellitus unresponsive to dietary measures and exercise

When NOT to use oral hypoglycemics

- Cirrhosis
- Allergies to sulfa drugs
- Heart failure

Topics for patient discussion

- Therapy regimen
- Signs and symptoms
- Blood glucose monitoring

TIME-OUT FOR TEACHING

Teaching about sulfonylureas

Include these topics in your teaching plan for the patient receiving a sulfonylurea:

- medication regimen, including the drug's name, dosage, frequency, duration, and possible adverse effects
- signs and symptoms to discuss with the practitioner, including hypo-

glycemia and hyperglycemia, and measures to correct them

- blood glucose monitoring
- avoidance of alcohol
- medical alert identification
- measures to deal with sun exposure
- follow-up care, including laboratory tests and practitioner visits.

- Used cautiously in pregnant and breast-feeding patients

● **Adverse reactions**

- Hypoglycemia, nausea, vomiting, heartburn, dizziness, drowsiness, headache, photosensitivity reactions (sulfonylureas), lactic acidosis (metformin), flatulence and diarrhea (alpha-glucoside inhibitors), upper respiratory tract infections (meglitinides), edema, and heart failure

● **Interactions**

- Concurrent use with beta-adrenergic blockers may mask signs and symptoms of hypoglycemia
- Anabolic steroids, alcohol, anticoagulants, chloramphenicol, fluconazole, cimetidine, gemfibrozil, MAO inhibitors, salicylates, and sulfonamides may cause hypoglycemia (necessitating reduced insulin dosage) and may increase hypoglycemic effects of oral hypoglycemics
- Hyperglycemia may occur with use of corticosteroids, rifampin, and thiazide diuretics

● **Nursing responsibilities**

- Instruct the patient to take alpha-glucoside inhibitors with first bite of food and to take meglitinides within 30 minutes of each meal
- Instruct the patient to contact the practitioner if he can't eat; inadequate intake increases the risk of hypoglycemia
- Instruct the patient taking a sulfonylurea to use sunscreen and protective clothing to prevent photosensitivity reactions (see *Teaching about sulfonylureas*)
- Assess for signs and symptoms of hypoglycemia or hyperglycemia
- Advise the patient to consult the practitioner before adjusting the dosage of an oral hypoglycemic
- Teach the patient how to recognize signs and symptoms of hypoglycemia and hyperglycemia
- Provide information about recommended dietary measures, exercise, foot care, and sick-day rules

Adverse reactions

- Hypoglycemia, nausea, vomiting, heartburn, dizziness, drowsiness, headache, photosensitivity reactions, lactic acidosis, flatulence and diarrhea, upper respiratory tract infections, edema, and heart failure

Key nursing actions

- Instruct patient to take alpha-glucoside inhibitors with the first bite of food and to take meglitinides within 30 minutes of each meal.
- Assess the patient for signs and symptoms of hypoglycemia or hyperglycemia.
- Provide information about recommended dietary measures, exercise, foot care, and sick-day rules.

- Teach the patient to follow recommended diabetic diet and to use the exchange system when planning meals
- Emphasize the importance of regular exercise, daily foot inspection, sick day rules, and alcohol restriction
- Know that stress, fever, trauma, infection, and surgery may increase insulin requirements or necessitate switching from an oral hypoglycemic to insulin
- Inform the patient that antidiabetics control but don't cure diabetes; emphasize the need for lifelong therapy
- Instruct the patient to carry sugar and identification describing the disease and drug regimen in case of hypoglycemic reaction

NCLEX CHECKS

It's never too soon to begin your NCLEX® preparation. Now that you've reviewed this chapter, carefully read each of the following questions and choose the best answer. Then compare your responses with the correct answers.

1. A client diagnosed with hypothyroidism is ordered levothyroxine (Synthroid). Which laboratory test must be closely monitored to evaluate the effectiveness of drug therapy?

- ☐ **1.** CD4+
- ☐ **2.** Glycosylated hemoglobin (Hb A_{1c})
- ☐ **3.** Prothrombin time
- ☐ **4.** T_4

2. A nurse is treating a child with primary nocturnal enuresis. Which pituitary agent is indicated for children with this disorder?

- ☐ **1.** Corticotropin
- ☐ **2.** Cosyntropin (Cortrosyn)
- ☐ **3.** Desmopressin (DDAVP)
- ☐ **4.** Somatropin (Humatrope)

3. A client diagnosed with hypoparathyroidism is ordered the vitamin D analogue calcitriol, 0.25 mcg by mouth daily. The nurse explains to the client that calcitriol increases the plasma level of calcium by:

- ☐ **1.** reducing bone resorption.
- ☐ **2.** decreasing osteoclastic activity.
- ☐ **3.** increasing GI absorption and bone resorption of calcium.
- ☐ **4.** stimulating the parathyroid gland to secrete parathyroid hormone.

4. Which type of insulin and route of administration should a nurse use in a medical emergency?

- ☐ **1.** NPH insulin I.M.
- ☐ **2.** NPH insulin subQ
- ☐ **3.** Regular insulin I.V.
- ☐ **4.** Regular insulin subQ

TOP 6

Items to study for your next test on drugs and the endocrine system

1. The mechanisms of action for pituitary, thyroid, and parathyroid drugs; insulin; and oral hypoglycemics

2. The rationale for using pituitary, thyroid, and parathyroid drugs; insulin; and oral hypoglycemics

3. Major adverse effects of pituitary, thyroid, and parathyroid drugs

4. Nursing responsibilities when administering pituitary, thyroid, and parathyroid drugs; insulin; and oral hypoglycemics

5. Patient teaching related to insulin and oral hypoglycemics

6. Purpose, mechanism of action, adverse reactions, and nursing considerations of antihypercalcemic drugs

5. A physician orders glipizide (Glucotrol) for a client with type 2 diabetes mellitus. The nurse appropriately instructs the client to take the drug:

- ☐ **1.** with meals.
- ☐ **2.** after meals.
- ☐ **3.** 30 minutes before bedtime.
- ☐ **4.** 30 minutes before breakfast.

6. A client in the endocrinology clinic has newly diagnosed Graves' disease. She reports tremors, diarrhea, heat intolerance, and palpitations. Which drug should the nurse plan to administer?

- ☐ **1.** Levothyroxine (Synthroid)
- ☐ **2.** Liothyronine (Cytomel)
- ☐ **3.** Propylthiouracil
- ☐ **4.** Thiothixene (Navane)

7. A client who was diagnosed with type 2 diabetes 5 years ago has controlled his blood glucose with diet and chlorpropamide (Diabinese). After a recent illness, his physician changed his drug to glyburide (DiaBeta). When teaching this client, the nurse should emphasize that glyburide:

- ☐ **1.** works in a similar way to chlorpropamide.
- ☐ **2.** is less potent than chlorpropamide, so he needs to take a larger dose.
- ☐ **3.** is more potent than chlorpropamide and can be taken every other day.
- ☐ **4.** stimulates insulin production, so he needs to eat soon after taking the drug.

8. A nurse is caring for a client who has received 40 units of NPH insulin and 10 units of regular insulin at 0800. The nurse suspects the client is experiencing a hypoglycemic reaction based on which response?

- ☐ **1.** Complaints of thirst
- ☐ **2.** Hot, dry skin
- ☐ **3.** Nervousness and agitation
- ☐ **4.** Dilute, pale urine

9. A client has an order for insulin glargine (Lantus) to be administered at 2200, but he requires sliding-scale coverage of regular insulin for his elevated blood glucose level now. The nurse should plan to:

- ☐ **1.** administer the regular insulin and withhold the Lantus insulin.
- ☐ **2.** administer the regular insulin and the Lantus insulin in separate syringes.
- ☐ **3.** combine the regular insulin and the Lantus insulin in one syringe and give one injection.
- ☐ **4.** administer the Lantus insulin, as ordered, and recheck the client's blood glucose level in 2 hours before administering the regular insulin.

10. An insulin-dependent client with diabetes has a blood glucose level of 279 mg/dl at 1630. Based on the following sliding scale coverage ordered by the physician, how much insulin should the nurse administer?

BLOOD GLUCOSE LEVEL	0700, 1200, AND 1630 INSULIN DOSE	2100 INSULIN DOSE
< 60 mg/dl	1 amp $D_{50}W$ and call physician	1 amp $D_{50}W$ and call physician
60 to 150 mg/ dl	3 units regular	2 units regular
151 to 200 mg/dl	5 units regular	4 units regular
201 to 250 mg/dl	8 units regular	6 units regular
251 to 300 mg/dl	10 units regular	8 units regular
301 to 350 mg/dl	14 units regular	10 units regular
351 to 400 mg/dl	16 units regular	12 units regular
> 400 mg/dl	Call physician	Call physician

☐ **1.** 3 units regular
☐ **2.** 4 units regular
☐ **3.** 8 units regular
☐ **4.** 10 units regular

ANSWERS AND RATIONALES

1. CORRECT ANSWER: 4
The nurse should monitor T_4 levels, which indicate thyroid function, to evaluate the effectiveness of levothyroxine therapy. CD4+ cell count is used to evaluate the progression of human immunodeficiency virus infection. Hemoglobin A_{1c} is used to measure a client's glucose levels over a 4-month period. Prothrombin time is used to measure clotting times for clients taking oral anticoagulants.

2. CORRECT ANSWER: 3
It's believed that children with primary nocturnal enuresis have insufficient antidiuretic hormone, so desmopressin is indicated. Cosyntropin and corticotropin stimulate the adrenal glands and won't help with enuresis. Somatropin is used for growth failure.

3. CORRECT ANSWER: 3
Calcitriol increases GI absorption and bone resorption of calcium and decreases renal calcium clearance, thereby increasing the serum calcium level. It isn't known to reduce bone resorption, decrease osteoclastic activity, or stimulate the parathyroid gland to secrete parathyroid hormone.

4. CORRECT ANSWER: 3
In a medical emergency, speed and onset of action are important. The I.V. route is the fastest route to action, and only regular insulin may be given by this route. Although regular insulin is fast-acting, the subQ route isn't the fastest route to

correct glycemic problems. If the goal is prolonged action, then NPH insulin given subQ would be the drug of choice; however, NPH insulin is never given I.M.

5. CORRECT ANSWER: 4

Glipizide is well absorbed; onset of action may be as soon as 30 minutes after intake, peaking within 2 to 3 hours. Taking the drug 30 minutes before breakfast ensures effectiveness at the first meal and throughout the day. Taking the drug with or after meals doesn't ensure effectiveness. Taking the drug before bedtime could result in nighttime hypoglycemia.

6. CORRECT ANSWER: 3

The client has hyperthyroidism. Propylthiouracil is an antithyroid drug that inhibits the synthesis of thyroid hormones. Levothyroxine and liothyronine are thyroid replacement hormones used to treat hypothyroidism. Thiothixene is an antipsychotic and wouldn't be used.

7. CORRECT ANSWER: 4

When taking glyburide, a second-generation oral antidiabetic agent, the client needs to eat soon after taking the drug. Glyburide works differently from chlorpropamide. It's more potent than chlorpropamide and requires a smaller dose, but still needs to be taken every day.

8. CORRECT ANSWER: 3

Signs and symptoms of hypoglycemia include complaints of hunger, restlessness, nervousness, agitation, headaches, confusion, and cool, clammy skin. Complaints of thirst; hot, dry skin; and dilute, pale urine are symptoms of hyperglycemia.

9. CORRECT ANSWER: 2

Both insulins should be given because the Lantus insulin provides 24-hour coverage and the regular insulin is needed to treat the client's elevated blood glucose. However, Lantus insulin can't be mixed with other insulins, so separate syringes are required.

10. CORRECT ANSWER: 4

According to the sliding scale, the correct dose of insulin for a 1630 blood glucose level of 279 mg/dl is 10 units of regular insulin.

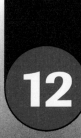

12

Drugs and the immune system

1. Which class of drugs works by inhibiting protein synthesis within fungal cells or altering the permeability of the cell membrane?

☐ 1. Cephalosporin
☐ 2. Antihistamines
☐ 3. Antifungals
☐ 4. Anthelmintics

CORRECT ANSWER: 3

2. A client is diagnosed with roundworm. The nurse anticipates that the physician will order:

☐ 1. mebendazole (Vermox).
☐ 2. acyclovir (Zovirax).
☐ 3. cefoxitin (Mefoxin).
☐ 4. rifapentine (Priftin).

CORRECT ANSWER: 1

3. A nurse is aware that a client taking a corticosteroid may experience:

☐ 1. hyperkalemia.
☐ 2. fluid retention.
☐ 3. hypoglycemia.
☐ 4. hair loss.

CORRECT ANSWER: 2

4. Before administering a penicillin-class drug, a nurse should first:

☐ 1. administer a fluid bolus.

☐ 2. insert an indwelling urinary catheter.

☐ 3. administer a test dose of the drug.

☐ 4. check the client's allergies.

CORRECT ANSWER: 4

5. When preparing discharge instructions for a client taking an immuno-suppressant, the nurse should advise him to:

☐ 1. avoid fresh fruits and vegetables.

☐ 2. go out into crowds as much as possible.

☐ 3. brush his teeth only once daily.

☐ 4. stop taking the drug as soon as he feels better.

CORRECT ANSWER: 1

LEARNING OBJECTIVES

After studying this chapter, you should be able to:

● Describe the general uses and mechanism of action for different classes of drugs used to treat the immune system.

● List the indications and common adverse effects of antihistamines, corticosteroids, immunosuppressants, antibacterials, antifungals, anthelmintics, antivirals, and antituberculotics.

● Identify important nursing responsibilities and patient teaching goals for administering immune system drugs.

● Discuss precautions that may help prevent infection in the immuno-suppressed patient.

CHAPTER OVERVIEW

Corticosteroids comprise two subgroups: glucocorticoids and mineralocorticoids. Glucocorticoids help decrease inflammation and immune response in various disorders. Mineralocorticoids cause reabsorption of sodium and water in the nephron and are used as replacement therapy in adrenocortical insufficiency. Immunosuppressants are used to prevent transplanted organ rejection and to treat certain autoimmune disorders, such as systemic lupus erythematosus (SLE) and idiopathic thrombocytopenic purpura.

Antibacterial drugs, including penicillins, cephalosporins, aminoglycosides, tetracyclines, fluoroquinolones, miscellaneous anti-infectives, and urinary tract antiseptics, are used to treat systemic microbial infections. Each class of drug kills (bactericidal) or inhibits (bacteriostatic) the growth of susceptible organisms. Before therapy begins, specimens for culture and sensitivity tests should be obtained.

Antifungals help treat fungal infections, including candidiasis, tinea, histoplasmosis, and aspergillosis. Infections may be local or systemic; systemic infections are more difficult to treat. Anthelmintics are used to treat parasitic worms of the intestinal tract and other organs.

Antivirals are used to treat herpes simplex I and II, genital herpes, herpes zoster varicella, certain influenza viruses, and human immunodeficiency virus (HIV). Replicating viruses invade the human cell and interfere with cellular metabolism, making them difficult to treat. Antituberculotics are used to treat tuberculosis (TB), an infection of the lung and other organs caused by *Mycobacterium tuberculosis*. Treatment for TB or for exposure to TB lasts 6 months to 2 years, making compliance difficult and contributing to the prevalence of resistant TB.

ANATOMY AND PHYSIOLOGY

● **Anatomy of the immune system**
  • Lymphatic system—consists of lymphocyte-containing (lymphoid) tissues, lymph, and a network of lymphatic vessels
  • Lymph tissues—found in lymph nodes, spleen, thymus, tonsils, adenoids, appendix, and intestinal Peyer's patches

● **Physiology**
  • Lymphatic system
    – Lymph
      · Carries foreign substances that enter tissue fluids to lymph nodes, where lymphocytes act on them
      · Is collected by lymphatic vessels, which return it to circulation
      · Flows through tiny lymphatic capillaries to progressively larger vessels reaching subclavian vein
    – Lymphocytes
      · Are white blood cells (WBCs) that develop from stem cells in bone marrow and differentiate into lymphocyte precursor cells
      · Have two types: T lymphocytes and B lymphocytes
      · Perform specific immune functions

A&P highlights

- The lymphatic system consists of lymphoid tissues, lymph, and a network of lymphatic vessels.
- Lymph carries foreign substances to the lymph nodes.
- Lymphatic vessels collect lymph and return it to circulation.
- Lymphocytes are WBCs that develop from stem cells in the bone marrow.
- There are two types of lymphocytes: T lymphocytes and B lymphocytes. Each performs specific immune functions.
- Two mechanisms—nonspecific resistance and acquired immunity—protect the body against microorganisms and other potentially harmful substances.
- Nonspecific resistance is a group of general protective mechanisms, such as skin, mucous membranes, antimicrobial substances, and inflammation, that ward off pathogens to which the body has not previously been exposed.
- Acquired immunity consists of specific immune responses (antibody formation or lymphatic activation) directed against specific organisms or toxins to which the body most likely has already been exposed.

- Mature and continuously recirculate between blood and various lymphatic tissues and organs
- Immunity
  - Refers to mechanisms that protect the body against microorganisms and other potentially harmful substances
  - Nonspecific resistance
    - Uses general protective mechanisms that function without prior exposure to harmful agents to ward off a wide range of pathogens
    - Includes skin and mucous membranes, antimicrobial substances, phagocytosis, inflammation, and fever
  - Acquired immunity
    - Consists of specific immune responses provided by the lymphatic system and directed against specific organisms or toxins
    - Usually requires previous exposure to foreign substance
    - Causes antibody formation (humoral immunity) or lymphatic activation (cell-mediated immunity)

● **Function**
- Serves as body's second circulatory system
  - Drains excess fluid from interstitial spaces and returns it to blood
  - Absorbs fats from GI tract and transports them to bloodstream
- Performs immune functions
  - B lymphocytes
    - Initially synthesize antibodies that rise to surface of lymphocyte (surface immunoglobulins), where they function as B-cell receptors
    - When mature, produce humoral immunity
      - Plasma cells—secrete antibodies
      - Memory cells—become plasma cells during subsequent exposure to an antigen
  - T lymphocytes
    - Initially seek, recognize, and attach to antigens that fit their surface receptors
    - Later, produce cell-mediated immunity
- Provides acquired immunity
  - Cell-mediated immunity
    - Relies on sensitized T lymphocytes
    - Serves as body's main defense against viruses, fungi, parasites, and some bacteria
    - Eliminates abnormal cells that may arise during cell division, which can develop into tumors if not destroyed
    - Causes organ transplant rejection
  - Humoral immunity
    - Relies on B-lymphocyte function
    - Provides major defense against many bacteria and bacterial toxins by producing immunoglobulin antibodies and an allergic response to the antigen

Functions of B lymphocytes

- Synthesize antibodies that function as B-cell receptors on the surface of the lymphocyte
- Produce humoral immunity (main defense against bacteria and bacterial toxins)
- Secrete antibodies

Functions of T lymphocytes

- Seek, recognize, and attach to antigens that fit their surface receptors
- Produce cell-mediated immunity (main defense against viruses, fungi, parasites, and some bacteria)

ANTIHISTAMINES

- **Mechanism of action**
  - Compete with histamine to bind to H_1 receptors throughout body
  - Block histamine's effects on body in hypersensitivity or allergic reactions

- **Pharmacokinetics**
  - Absorption: Well absorbed after oral and parental administration
  - Distribution: Widely distributed throughout body
  - Metabolism: Metabolized in liver
  - Excretion: Excreted in urine; fexofenadine excreted in feces

- **Drug examples**
  - Cetirizine (Zyrtec), clemastine (Dayhist-1), dimenhydrinate (Dimetabs), diphenhydramine (Benadryl), fexofenadine (Allegra), loratadine (Claritin), promethazine (Phenergan)

- **Indications**
  - Symptomatic relief of symptoms of seasonal allergic rhinitis in adults and children
  - Treatment of chronic, idiopathic urticaria
  - Adjunctive therapy in treatment of anaphylactic reactions (dimenhydrinate, diphenhydramine and promethazine)
  - Treatment and prevention of motion sickness (diphenhydramine and promethazine)

- **Contraindications and precautions**
  - Contraindicated in patients with previous history of allergic reaction to antihistamines and patients who are in third trimester of pregnancy or breast-feeding
  - Cetirizine shouldn't be used in patients with allergy to hydroxyzine
  - Promethazine shouldn't be used in patients with severe central nervous system (CNS) depression or bone marrow depression and those taking monoamine oxidase (MAO) inhibitors
  - Used cautiously in patients with narrow-angle glaucoma, symptomatic benign prostatic hyperplasia, or asthma
  - Dimenhydrinate used cautiously in patients with arrhythmias
  - Fexofenadine used cautiously in patients with hepatic or renal impairment

- **Adverse reactions**
  - CNS depression and other CNS effects (disturbed coordination and muscle weakness); GI upset (epigastric distress, loss of appetite [loratadine may increase appetite], nausea and vomiting, and constipation); dryness of mouth, nose, and throat; increased respiratory secretions; hypotension or hypertension; increased heart rate; arrhythmias; fever; photosensitivity; rash; myalgia; and angioedema
  - Possible CNS stimulation (excitation, restlessness, insomnia, and palpitations) in elderly patients

- Possible anaphylactic shock (clemastine, dimenhydrinate, and diphenhydramine)

● **Interactions**
- Methohexital, phenobarbital anesthetic, and thiopental increase the frequency and severity of neuromuscular excitation and hypotension when administered with promethazine
- Use with alcohol or other CNS depressants increases depressant effects
- MAO inhibitors increase the anticholinergic effects of clemastine and diphenhydramine
- Ketoconazole and erythromycin increase the levels of fexofenadine
- Antacids decrease the effects of fexofenadine

● **Nursing responsibilities**
- Observe for signs and symptoms of hypersensitivity reaction (urticaria, drug rash, and photosensitivity)
- Administer drug with food or milk to decrease GI irritation
- Withhold drug if the patient is scheduled to receive an allergy skin test; drug could mask positive result
- Use Z-track method if giving drug parenterally
- Monitor for sedation and other CNS depressive effects

CORTICOSTEROIDS (ADRENOCORTICOIDS)

● **Mechanism of action**
- Glucocorticoids: Produce various metabolic effects, suppress inflammation, and alter normal immune response; also promote sodium and water retention and potassium excretion
- Mineralocorticoids: Enhance reabsorption of sodium and chloride and promote excretion of potassium and hydrogen from renal tubules, thereby helping to maintain fluid and electrolyte balance

● **Pharmacokinetics**
- Absorption: Readily absorbed from GI tract
- Distribution: Widely distributed
- Metabolism: Metabolized in liver
- Excretion: Excreted in urine

● **Drug examples**
- Glucocorticoids: betamethasone (Celestone), cortisone (Cortone), dexamethasone (Decadron, Hexadrol), hydrocortisone (Cortef, Hydrocortone, Solu-Cortef), methylprednisolone (Depo-Medrol, Medrol, Solu-Medrol), prednisolone (Delta-Cortef), prednisone (Orasone), triamcinolone (Aristocort, Azmacort, Kenalog)
- Mineralocorticoids: fludrocortisone (Florinef)

● **Indications**
- Replacement therapy for adrenocortical insufficiency (glucocorticoids)

Key nursing actions

- Observe for hypersensitivity reaction.
- Administer with food or milk.
- Withhold before allergy skin test.

Key facts about corticosteroids

- Also called *adrenocorticoids*
- Two types: glucocorticoids and mineralocorticoids
- Glucocorticoids produce various metabolic effects, suppress inflammation, alter normal immune response, and promote sodium and water retention and potassium excretion.
- Mineralocorticoids enhance reabsorption of sodium and chloride and promote excretion of potassium and hydrogen (to help maintain fluid and electrolyte balance).
- Metabolized in liver
- Excreted in urine

- Treat neoplastic diseases, septic shock, autoimmune diseases, cerebral edema, and inflammation of joints, GI tract, respiratory tract, and skin (glucocorticoids)
- Replacement therapy in primary or secondary adrenal insufficiency (mineralocorticoids)

Contraindications and precautions
- Glucocorticoids used with extreme caution in patients with serious infection; may mask signs and symptoms of infection
- Mineralocorticoids used cautiously in patients with cardiovascular disease and hypertension

Adverse reactions
- Glucocorticoids: Muscle wasting, osteoporosis, growth retardation (in children), peptic ulcer, increased serum glucose level, hypertension, seizures, mood swings, cataracts, glaucoma, fragile skin, hirsutism, increased appetite, altered fat distribution, possible masking of signs and symptoms of infection (more likely to occur when given in doses above normal body levels for nonendocrine disorders than when given as replacement therapy)
- Mineralocorticoids: Sodium and fluid retention, hypokalemia, euphoria, depression, hyperglycemia, acute adrenal insufficiency after abrupt withdrawal, redistribution of fat, insomnia, hirsutism, and GI distress or ulcers

Interactions
- Concurrent use with drugs that induce hypokalemia (such as potassium depleting diuretics) causes additive hypokalemia
- Concurrent use with insulin or oral hypoglycemics may increase blood glucose levels, thereby increasing insulin or oral hypoglycemic requirements
- Phenobarbital, phenytoin, and rifampin may enhance metabolism of glucocorticoids, decreasing effects of glucocorticoids
- Hormonal contraceptives may block metabolism of glucocorticoids

Nursing responsibilities
- Administer daily doses in morning to mimic body's normal pattern of cortisol secretion
- Assess for symptomatic improvement and adverse effects
- Know that additional doses may be needed during periods of stress or infection
- Monitor regularly for weight changes and fluid and electrolyte imbalances, especially hypokalemia; promote increased intake of high-potassium foods to prevent hypokalemia
- Monitor the patient taking a mineralocorticoid for signs of fluid retention by taking daily weights, assessing breath sounds, and checking for peripheral edema
- Warn the patient not to stop drug abruptly; doing so may cause life-threatening adrenal insufficiency

When to use corticosteroids
- Replacement therapy for adrenocortical insufficiency
- Neoplastic diseases
- Septic shock
- Autoimmune diseases
- Cerebral edema
- Inflammation of the joints, GI tract, respiratory tract, or skin

When NOT to use corticosteroids
- Serious infection

Adverse reactions
- Muscle wasting, osteoporosis, growth retardation, peptic ulcer, increased serum glucose level, hypertension, seizures, mood swings, cataracts, glaucoma, fragile skin, hirsutism, increased appetite, altered fat distribution, sodium and fluid retention, hypokalemia, euphoria, depression, hyperglycemia, acute adrenal insufficiency after abrupt withdrawal, redistribution of fat, insomnia, hirsutism, GI distress or ulcers

Key nursing actions
- Administer daily doses in the morning.
- Assess patient for symptomatic improvement and adverse effects.
- Administer additional doses during periods of stress or infection, as ordered.
- Monitor regularly for weight changes and fluid and electrolyte imbalances.
- Instruct the patient to consult with practitioner before receiving vaccinations.

Topics for patient discussion

- Medication regimen, including guidelines for missed doses
- Signs and symptoms to discuss with the practitioner
- Avoidance of abrupt drug discontinuation
- Avoidance of alcohol, cigarettes, caffeine, and aspirin-containing products
- Possible mood alterations
- Dietary restrictions and allowances
- Follow-up care

Key facts about immunosuppressants

- Azathioprine suppresses cell-mediated immunity and alters antibody formation.
- Basiliximab and daclizumab inhibit activation of lymphocytes.
- Cyclosporine and sirolimus inhibit proliferation and function of T lymphocytes.
- Muromonab-CD3 blocks T-cell function.
- Mycophenolate mofetil inhibits proliferation of T and B lymphocytes, inhibits recruitment of leukocytes to sites of inflammation, and suppresses B lymphocyte antibody formation.
- Prednisone inhibits macrophage formation and hinders migration of macrophages and leukocytes to inflamed areas.
- Tacrolimus inhibits T-lymphocyte activation.
- Metabolized in liver
- Excreted in urine and feces

 TIME-OUT FOR TEACHING

Teaching about glucocorticoids

Include these topics in your teaching plan for the patient receiving a glucocorticoid:
- medication regimen, including the drug's name, dosage, frequency, duration, and possible adverse effects
- signs and symptoms to discuss with the practitioner
- avoidance of abrupt drug discontinuation
- consistent dosing
- guidelines for missed doses
- avoidance of alcohol, cigarettes, caffeine, and aspirin-containing products
- possible mood alterations
- dietary restrictions and allowances
- follow-up care, including practitioner visits.

- Instruct the patient to consult the practitioner before receiving vaccinations
- Advise the patient to avoid fresh fruits and raw vegetables, which tend to have higher levels of bacteria than cooked foods; may increase risk of infection in an immunosuppressed patient
- Teach the patient the importance of complying with therapy (see *Teaching about glucocorticoids*)
- Instruct the patient to carry identification describing disease and drug regimen

IMMUNOSUPPRESSANTS

Mechanism of action

- Azathioprine: Suppresses cell-mediated immunity and alters antibody formation
- Basiliximab and daclizumab: Inhibit activation of lymphocytes; both are monoclonal antibodies
- Cyclosporine and sirolimus: Inhibit proliferation and function of T lymphocytes
- Muromonab-CD3: Reacts with T_3 complex, blocking T-cell function
- Mycophenolate mofetil: Inhibits proliferation of T lymphocytes and B lymphocytes and the recruitment of leukocytes to inflamed areas; also suppresses antibody formation by B lymphocytes
- Prednisone: Inhibits macrophage formation and hinders migration of macrophages and leukocytes to inflamed areas
- Tacrolimus: Inhibits T-lymphocyte activation

Pharmacokinetics

- Absorption: Varies widely with each drug
- Distribution: Varies widely with each drug
- Metabolism: Metabolized in liver
- Excretion: Excreted in urine and feces

Drug examples

- Antilymphocyte globulin, antilymphocyte serum, antithymocyte globulin (Atgam), azathioprine (Imuran), basiliximab (Simulect), cyclosporine (Sandimmune, Neoral), daclizumab (Zenapax), muromonab-CD3 (Orthoclone OKT3), mycophenolate mofetil (CellCept), prednisone (Deltasone), sirolimus (Rapamune), tacrolimus (Prograf)

Indications

- Prevent organ transplant rejection

Contraindications and precautions

- All drugs used cautiously in patients with bone marrow depression, infection, or cancer
- Mycophenolate mofetil used cautiously in patients with GI disorders or bone marrow depression
- Tacrolimus contraindicated in patients with hypersensitivity to castor oil derivatives (I.V. form); used cautiously in pregnant and breast-feeding patients and those with impaired liver or kidney function or lymphomas
- Sirolimus used cautiously in patients with hyperlipidemia or impaired liver or kidney function

Adverse reactions

- Peptic ulcer, edema, altered fat distribution, increased serum glucose levels, mood swings, hirsutism, fragile skin, nausea, vomiting, diarrhea, anorexia, anemia, leukopenia, thrombocytopenia, and hepatotoxicity
- Bone marrow suppression and liver toxicity (azathioprine)
- Anaphylaxis, respiratory depression, hypertension, hypotension, chest pain, tachycardia, pulmonary edema, and renal tubular necrosis (basiliximab and daclizumab)
- Gingival hyperplasia, infection, nephrotoxicity, and hyperkalemia (cyclosporine)
- Headache, tremor, weakness, chest pain, and urinary tract infection (UTI) (mycophenolate mofetil)
- Nephrotoxicity, tremor, hyperlipidemia, hypertension, arthralgia, and myalgia (sirolimus and tacrolimus)

Interactions

- Allopurinol increases the risk of azathioprine toxicity
- Concurrent use of cyclosporine with other nephrotoxic drugs causes additive nephrotoxicity
- Cimetidine, calcium channel blockers, hormonal contraceptives, erythromycin, and ketoconazole increase the risk of cyclosporine toxicity
- Phenobarbital, phenytoin, rifampin, and co-trimoxazole (sulfamethoxazole-trimethoprim) I.V. decrease effects of cyclosporine
- Sirolimus may interact with many drugs, possibly increasing the risk of nephrotoxicity and neurotoxicity; may increase cholesterol and triglyceride levels
- Tacrolimus may interact with many drugs, possibly increasing the risk of nephrotoxicity and neurotoxicity; may alter glucose and potassium levels

When to use immunosuppressants

- Organ or bone marrow transplant

When NOT to use immunosuppressants

- Hypersensitivity to castor oil derivatives
- GI disorders
- Bone marrow depression, infection, or cancer
- Hypersensitivity to castor oil derivatives
- Impaired liver or kidney function
- Lymphomas
- Pregnancy or breast-feeding
- Hyperlipidemia

Adverse reactions

- Peptic ulcer, edema, altered fat distribution, increased serum glucose levels, mood swings, hirsutism, fragile skin, nausea, vomiting, diarrhea, anorexia, anemia, leukopenia, thrombocytopenia, hepatotoxicity, anaphylaxis, hypertension, infection, nephrotoxicity, tremor

Key nursing actions

- Monitor for adverse effects, toxicity, and signs and symptoms of infection.
- Maintain isolation precautions, as indicated.
- Monitor fluid intake and output.
- Instruct patient to report unusual bleeding or signs and symptoms of infection or transplant rejection.
- Urge the patient to use contraception to prevent pregnancy.
- Teach the patient to avoid flowers, plants, fresh fruit, and raw vegetables because they increase the risk of infection.
- Teach the patient about the importance of lifelong compliance with immunosuppressive therapy to prevent organ rejection.

Key facts about penicillins

- Usually bactericidal
- Partially metabolized in liver
- Mostly excreted in urine

● **Nursing responsibilities**
- Monitor for anaphylaxis when administering a monoclonal antibody (basiliximab or daclizumab)
- Monitor for signs of rejection, nephrotoxicity, or neurotoxicity when giving sirolimus or tacrolimus
- Monitor the serum drug level to prevent toxicity; instruct the patient to maintain proper oral hygiene to prevent gingival hyperplasia when administering cyclosporine
- Know that Sandimmune and Neoral aren't interchangeable
- Protect the patient from visitors and staff with infections after organ transplantation; as indicated, maintain isolation precautions
- Monitor WBC counts; notify the practitioner if they fall below 3,000/mm³
- Assess for signs and symptoms of infection (fever, tachycardia, malaise, redness, and inflammation)
- Monitor fluid intake and output during immunosuppressive therapy to prevent nephrotoxicity; decreased urine output may lead to azathioprine toxicity
- Instruct the patient to report immediately any signs and symptoms of infection, unusual bleeding, or transplant rejection (fever, graft tenderness, decreased urine output, and edema)
- Inform the patient about potential teratogenic drug effects during pregnancy; urge the patient to use contraception
- Teach the patient to avoid flowers and plants and eating fresh fruit and raw vegetables, which have higher levels of bacteria than cooked foods; may increase risk of infection in an immunosuppressed patient
- Instruct the patient on importance of lifelong compliance with immunosuppressive therapy to prevent organ transplant rejection

ANTIBACTERIAL DRUGS

PENICILLINS

● **Mechanism of action**
- Bactericidal; inhibit synthesis of bacterial cell wall and cause rapid cell lysis

● **Pharmacokinetics**
- Absorption: Varies with oral forms
- Distribution: Widely distributed
- Metabolism: Partially metabolized in liver
- Excretion: Excreted in urine

● **Drug examples**
- Aminopenicillins: amoxicillin (Amoxil), amoxicillin/clavulanate (Augmentin, Augmentin XR), ampicillin (Principen), ampicillin and sulbactam (Unasyn)

- Extended-spectrum penicillins: carbenicillin (Geocillin), piperacillin (Pipracil), piperacillin/tazobactam sodium (Zosyn), ticarcillin (Ticar), ticarcillin/clavulanate (Timentin)
- Natural penicillins: procaine penicillin G, penicillin G potassium, penicillin V (Pen-Vee K)
- Penicillinase-resistant penicillins: dicloxacillin, nafcillin, oxacillin

Indications

- Treat infections by gram-positive cocci and bacilli and some gram-negative cocci; also effective against some anaerobes
- Treat enterococcal infections (aminopenicillins)
- Treat infections by gram-negative bacteria (extended-spectrum penicillins)
- Treatment of choice for gonorrhea (natural penicillins)
- Treat infections caused by staphylococci that synthesize the enzyme penicillinase (penicillinase-resistant penicillins)

Contraindications and precautions

- Contraindicated in patients allergic to any penicillin or cephalosporin; may have up to a 10% cross-sensitivity to other penicillins in this group
- Procaine penicillin G contraindicated in patients allergic to "caine"-type local anesthetics

Adverse reactions

- Nausea, vomiting, diarrhea, epigastric distress, rash, allergic reaction, serum sickness, pain at I.M. injection site, phlebitis at I.V. infusion site, resistant bacterial and fungal superinfections (with broad-spectrum drugs)

Interactions

- Penicillins may decrease the effectiveness of aminoglycosides
- Use of penicillins with a hormonal contraceptive increases the risk of breakthrough bleeding; may diminish efficacy of contraceptive
- Large doses of I.V. penicillin can prolong bleeding time and increase the bleeding risk when used with anticoagulants
- Probenecid decreases renal excretion of penicillin, thereby increasing penicillin levels and enhancing penicillin's effectiveness
- Penicillins decrease tubular secretion of methotrexate, increasing the risk of toxicity
- Tetracyclines may decrease bactericidal effects of penicillins

Nursing responsibilities

- Obtain the patient's allergy history before administering drug
- Know that an allergic reaction to penicillin may occur even in a patient with no history of allergic reactions
- Obtain appropriate specimens for culture and sensitivity before initiating drug therapy; however, first dose may be given pending results
- Observe for signs and symptoms of allergic reaction after administering drug; if reactions occur, discontinue drug and notify the practitioner

When to use penicillins

- Gram-positive cocci and bacilli infections
- Some gram-negative cocci infections
- Some anaerobe infections
- Enterococcal infections
- Gram-negative bacterial infections
- Gonorrhea
- Staphylococci infections

When NOT to use penicillins

- Allergy to penicillin or cephalosporin
- Allergy to caine-type local anesthetics

Adverse reactions

- Nausea, vomiting, diarrhea, epigastric distress, rash, allergic reaction, pain at I.M. injection site, phlebitis at I.V. infusion site, resistant bacterial and fungal superinfections

Key nursing actions

- Obtain an allergy history.
- Obtain appropriate specimens for culture and sensitivity.
- Watch for signs and symptoms of an allergic reaction; if any occur, discontinue the drug and notify the practitioner.
- Instruct the patient to avoid taking oral penicillin with acidic juices or carbonated beverages.
- Assess for signs and symptoms of superinfection.
- Instruct in use of alternative contraception methods.

- Instruct the patient to avoid taking oral penicillin with acidic juices or carbonated beverages; may reduce drug absorption
- Assess the patient (especially if elderly or debilitated) for signs and symptoms of superinfection, particularly if he's on prolonged therapy
- Instruct the female patient taking hormonal contraceptives to use an alternative contraceptive method (barrier method) during entire course of penicillin therapy
- Administer drug 1 hour before or 2 hours after meals
- Instruct the patient to notify practitioner if signs of superinfection (black, furry overgrowth on tongue, loose or foul-smelling stools, and [in females] vaginal itching or discharge) occur
- Instruct the patient on importance of complying with therapy and completing the full therapeutic course, even if feeling better; inadequate dosage or premature discontinuation of therapy may exacerbate infection and lead to resistant organisms

CEPHALOSPORINS

- **Mechanism of action**
  - Chemically and pharmacologically similar to penicillins
  - Bactericidal; kill or inhibit many gram-positive and gram-negative bacteria and some anaerobic bacteria

- **Pharmacokinetics**
  - Absorption: Oral absorption of cephalosporins varies widely; many are given I.V.
  - Distribution: Widely distributed
  - Metabolism: Varies widely
  - Excretion: Excreted primarily in urine

- **Drug examples**
  - First-generation cephalosporins: cefadroxil (Duricef), cefazolin (Ancef), cephalexin (Keflex, Keftab), cephapirin
  - Second-generation cephalosporins: cefaclor (Ceclor, Ceclor CD), cefoxitin (Mefoxin), cefprozil (Cefzil), cefuroxime (Ceftin), loracarbef (Lorabid)
  - Third-generation cephalosporins: cefdinir (Omnicef), cefditoren (Spectracef), cefoperazone (Cefobid), cefotaxime (Claforan), cefpodoxime (Vantin), ceftazidime (Fortaz, Tazicef, Tazidime), ceftibuten (Cedax), ceftizoxime (Cefizox), ceftriaxone (Rocephin)
  - Fourth-generation cephalosporin: cefepime (Maxipime)

- **Indications**
  - Treat infections caused by gram-positive and gram-negative bacteria
    - First-generation cephalosporins are active against infections caused by most gram-positive cocci and certain gram-negative bacilli
    - Each subsequent generation has increased activity against gram-negative organisms and reduced activity against gram-positive organisms

Key facts about cephalosporins

- Chemically and pharmacologically similar to penicillins
- Bactericidal (not antifungal or antiviral)
- Metabolism varies by drug
- Excreted primarily in urine

When to use cephalosporins

- Gram-positive and gram-negative bacterial infections
- Gram-positive and gram-negative cocci infections
- Certain gram-negative bacilli infections

Contraindications and precautions
- Used cautiously in patients allergic to penicillins (to prevent cross-sensitivity), pregnant or breast-feeding patients, and those with a history of GI disease (particularly colitis)

Adverse reactions
- Nausea, vomiting, diarrhea, rash, anaphylaxis, seizures, pain at I.M. injection site, phlebitis at I.V. infusion site, and pseudomembranous colitis

Interactions
- Probenecid decreases excretion of cephalosporins, increasing cephalosporin levels
- Use of cefoperazone with alcohol may cause a disulfiram-like reaction (flushing, headache, and tachycardia)

Nursing responsibilities
- Obtain the patient's allergy history before administering drug
- Know that an allergic reaction to cephalosporin may occur even in a patient with no history of allergic reactions
- Observe for signs and symptoms of allergic reaction after administering drug; discontinue drug and notify the practitioner if reactions occur

AMINOGLYCOSIDES

Mechanism of action
- Bactericidal; exact mechanism unclear
- Thought to bind to ribosomal subunits, inhibiting bacterial protein synthesis

Pharmacokinetics
- Absorption: Poor oral absorption; most drugs given parenterally
- Distribution: Widely distributed
- Metabolism: Most drugs not metabolized
- Excretion: Excreted unchanged in urine

Drug examples
- Amikacin (Amikin), gentamicin (Garamycin), kanamycin (Kantrex), neomycin (Mycifradin), streptomycin, tobramycin

Indications
- Treat infections caused by aerobic gram-negative bacilli and some gram-positive bacteria
- Treat septicemia; postoperative pulmonary, intra-abdominal, and serious recurrent UTIs; infections of bones, skin, soft tissues, and joints; and ammonia-forming bacteria in GI tract of patients with hepatic encephalopathy
- Adjunct to other antibacterials in treatment of serious staphylococcal infections, serious *Pseudomonas aeruginosa* infections, enterococcal infections, nosocomial pneumonia, TB, pelvic inflammatory disease, and serious *Klebsiella* infections

When NOT to use aminoglycosides

- Pregnancy
- Breast-feeding

Adverse reactions

- Vestibular and cochlear ototoxicity, nephrotoxicity, and neurotoxicity; nausea; vomiting; diarrhea; hypersensitivity reactions; hemolytic anemia; transient neutropenia; leukopenia; thrombocytopenia; elevated liver enzyme levels; vein irritation, phlebitis, and sterile abscess

Key nursing actions

- Assess eighth cranial nerve function to detect vertigo and hearing loss.
- Monitor renal function for evidence of nephrotoxicity.
- Promote fluid intake of 1,500 to 2,000 ml/day.
- Monitor peak and trough levels to evaluate drug effectiveness and prevent toxicity.

Key facts about tetracyclines

- Bacteriostatic (may be bactericidal with certain organisms)
- Bind reversibly to 30S and 50S ribosomal units, inhibiting bacterial protein synthesis
- Metabolized in kidneys or not metabolized at all
- Excreted in urine

● **Contraindications and precautions**
- Contraindicated in pregnant or breast-feeding patients
- Used cautiously in patients with renal failure or neuromuscular disease and in elderly or debilitated patients

● **Adverse reactions**
- Vestibular and cochlear ototoxicity, nephrotoxicity, and neurotoxicity (paresthesia, respiratory depression, and neuromuscular weakness); ototoxicity and nephrotoxicity reversible only if detected early and drug is discontinued immediately
- Nausea, vomiting, and diarrhea (most common)
- Hypersensitivity reactions, hemolytic anemia, transient neutropenia, leukopenia, thrombocytopenia, elevated liver enzyme levels; and vein irritation, phlebitis, and sterile abscess (with I.V. form of aminoglycosides)

● **Interactions**
- Use with another aminoglycoside or a loop diuretic may cause additive ototoxicity
- Inactivation occurs when aminoglycosides are mixed with penicillins
- Administration with cephalosporins in the same site may cause inactivation
- Use with certain inhalation anesthetics or neuromuscular blockers may cause respiratory paralysis

● **Nursing responsibilities**
- Assess eighth cranial nerve function to detect vertigo and hearing loss (usually involves high frequencies) before starting drug therapy and during treatment; permanent damage may occur without immediate intervention
- Monitor renal function for evidence of nephrotoxicity
- Make sure patient is well hydrated during treatment; promote fluid intake of 1,500 to 2,000 ml/day to maintain adequate renal function
- Monitor peak and trough levels to evaluate drug effectiveness and prevent toxicity; drug must be given at proper administration times so that accurate blood levels are drawn

TETRACYCLINES

● **Mechanism of action**
- Bacteriostatic; may be bactericidal with certain organisms
- Bind reversibly to 30S and 50S ribosomal units, inhibiting bacterial protein synthesis

● **Pharmacokinetics**
- Absorption: Absorbed systemically after oral administration
- Distribution: Widely distributed
- Metabolism: Metabolized in kidneys; may not be metabolized
- Excretion: Excreted in urine

● **Drug examples**
  • Demeclocycline (Declomycin), doxycycline (Vibramycin), minocycline (Minocin), oxytetracycline (Terramycin), tetracycline (Sumycin)

● **Indications**
  • Treat some gram-positive and gram-negative organisms; many such organisms are resistant to tetracyclines
  • Treat Lyme disease, gonorrhea, and syphilis in penicillin-allergic patients; also infections by unusual organisms (*Mycoplasma, Chlamydia, Rickettsia*)
  • Treat acne (occasionally)
  • Diuretic treatment of syndrome of inappropriate antidiuretic hormone (demeclocycline)

● **Contraindications and precautions**
  • Contraindicated in pregnant and breast-feeding patients and those with hypersensitivity to tetracyclines
  • Not for use in children younger than age 8 unless no alternatives exist; may cause permanent tooth discoloration
  • Used cautiously in elderly patients

● **Adverse reactions**
  • GI symptoms (most common), including anorexia, GI upset, flatulence, nausea, vomiting, bulky and loose stools, and epigastric burning
  • Hypersensitivity reactions, pancreatitis, hepatotoxicity, photosensitivity reaction, rash, pain at I.M. injection site, phlebitis at I.V. infusion site, and mild increase in blood urea nitrogen (BUN) levels

● **Interactions**
  • Antacids, calcium supplements, iron supplements, laxatives containing magnesium, and milk and dairy products reduce absorption of tetracyclines
  • Tetracyclines may increase effects of oral anticoagulants
  • Tetracyclines decrease effectiveness of hormonal contraceptives
  • Tetracyclines decrease effectiveness of penicillins

● **Nursing responsibilities**
  • Obtain urine specimen for culture and sensitivity before starting drug therapy; first dose may be given with results pending
  • Give doxycycline and minocycline I.V. only because of the risk of thrombophlebitis and hepatotoxicity; if giving drug I.V., monitor I.V. sites often for phlebitis
  • Instruct the patient not to take antacids, calcium supplements, iron supplements, laxatives containing magnesium, or milk or dairy products within 2 to 3 hours of taking drug (see *Teaching about tetracyclines*, page 248)
  • Advise the patient to use sunscreen and protective clothing to prevent photosensitivity reactions
  • Instruct the patient to discard outdated or decomposed tetracycline; may be toxic

---

When to use tetracyclines

● Gram-positive and gram-negative infections
● Lyme disease
● Gonorrhea
● Syphilis
● *Mycoplasma, Chlamydia*, and *Rickettsia* infection
● Acne
● Syndrome of inappropriate antidiuretic hormone

When NOT to use tetracyclines

● Pregnancy
● Breast-feeding
● Hypersensitivity to tetracyclines
● Children younger than age 8

Adverse reactions

● GI-related effects, such as anorexia, GI upset, flatulence, nausea, vomiting, bulky and loose stools, epigastric burning; hypersensitivity reactions; pancreatitis; hepatotoxicity; photosensitivity reaction; rash; pain at I.M. injection site; phlebitis at I.V. infusion site; mild increase in BUN levels

Key nursing actions

● Obtain urine specimen for culture and sensitivity before starting drug therapy.
● If giving drug I.V., monitor I.V. sites for phlebitis.

Topics for patient discussion

- Medication regimen
- Signs and symptoms to discuss with practitioner
- Avoidance of milk products and drugs containing calcium, magnesium, aluminum, or iron
- Administration on an empty stomach
- Measures to take for sun exposure
- Importance of completing therapy
- Use of alternative contraception during therapy and for 1 week afterward
- Follow-up care
- Importance of discarding outdated or decomposed drug

Key facts about fluoroquinolones

- Broad-spectrum, systemic antibacterials
- Active against wide range of organisms
- Produce a bactericidal effect by inhibiting intracellular enzymes
- Most unmetabolized
- Excreted primarily in urine

When to use fluoroquinolones

- Aerobic gram-positive and gram-negative infections
- Bone and joint infections
- Skin and soft-tissue infections
- Intra-abdominal infections
- Urinary tract infections
- Pyelonephritis
- Pneumonia
- Acute sinusitis
- Chronic bronchitis
- Gonorrhea
- Endocervical and urethral chlamydial infections
- Pelvic inflammatory disease

TIME-OUT FOR TEACHING

Teaching about tetracyclines

Include these topics in your teaching plan for the patient receiving a tetracycline:
- medication regimen, including the drug's name, dosage, frequency, duration, and possible adverse effects
- signs and symptoms to discuss with the practitioner
- avoidance of milk products and drugs containing calcium, magnesium, aluminum, or iron

- administration on an empty stomach
- avoidance of direct sunlight and measures to take for sun exposure
- importance of completing therapy
- use of alternative contraception during therapy and for 1 week afterward
- follow-up care, including practitioner visits.

- Inform the patient that tetracyclines may cause staining of soft contact lenses
- Instruct the female patient taking hormonal contraceptives to use alternative contraceptive method (barrier method) during entire course of tetracycline therapy

FLUOROQUINOLONES

● Mechanism of action
- Broad-spectrum, systemic antibacterial action; active against a wide range of organisms
- Produce bactericidal effect by inhibiting intracellular enzymes essential for the duplication, transcription, and repair of bacterial deoxyribonucleic acid (DNA)

● Pharmacokinetics
- Absorption: Absorbed rapidly from GI tract
- Distribution: Widely distributed
- Metabolism: Some drugs undergo partial hepatic metabolism; others aren't metabolized
- Excretion: Excreted primarily in urine

● Drug examples
- Ciprofloxacin (Cipro), gatifloxacin (Tequin), gemifloxacin (Factive), levofloxacin (Levaquin), lomefloxacin (Maxaquin), moxifloxacin (Avelox), norfloxacin (Noroxin), sparfloxacin (Zagam)

● Indications
- Treat many aerobic gram-positive and gram-negative organisms
- Treat bone and joint infections, skin and soft-tissue infections, intra-abdominal infections, UTIs, pyelonephritis, pneumonia, acute sinusitis, and chronic bronchitis

- Treat gonorrhea, endocervical and urethral chlamydial infections, and pelvic inflammatory disease
- Prevention of bacterial UTIs

● **Contraindications and precautions**
  - Contraindicated in children
  - Used with extreme caution in patients with cardiovascular disorders, CNS disorders, seizures, renal insufficiency, cerebral ischemia, or severe hepatic dysfunction

● **Adverse reactions**
  - Nausea, crystalluria, phototoxicity, diarrhea, rash, and dizziness

● **Interactions**
  - May increase serum levels of methylxanthines, causing methylxanthine toxicity
  - Antacids may reduce effectiveness of fluoroquinolones when given within 2 to 8 hours of fluoroquinolone administration
  - Increase QT interval of drugs known to prolong the QT interval; should be used cautiously together
  - Probenecid may decrease renal excretion and increase serum levels of fluoroquinolones

● **Nursing responsibilities**
  - Obtain urine for culture and sensitivity testing before starting drug therapy; first dose may be given pending results
  - Separate administration times of drug and antacids, calcium, and iron by at least 2 hours
  - Instruct the patient to take drug with 8 ounces of water
  - Teach the patient to use sunblock and protective clothing to prevent photosensitivity reactions
  - Monitor renal function
  - Explain importance of completing full course of therapy as prescribed, even if feeling better

MISCELLANEOUS ANTI-INFECTIVES

● **Mechanism of action**
  - May be bactericidal or bacteriostatic
  - Block protein synthesis; may block synthesis of the cell wall, causing cell lysis and cell death

● **Pharmacokinetics**
  - Absorption: Varies with drug
  - Distribution: Rapidly distributed throughout body
  - Metabolism: Varies with drug
  - Excretion: Varies with drug

When NOT to use fluoroquinolones

- Children
- Cardiovascular disorders
- CNS disorders
- Seizures
- Renal insufficiency
- Cerebral ischemia
- Severe hepatic dysfunction

Adverse reactions

- Nausea, crystalluria, phototoxicity, diarrhea, and rash

Key nursing actions

- Obtain urine for culture and sensitivity testing before starting drug therapy.
- Administer with 8 ounces of water at least 2 hours before or after patient takes antacid, calcium, or iron.
- Monitor the patient's renal function.
- Explain to the patient the importance of completing the full course of therapy as prescribed.

Key facts about other anti-infectives

- Bactericidal or bacteriostatic
- Block protein synthesis or synthesis of cell wall
- Metabolism varies with drug
- Excretion varies with drug

When to use other anti-infectives

- Gram-negative and gram-positive aerobic and anaerobic infections
- Severe infections
- Ampicillin-resistant *H. influenzae* infections
- Pneumococci
- Group A streptococci
- *Pneumocystis carinii* pneumonia
- Penicillin-resistant staphylococcal infections

When NOT to use other anti-infectives

- Hypersensitivity to macrolide antibiotics
- Pimozide use
- Allergy to anti-infectives
- Pregnancy (first trimester)

Adverse reactions

- Bone marrow depression, pseudomembranous colitis, GI upset, hepatotoxicity, ototoxicity, nephrotoxicity, seizures, nausea, vomiting, diarrhea, thrombophlebitis at infusion site, bronchospasm, cough, neuromuscular reactions, headache, dry mouth, metallic taste

● **Drug examples**
- Azithromycin (Zithromax), aztreonam (Azactam), chloramphenicol (Chloromycetin), clarithromycin (Biaxin, Biaxin XL), clindamycin (Cleocin), erythromycin (E-Mycin, Erythrocin), imipenem and cilastatin (Primaxin), metronidazole (Flagyl), pentamidine (NebuPent, Pentam), vancomycin (Vancocin)

● **Indications**
- Treat infections caused by gram-negative aerobic bacteria (aztreonam)
- Treat severe infections and ampicillin-resistant *Haemophilus influenzae* infections (chloramphenicol)
- Treat infections caused by most aerobic gram-positive organisms (clindamycin)
- Treat infections caused by most gram-positive and gram-negative organisms, pneumococci, and group A streptococci (erythromycin)
- Treat infections caused by gram-positive, gram-negative, and anaerobic organisms (imipenem and cilastatin)
- Treat infection caused by anaerobic organisms, including *Bacteroides* and *Trichomonas vaginalis* (metronidazole)
- Prevent and treat *Pneumocystis carinii* pneumonia in patients who test positive for HIV or who have acquired immunodeficiency syndrome (pentamidine)
- Treat penicillin-resistant staphylococcal infections (vancomycin)

● **Contraindications and precautions**
- Azithromycin, clarithromycin, and erythromycin contraindicated in patients hypersensitive to macrolide antibiotics and those receiving pimozide; used cautiously in patients with renal or hepatic dysfunction
- Aztreonam contraindicated in patients allergic to drug; used cautiously in elderly patients and those with renal or hepatic dysfunction
- Chloramphenicol contraindicated in patients allergic to drug; used cautiously in patients with impaired renal or hepatic function, acute intermittent porphyria, or glucose-6-phosphate dehydrogenase (G6PD) deficiency and in those taking drugs that cause bone marrow suppression or blood disorders
- Metronidazole contraindicated in patients allergic to drug and during first trimester of pregnancy; used cautiously in patients with a history of blood dyscrasias or CNS disorder, patients with hepatic disease or alcoholism, and those taking hepatotoxic drugs

● **Adverse reactions**
- Bone marrow depression (chloramphenicol)
- Pseudomembranous colitis (clindamycin)
- GI upset and hepatotoxicity (erythromycin)
- Ototoxicity and nephrotoxicity (vancomycin)
- Seizures, nausea, vomiting, diarrhea, and thrombophlebitis at infusion site (aztreonam or imipenem and cilastatin)

- Nephrotoxicity, bronchospasm, cough (with nebulizer use), and thrombophlebitis at infusion site (pentamidine)
- Neuromuscular reactions, nausea, headache, dry mouth, and metallic taste (metronidazole)

● **Interactions**
- Use of metronidazole with alcohol may cause a disulfiram-like reaction (nausea, vomiting, tachycardia, flushing, and sweating); use with warfarin may prolong bleeding
- Use of vancomycin with other ototoxic and nephrotoxic drugs may cause additive ototoxicity and nephrotoxicity

● **Nursing responsibilities**
- Institute seizure precautions if the patient is receiving aztreonam or imipenem and cilastatin
- Monitor renal status (urine output and serum BUN and creatinine levels) before, during, and after pentamidine therapy; maintain adequate hydration to minimize risk of nephrotoxicity
- Monitor I.V. infusion site for thrombophlebitis
- Caution the patient to avoid alcohol when taking metronidazole to prevent disulfiramlike reaction
- Assess for cough or shortness of breath after pentamidine inhalation therapy

URINARY TRACT ANTISEPTICS

● **Mechanism of action**
- Bacteriostatic; inhibit growth of many species of bacteria in urine
- Form high concentrations in urine, providing local antibacterial effect within the urinary tract

● **Pharmacokinetics**
- Absorption: Well absorbed from GI tract
- Distribution: Widely distributed
- Metabolism: Metabolized in liver
- Excretion: Excreted in urine

● **Drug examples**
- Sulfonamides: co-trimoxazole (Bactrim, Bactrim DS, Septra), sulfadiazine, sulfisoxazole
- Miscellaneous: methenamine (Hiprex), nalidixic acid, nitrofurantoin (Furadantin, Macrodantin)

● **Indications**
- Treat infections caused by susceptible organisms in urinary tract (sulfonamides); use may be limited in systemic infections because safe doses of drugs don't reach effective levels in plasma
- Prevent recurrent UTIs (methenamine)

When NOT to use urinary tract antiseptics

- Pregnancy
- Breast-feeding
- Children younger than age 2
- Hypersensitivity to sulfa drugs
- Severe renal or hepatic disease
- Porphyria
- History of Stevens-Johnson syndrome

Adverse reactions

- Fever, nausea, vomiting, rash, crystalluria, photosensitivity reaction, blood dyscrasias, Stevens-Johnson syndrome, erythema multiforme, toxic epidermal necrolysis

Key nursing actions

- Assess for signs and symptoms of urinary tract infection.
- Before therapy, obtain specimens for culture and sensitivity tests.
- Make sure the patient maintains a fluid intake of 2 to 3 qt/day to reduce crystalluria.
- Teach about proper hygiene measures to reduce the chance of reinfection.
- Monitor the patient's urinary elimination patterns.
- Teach the patient about the importance of complying with the full course of therapy, even if feeling better.
- Instruct a woman taking hormonal contraceptives to use an alternative contraceptive method (barrier method) during the entire course of therapy.

Contraindications and precautions

- Sulfonamides contraindicated in pregnant and breast-feeding patients, children younger than age 2, patients hypersensitive to sulfa drugs, and those with severe renal or hepatic disease, porphyria, or a history of Stevens-Johnson syndrome
- Sulfonamides used cautiously in patients with mild to moderate renal or hepatic disease, severe allergies, asthma, blood dyscrasias, G6PD deficiency, or urinary obstruction

Adverse reactions

- Fever, nausea, vomiting, rash, crystalluria, photosensitivity reaction, blood dyscrasias (such as agranulocytosis and aplastic anemia), Stevens-Johnson syndrome, erythema multiforme, and toxic epidermal necrolysis (sulfonamides)
- GI upset, hypersensitivity, peripheral neuropathy, and photosensitivity (nitrofurantoin)
- Blood dyscrasias (nalidixic acid and nitrofurantoin)

Interactions

- Sulfonamides may increase effects of oral hypoglycemics, decrease effectiveness of hormonal contraceptives, and increase the risk of bleeding in patients taking oral anticoagulants
- Use of antacids with nitrofurantoin may decrease extent and rate of nitrofurantoin absorption
- Use of probenecid or sulfinpyrazone with nitrofurantoin may inhibit renal excretion of nitrofurantoin, reduce its efficacy, and increase its toxic potential

Nursing responsibilities

- Assess for signs and symptoms of UTI (urinary frequency and urgency, burning on urination, and flank pain)
- Obtain specimens for culture and sensitivity tests before initiating therapy; first dose may be given while results are pending
- Instruct the patient to take nitrofurantoin with food or milk to minimize GI irritation
- Make sure the patient maintains a fluid intake of 2 to 3 qt (2 to 3 L)/day to reduce crystalluria
- Instruct the patient on proper hygiene measures to reduce the chance of reinfection
- Advise the patient to use sunscreen and protective clothing to prevent photosensitivity reactions
- Monitor urinary elimination patterns for changes in quantity or frequency and for dysuria
- Inform the patient that nitrofurantoin may turn urine rusty yellow
- Explain importance of complying with the full course of therapy, even if feeling better; inadequate dosage or premature discontinuation of therapy may exacerbate infection and lead to resistant organisms

- Emphasize that sharing antibacterial drugs may be dangerous
- Instruct the female patient taking hormonal contraceptives to use alternative contraceptive method (barrier method) during entire course of sulfonamide therapy

ANTIFUNGALS

● **Mechanism of action**
  - Kill or inhibit fungal growth by inhibiting protein synthesis within fungal cells or altering the permeability of cell membrane

● **Pharmacokinetics**
  - Absorption: Varies widely; usually well absorbed
  - Distribution: Widely distributed
  - Metabolism: Varies widely
  - Excretion: Varies widely

● **Drug examples**
  - Amphotericin B (Amphocin, Abelcet, Amphotec, AmBisome, Fungizone), caspofungin acetate (Cancidas), clotrimazole (Gyne-Lotrimin, Mycelex), econazole (Spectazole), fluconazole (Diflucan), flucytosine (5-FC [Ancobon]), itraconazole (Sporanox), ketoconazole (Nizoral), miconazole (Micatin, Monistat), nystatin (Mycostatin), terbinafine hydrochloride (Lamisil), voriconazole (Vfend)

● **Indications**
  - Treat serious systemic fungal infections (amphotericin B, caspofungin acetate, fluconazole, flucytosine, and voriconazole)
  - Treat oral and vaginal *Candida* infections (clotrimazole, fluconazole, itraconazole, miconazole, and nystatin)
  - Treat ringworm, athlete's foot, and jock itch (econazole)
  - Treat pulmonary, subcutaneous, and systemic fungal infections (ketoconazole and itraconazole)
  - Treat toenail or fingernail fungus (terbinafine hydrochloride and itraconazole)

● **Contraindications and precautions**
  - Contraindicated in pregnant or breast-feeding patients and those with hypersensitivity to drugs or its components

● **Adverse reactions**
  - Hypersensitivity reactions, nausea, and vomiting
  - Headache, hypotension, hypokalemia, fever, chills, dyscrasias, phlebitis, and nephrotoxicity (amphotericin B)
  - Blood dyscrasias (amphotericin B and flucytosine)
  - Fever, tachycardia, tachypnea, and muscle ache (caspofungin acetate)
  - Possible pruritus and skin irritation (miconazole and econazole)

Key facts about antifungals

- Kill or inhibit fungal growth
- Metabolism and excretion vary by drug

When to use antifungals

- Serious systemic fungal infections
- Oral and vaginal *Candida* infections
- Ringworm
- Athlete's foot
- Jock itch
- Pulmonary, subcutaneous, and systemic fungal infections
- Toenail or fingernail fungus

When NOT to use antifungals

- Hypersensitivity to antifungal drugs or their components
- Pregnancy
- Breast-feeding

Adverse reactions

- Hypersensitivity reactions, nausea, vomiting, headache, hypotension, hypokalemia, fever, chills, dyscrasias, phlebitis, nephrotoxicity, tachycardia, tachypnea, muscle ache, pruritus, skin irritation, rash, diarrhea, dyspepsia, abnormal vision, photosensitivity reactions

Topics for patient discussion

- Medication regimen and administration
- Signs and symptoms to discuss with the practitioner
- Avoidance of occlusive dressings
- Importance of compliance with therapy
- Importance of washing personal articles and kitchen utensils in hot, soapy water to prevent the spread of parasites
- Follow-up care

Key nursing actions

- Before initiating therapy, obtain specimens for culture and sensitivity tests.
- Administer amphotericin B by infusion pump, as ordered, to ensure an accurate rate.
- Monitor the patient closely for reactions, such as fever, chills, nausea, vomiting, headache, and phlebitis.
- Assess infected areas for improvement.
- Monitor the patient's renal and electrolyte status.

- Rash, pruritus, diarrhea, dyspepsia, and headache (terbinafine hydrochloride)
- Fever, rash, abnormal vision, and photosensitivity reactions (voriconazole)

● **Interactions**
- Use of antifungals with other nephrotoxic drugs may cause additive nephrotoxicity
- Use of amphotericin B with diuretics may cause additive hypokalemia
- Use of flucytosine with other bone marrow depressants may cause additive bone marrow depression
- Fluconazole, itraconazole, ketoconazole, and voriconazole may increase effects of oral anticoagulants by increasing prothrombin time
- Use of itraconazole with antidiabetics may increase the risk of hypoglycemia
- Use of ketoconazole with alcohol may increase hepatotoxicity
- Use of itraconazole or voriconazole with pimozide or quinidine may cause prolongation of the QT interval

● **Nursing responsibilities**
- Obtain specimens for culture and sensitivity tests before initiating therapy; first dose may be given pending test results
- Know that amphotericin B is administered only to hospitalized patients or those under close medical supervision
- Administer amphotericin B by infusion pump, as ordered, to ensure accurate rate; many practitioners order a test dose before full infusion to determine patient tolerance
- Monitor closely for drug infusion reaction (fever, chills, nausea, vomiting, headache, and phlebitis) for 1 to 2 hours after each I.V. amphotericin B dose
- Assess infected areas during therapy for improvement in patient's condition
- Monitor renal and electrolyte status
- Instruct the patient not to use an occlusive dressing with topical preparations unless otherwise ordered
- Provide appropriate teaching if the patient is receiving vaginal cream, ointment, tablets, or suppositories
  - Teach her how to apply the preparation
  - Recommend using sanitary napkins to help prevent clothing stains
  - Instruct her to continue treatment during menstruation
  - Advise her to avoid sexual contact or to have her partner wear a condom to prevent reinfection until infection disappears
- Explain that if one family member has a parasitic infection, the entire family must be evaluated
- Instruct the patient and family to wash all personal articles and kitchen utensils in hot, soapy water to prevent spread of parasites

TIME-OUT FOR TEACHING

Teaching about antifungals

Include these topics in your teaching plan for the patient receiving an antifungal:
- medication regimen, including the drug's name, dosage, frequency, duration, and possible adverse effects
- signs and symptoms to discuss with the practitioner, including those related to infection or adverse effects
- proper procedure for administration
- avoidance of occlusive dressings
- importance of compliance with therapy
- follow-up care, including practitioner visits.

- Advise the patient receiving voriconazole to use sunscreen and protective clothing to prevent photosensitivity reactions
- Inform the patient that therapy could take weeks to months
- Explain the importance of complying with therapeutic regimen (see *Teaching about antifungals*)

ANTHELMINTICS

● **Mechanism of action**
- Paralyze parasitic worm (helminth), suppressing egg and larva production and causing its head to detach from the intestinal wall; may also interfere with parasite's cellular function
- Ivermectin: Paralyzes and kills worm
- Praziquantel and pyrantel: Paralyze worm, allowing for its expulsion in stools
- Albendazole and mebendazole: Interfere with worm's glucose use and cellular processes
- Thiabendazole: Interferes with worm's enzyme systems; suppresses egg and larva production in pork roundworm (trichinella)

● **Pharmacokinetics**
- Absorption: Varies with drug
- Distribution: Widely distributed
- Metabolism: Varies with drug
- Excretion: Excreted in urine or feces

● **Drug examples**
- Albendazole (Albenza), ivermectin (Stromectol), mebendazole (Vermox), praziquantel (Biltricide), pyrantel (Pin-Rid, Pin-X), thiabendazole (Mintezol)

● **Indications**
- Treat parasitic worm (helminthic) infections

Key facts about anthelmintics

- Paralyze or kill the worm or interfere with its processes
- Metabolism varies by drug
- Excreted in urine or feces

When to use anthelmintics

- Parasitic worm infections

When NOT to use anthelmintics

- Hepatic disease
- Pregnancy
- Breast-feeding
- Children younger than age 4

Adverse reactions

- Abdominal pain, anorexia, nausea, vomiting, diarrhea, dizziness, drowsiness, headache, and elevated liver enzyme levels

Key nursing actions

- Explain that all family members should be evaluated.
- Teach the patient and family to wash all personal articles and food preparation articles and utensils in hot, soapy water to prevent spread of the parasite.
- Teach the patient and family members to wash hands well, use disposable towels to dry hands, and keep hands away from the mouth.
- Advise the patient to complete the full course of therapy, even if symptoms subside.

Key facts about antivirals

- Inhibit viral replication or prevent viral penetration of host cell
- Metabolism varies by drug
- Excretion varies by drug

● Contraindications and precautions

- Pyrantel contraindicated in patients with hepatic disease and during pregnancy
- Praziquantel used cautiously in pregnant or breast-feeding patients and children younger than age 4
- Mebendazole used cautiously in children younger than age 2

● Adverse reactions

- Abdominal pain, anorexia, nausea, vomiting, diarrhea, dizziness, drowsiness, headache, and elevated liver enzyme levels

● Interactions

- Varies with drug

● Nursing responsibilities

- Be aware that a purgative to facilitate bowel movements may follow administration of these drugs
- Explain why all family members should be evaluated if one member has a parasitic infection
- Instruct the patient and family to wash all personal articles (including sheets and clothes) and food preparation articles and utensils (including cutting boards and knives) in hot, soapy water to prevent spread of parasite
- Instruct the patient and family to wash hands well, use disposable towels to dry hands, and keep hands away from the mouth
- Advise the patient that dizziness and drowsiness may occur; caution against performing hazardous activities until drug's effects are known
- Advise the patient to complete the full course of therapy and not to discontinue drug when symptoms subside
- Instruct the patient not to use drug to treat symptoms of other infections
- Inform the patient that reevaluation will be performed at the recommended interval and that a second course of treatment may be required

ANTIVIRALS

● Mechanism of action

- Inhibit viral replication or prevent viral penetration into host cell; most antivirals inhibit reverse transcriptase (enzyme essential for retroviral DNA synthesis), thereby inhibiting viral replication
- Acyclovir, cidofovir, famciclovir, ganciclovir, valacyclovir, and valganciclovir hydrochloride: Inhibit viral DNA replication
- Amantadine and rimantadine: Prevent penetration of virus into host cells
- Vidarabine and trifluridine: Interfere with DNA synthesis, blocking viral reproduction
- Saquinavir, ritonavir, indinavir sulfate, nelfinavir mesylate, and amprenavir: Protease inhibitors; prevent division of viral polyproteins, which are essential to HIV maturation

- Zanamivir and oseltamivir: Inhibits neuroaminidase on surface of influenza virus, which alters virus particle aggregation and release

● **Pharmacokinetics**
- Varies with drug

● **Drug examples**
- Abacavir sulfate (Ziagen), abacavir sulfate/lamivudine/zidovudine (Trizivir), acyclovir (Zovirax), amantadine (Symmetrel), amprenavir (Agenerase), cidofovir (Vistide), delavirdine mesylate (Rescriptor), didanosine, efavirenz (Sustiva), famciclovir (Famvir), fomivirsen (Vitravene), fosamprenavir (Levixa), foscarnet (Foscavir), ganciclovir (DHPG [Cytovene]), indinavir (Crixivan), lamivudine (3TC [Epivir]), lamivudine/zidovudine (Combivir), lopinavir/ritonavir (Kaletra), nelfinavir (Viracept), nevirapine (Viramune), oseltamivir (Tamiflu), rimantadine (Flumadine), ritonavir (Norvir), saquinavir (Fortovase, Invirase), stavudine (d4T [Zerit]), tenofovir disoproxil fumarate (Viread), tipranavir (Aptivus), trifluridine (Viroptic), valacyclovir (Valtrex), valganciclovir (Valcyte), zalcitabine (ddC [Hivid]), zanamivir (Relenza), zidovudine (AZT [Retrovir])

● **Indications**
- Treat genital herpes simplex, localized cutaneous herpes zoster infections (shingles), and chickenpox (varicella) (acyclovir and valacyclovir)
- Treat herpes simplex encephalitis and serious herpesvirus infections (acyclovir)
- Prevent influenza A viral infection (amantadine and rimantadine)
- Treat ophthalmic herpes simplex (fomivirsen sodium, ganciclovir, and trifluridine)
- Treat cytomegalovirus retinitis (cidofovir, ganciclovir, foscarnet, and valganciclovir)
- Virustatic action in treatment of HIV infection (zidovudine, saquinavir, ritonavir, indinavir sulfate, nelfinavir mesylate, amprenavir, and didanosine)
- Treat advanced HIV infection (zalcitabine used with zidovudine, tenofovir disoproxil fumarate, lamivudine, stavudine, or abacavir sulfate)
- Treat influenza A and B viral infections (zanamivir and oseltamivir phosphate)
- Prevent influenza A and B viral infections (oseltamivir)
- Seroconverting Hepatitis C patients to negative titers (interferon and ribavirin combination is 60% effective)

● **Contraindications and precautions**
- Contraindicated in patients with known or suspected hypersensitivity to these drugs or their components
- Used cautiously in patients with underlying neurologic disease, renal disease, or dehydration and those receiving nephrotoxic drugs

When to use antivirals

- Genital herpes simplex
- Localized cutaneous herpes zoster infections (shingles)
- Chickenpox (varicella)
- Herpes simplex encephalitis
- Influenza A and B viral infection prevention or treatment
- Ophthalmic herpes simplex
- Cytomegalovirus retinitis
- HIV infection

When NOT to use antivirals

- Hypersensitivity to antivirals or their components

Adverse reactions

- Dizziness; ataxia; headache; diarrhea; nausea; vomiting; renal failure; phlebitis at I.V. infusion site; hypotension; anemia; bone marrow depression; granulocytopenia; thrombocytopenia; rash; fever; abnormal liver function test results; vision changes; eye pain; uveitis; vitreitis; pancreatitis; increased intraocular pressure; burning, stinging, tearing, or edema of the eyelid

Key nursing actions

- Administer I.V. infusions by infusion pump, as prescribed.
- Make sure the patient maintains an adequate fluid intake to prevent crystalluria when administering acyclovir
- Monitor the patient's neurologic status.
- Teach the patient how to apply the prescribed topical or ophthalmic drug, as appropriate.
- Caution the patient with infectious skin lesions not to use over-the-counter preparations because they may delay healing.
- Promote abstinence or condom use while lesions are present.

● Adverse reactions

- Dizziness, ataxia, headache, diarrhea, nausea, vomiting, renal failure, and phlebitis at I.V. infusion site (acyclovir)
- Dizziness, ataxia, headache, and hypotension (amantadine)
- Anemia and bone marrow depression (zidovudine)
- Granulocytopenia, thrombocytopenia, anemia, rash, fever, diarrhea, headache, and abnormal liver function test results (ganciclovir and valganciclovir)
- Vision changes, eye pain, uveitis, vitreitis, vomiting, bone marrow suppression, pancreatitis, and increased intraocular pressure (fomivirsen sodium)
- Burning, stinging, tearing, edema of the eyelid, and increased intraocular pressure (trifluridine)
- Fever, nausea, anemia, diarrhea, renal toxicity, headache, and seizures (cidofovir and foscarnet)
- Headache, diarrhea, peripheral neuropathy, and rash (didanosine)
- Neuropathy and pancreatitis (zalcitabine)
- Nausea, bone marrow suppression, rash, fever, paresthesia, peripheral neuropathy, dizziness, and diarrhea (saquinavir, ritonavir, nelfinavir, amprenavir, tenofovir, lamivudine, stavudine, abacavir sulfate, nevirapine, delavirdine, and efavirenz)

● Interactions

- Use of acyclovir, foscarnet, ganciclovir, or cidofovir with similar-acting drugs may cause additive nephrotoxicity
- Use of amantadine with similar-acting drugs may cause additive anticholinergic effects
- Probenecid increases serum levels of acyclovir, ganciclovir, valganciclovir, valacyclovir, and zidovudine, possibly causing toxicity
- Alcohol may increase levels of antivirals, resulting in increased risk of toxicity

● Nursing responsibilities

- Administer I.V. infusions around the clock by infusion pump, as prescribed, to ensure accuracy
- Make sure the patient maintains an adequate fluid intake to prevent crystalluria when administering acyclovir
- Assess lesions daily for changes in color or amount of drainage
- Monitor neurologic status, including level of consciousness, for CNS adverse effects
- Teach the patient how to apply prescribed topical or ophthalmic drug, as appropriate
- Instruct the patient to use gloves when applying topical preparations to prevent the spread of infection and to use strict hand-washing technique
- Caution the patient with infectious skin lesions not to use over-the-counter preparations because they may delay healing

- Advise the patient with genital herpes that acyclovir isn't a cure and won't prevent the spread of infection to others; promote abstinence or condom use while lesions are present (open lesions are contagious)

ANTITUBERCULOTICS

● **Mechanism of action**
- Kill or inhibit growth of *Mycobacterium* organisms that cause TB

● **Pharmacokinetics**
- Varies with drug

● **Drug examples**
- Aminosalicylate (para-amino salicylate, PAS [Paser]), capreomycin (Capastat), cycloserine (Seromycin), ethambutol (Myambutol), ethionamide (Trecator-SC), isoniazid (INH [Nydrazid]), pyrazinamide, rifampin (Rifadin, Rimactane), rifampin/isoniazid (Rifamate), rifampin/isoniazid/pyrazinamide (Rifater), rifapentine (Priftin), streptomycin

● **Indications**
- Firstline treatment of TB (isoniazid and rifampin)
- Adjunct to first-line drugs in treatment of TB when patient is resistant or allergic to less toxic drugs (cycloserine, pyrazinamide, streptomycin, aminosalicylate sodium, capreomycin, ethionamide, rifapentine, and ethambutol)

● **Contraindications and precautions**
- Contraindicated in patients hypersensitive to drug and those with severe liver disease

● **Adverse reactions**
- Nausea, vomiting, and hepatitis
- Neurotoxicity and deficiencies of vitamin B_{12} and folic acid (cycloserine)
- Optic neuritis (ethambutol)
- Peripheral neuropathy (isoniazid)
- Abdominal cramps, diarrhea, headache, hyperuricemia, and ataxia; may turn body fluids red-orange (rifampin and rifapentine)
- Hepatotoxicity (pyrazinamide)
- Ototoxicity (streptomycin)

● **Interactions**
- Antacids delay absorption of isoniazid
- Use of isoniazid with other antituberculotics may cause additive neurotoxicity
- Isoniazid inhibits metabolism of phenytoin and certain other drugs, increasing the risk of toxicity
- Rifampin and rifapentine decrease effectiveness of estrogens, opioid analgesics, oral anticoagulants, hormonal contraceptives, and oral hypoglycemics by increasing hepatic drug metabolizing enzyme activity
- Concurrent use with alcohol increases the risk of hepatotoxicity

Key facts about antituberculotics

- Kill or inhibit growth of *Mycobacterium* organisms that cause TB
- Metabolism varies by drug
- Excretion varies by drug

When to use antituberculotics

- TB

When NOT to use antituberculotics

- Hypersensitivity to antituberculotics
- Severe liver disease

Adverse reactions

- Nausea, vomiting, hepatitis, neurotoxicity, vitamin B_{12} and folic acid deficiencies, optic neuritis, peripheral neuropathy, abdominal cramps, diarrhea, headache, hyperuricemia, ataxia, body fluid color changes, hepatotoxicity, ototoxicity

Topics for patient discussion

- Medication regimen
- Signs and symptoms to discuss with the practitioner
- Body secretion color changes
- Infection-control and safety measures
- Need for long-term compliance
- Importance of avoiding alcohol
- Follow-up care

Key nursing actions

- Assess breath sounds.
- Evaluate sputum for character and amount.
- Before initiating therapy, obtain specimens for culture and sensitivity tests.
- Instruct women to use an effective barrier method of contraception, as appropriate.
- Emphasize the need to comply with therapy, even after the patient feels better.

TIME-OUT FOR TEACHING

Teaching about antituberculotics

Include these topics in your teaching plan for the patient receiving an antituberculotic:
- medication regimen, including the drug's name, dosage, frequency, duration, and possible adverse effects
- signs and symptoms to discuss with the practitioner
- possible changes in color of body secretions
- infection control measures
- need for long term compliance
- safety measures
- follow-up care, including laboratory tests and practitioner visits.

● Nursing responsibilities

- Assess breath sounds, and evaluate sputum for character and amount
- Obtain specimens for culture and sensitivity tests; first dose may be given pending results before initiating therapy
- Instruct the patient to avoid alcohol during drug therapy to prevent hepatotoxicity
- Know that isoniazid is commonly given with pyridoxine (vitamin B6) to reduce peripheral neuropathy
- Assess the patient taking ethambutol for vision changes frequently; vision impairment may be permanent unless identified early
- Warn the patient taking rifampin that drug may color feces, saliva, sputum, sweat, tears, and urine red-orange to red-brown; may also permanently discolor soft contact lenses
- Instruct the female patient taking rifampin to use an effective barrier method of contraception
- Emphasize importance of complying with therapy, even after the patient feels better; 1 to 2 years of therapy may be necessary (see *Teaching about antituberculotics*)

NCLEX CHECKS

It's never too soon to begin your NCLEX® preparation. Now that you've reviewed this chapter, carefully read each of the following questions and choose the best answer. Then compare your responses with the correct answers.

1. A nurse is caring for a client diagnosed with SLE. The client is ordered prednisone, 20 mg four times daily. When giving discharge instructions, the nurse should teach the client to avoid eating:
- ☐ **1.** cold cuts and hot dogs.
- ☐ **2.** canned peaches and beans.
- ☐ **3.** white bread and cooked rice.
- ☐ **4.** fresh fruits and raw vegetables.

2. A client has been ordered oral tetracycline (Sumycin) for a skin infection. The nurse should instruct the client to:

- ☐ **1.** eat fresh fruit to prevent constipation.
- ☐ **2.** stay in direct sunlight as much as possible.
- ☐ **3.** reduce fluid intake to prevent renal failure.
- ☐ **4.** avoid taking the drug with milk or antacids.

3. A nurse knows that a client who's allergic to penicillin may also have a cross-allergy to which class of antibiotics?

- ☐ **1.** Aminoglycosides
- ☐ **2.** Cephalosporins
- ☐ **3.** Macrolides
- ☐ **4.** Sulfas

4. A physician orders co-trimoxazole (Bactrim) for 10 days for a client with a UTI. The client also has diabetes and is taking an oral sulfonylurea. Which instruction by the nurse is appropriate?

- ☐ **1.** Limit fluid intake to 1 qt (1 L) daily.
- ☐ **2.** Take co-trimoxazole with an antacid.
- ☐ **3.** Continue to take the oral antidiabetic as usual.
- ☐ **4.** Drink at least eight 8-oz glasses (240-ml) of fluid daily.

5. A client is receiving amphotericin B (Fungizone) I.V. for a severe systemic fungal infection. Which adverse reaction is most common?

- ☐ **1.** Anuria
- ☐ **2.** Coagulation defects
- ☐ **3.** Peripheral neuropathies
- ☐ **4.** Normochromic or normocytic anemia

6. A client who was diagnosed recently with pulmonary TB is ordered a drug regimen of isoniazid (INH), 300 mg by mouth (P.O.) daily; rifampin (Rifadin), 600 mg P.O. daily; pyridoxine (vitamin B$_6$), 10 mg P.O. daily; ethambutol (Myambutol), 400 mg P.O. daily; and pyrazinamide, 1.5 g P.O. daily. Which statement best explains the rationale for giving these drugs at the same time to treat active TB?

- ☐ **1.** The drugs are bacteriostatic in usual doses.
- ☐ **2.** Rifampin increases the activity of isoniazid.
- ☐ **3.** They're second-line agents and only effective together.
- ☐ **4.** Combination therapy can prevent or delay bacterial resistance.

7. A client with HIV is beginning an antiretroviral regimen. To reduce the risk of developing HIV infection that's resistant to the drug, he would need to take which drug without missing doses?

- ☐ **1.** Didanosine
- ☐ **2.** Nevirapine (Viramune)
- ☐ **3.** Ritonavir (Norvir)
- ☐ **4.** Zidovudine (AZT)

TOP 8

Items to study for your next test on drugs and the immune system

1. Mechanism of action of corticosteroids, immunosuppressants, antibacterials, antifungals, anthelmintics, antivirals, and antituberculotics

2. General characteristics of penicillins, cephalosporins, aminoglycosides, tetracyclines, fluoroquinolones, and urinary tract antiseptics

3. Indications for corticosteroids, immunosuppressants, antibacterials, antifungals, anthelmintics, antivirals, and antituberculotics

4. Common adverse effects of corticosteroids, immunosuppressants, the various classes of antibacterials, antifungals, anthelmintics, antivirals, and antituberculotics

5. Nursing responsibilities when administering corticosteroids, immunosuppressants, antibacterials, antifungals, anthelmintics, antivirals, and antituberculotics

6. Teaching for patients receiving corticosteroids, immunosuppressants, antibacterials, antifungals, antivirals, or antituberculotics

7. Precautions for preventing infection in immunosuppressed patients

8. Teaching for patients infected with helminths and their families

8. After undergoing small-bowel resection, a client is ordered metronidazole (Flagyl) 500 mg I.V. The mixed I.V. solution contains 100 ml. The nurse is to run the drug over 30 minutes. The drip factor of the available I.V. tubing is 15 gtt/ml. What's the drip rate? Record your answer as a whole number.

_____ gtt/minute

9. A client is being discharged on 60 mg of prednisone (Orasone) daily. Which instruction should the nurse give the client?
- ☐ **1.** Stop taking the medication if you experience heartburn.
- ☐ **2.** Take the medication at bedtime.
- ☐ **3.** Eat a high-protein, low-sodium diet.
- ☐ **4.** Restrict your intake of potassium-rich foods.

10. Which client should a nurse expect to be a candidate for aminoglycoside therapy?
- ☐ **1.** A pregnant client with a UTI
- ☐ **2.** A 5-year-old child with meningitis
- ☐ **3.** A client with an infected diabetic foot ulcer and renal failure
- ☐ **4.** A client who's scheduled for intestinal surgery

ANSWERS AND RATIONALES

1. CORRECT ANSWER: 4
Because of the immunosuppressive effects of prednisone, the client is more susceptible to infection. Fresh fruits and raw vegetables tend to have higher levels of bacteria than cooked foods, thereby increasing the client's risk of infection. Cold cuts and hot dogs have high levels of sodium, which will increase the fluid retention commonly associated with prednisone, but this effect isn't as serious as the potential for life-threatening infections. Canned peaches and beans, white bread, and cooked rice aren't contraindicated with prednisone therapy.

2. CORRECT ANSWER: 4
Milk and antacids reduce the absorption of tetracyclines. Therefore, tetracyclines should be given 1 hour before or 2 hours after ingesting a dairy product or an antacid. Diarrhea, not constipation, is an adverse reaction to tetracyclines. Sunlight should be avoided because tetracycline can cause photosensitivity. Fluid intake should be increased, not reduced, to prevent renal failure.

3. CORRECT ANSWER: 2
Cephalosporins and penicillins are chemically related. Cephalosporins have a cross-allergy rate of about 10%. Aminoglycosides, macrolides, and sulfas aren't chemically related to penicillins.

4. CORRECT ANSWER: 4
Sulfonamides such as co-trimoxazole may cause crystalluria. Increasing fluid intake to 64 ounces daily will increase urine output (which should be 1,500 ml daily), possibly preventing crystalluria. Limiting fluid intake is just the opposite of what should be recommended. Co-trimoxazole interacts with sulfonylureas to

produce increased hypoglycemic effects, so the dose of the oral antidiabetic may have to be adjusted and the client's glucose level carefully monitored. Co-trimoxazole doesn't need to be taken with an antacid.

5. CORRECT ANSWER: 4
Most clients receiving I.V. amphotericin B develop normochromic or normocytic anemia that will significantly decrease hemoglobin level and hematocrit. Although up to 80% of clients receiving amphotericin B may develop some degree of nephrotoxicity, anuria isn't a common complication. Amphotericin B isn't known to cause coagulation defects or peripheral neuropathies.

6. CORRECT ANSWER: 4
Mycobacterium tuberculosis can rapidly develop bacterial resistance to isoniazid and rifampin, so they're given with other antituberculotics in combination to prevent or delay bacterial resistance. Rifampin doesn't increase the activity of isoniazid. All of the drugs listed are bactericidal, except for ethambutol, which is the only one that's bacteriostatic in usual doses. Not all of the drugs listed are second-line agents.

7. CORRECT ANSWER: 3
Ritonavir, a protease inhibitor, requires maximum compliance and must be taken consistently. HIV can easily become resistant in the presence of low concentrations of drug, and clients who don't take all doses are at risk for developing a resistant organism. Although resistance can develop with didanosine, nevirapine, and zidovudine, these drugs aren't as concentration-dependent as protease inhibitors.

8. CORRECT ANSWER: 50
To determine the drip rate, use this equation:
$$100 \text{ ml}/30 \text{ minutes} \times 15 \text{ gtt}/1 \text{ ml} = 49.9 \text{ gtt/minute (50 gtt/minute)}.$$

9. CORRECT ANSWER: 3
Glucocorticoids cause protein catabolism and stimulate aldosterone secretion, which causes sodium retention and potassium secretion. Therefore, a diet high in protein and low in sodium is needed. Prednisone should never be abruptly stopped. It should be taken in the early morning to mimic the normal body secretion of cortisol. Potassium-rich foods should be encouraged, not restricted.

10. CORRECT ANSWER: 4
Aminoglycosides, such as kanamycin or neomycin, may be used before surgery to reduce the normal flora content of the intestinal tract. At therapeutic doses, aminoglycosides can cross the placenta but not the blood-brain barrier; therefore, their use is contraindicated during pregnancy. Aminoglycosides aren't the treatment of choice for meningitis in children; they're more commonly used for treating *Pseudomonas* and *Escherichia coli* infections. Because the major organ of elimination of aminoglycosides is the kidney, these drugs shouldn't be given to a client with renal failure.

13

Drugs and cancer

PRETEST

1. Nitrogen mustards belong to which antineoplastic drug group?

- ☐ 1. Alkylating agents
- ☐ 2. Antibiotic antineoplastics
- ☐ 3. Antimetabolites
- ☐ 4. Hormonal antineoplastics

CORRECT ANSWER: 1

2. Which adverse reaction is most commonly associated with antineoplastic therapy?

- ☐ 1. Anemia
- ☐ 2. Leukopenia
- ☐ 3. Thrombocytopenia
- ☐ 4. Bone marrow suppression

CORRECT ANSWER: 4

3. Which laboratory value should a nurse closely monitor in any client receiving an antineoplastic?

- ☐ 1. Potassium
- ☐ 2. Sodium
- ☐ 3. White blood cell count
- ☐ 4. Creatinine

CORRECT ANSWER: 3

4. While spiking a piggyback drug bag that contains a chemotherapy agent, the nurse splashes some of the drug on her hand and arm. Her first action should be to:

- ☐ 1. finish hanging the I.V., then call the practitioner.
- ☐ 2. rinse the area with water, then call the practitioner.
- ☐ 3. pat the area with a gauze pad before rinsing it.
- ☐ 4. wipe off the fluid and get a new piggyback bag because the old one was contaminated.

CORRECT ANSWER: 2

5. A nurse should instruct a client taking imatinib (Gleevec) to take the medication:

- ☐ 1. with food.
- ☐ 2. on an empty stomach.
- ☐ 3. at bedtime.
- ☐ 4. with water only.

CORRECT ANSWER: 1

LEARNING OBJECTIVES

After studying this chapter, you should be able to:

- Identify major classifications and mechanisms of action of drugs used to treat cancer.
- List major adverse effects of alkylating drugs, antitumor antibiotics, antimetabolites, hormonal drugs, drugs alternating hormone response, vinca alkaloids and natural products, monoclonal antibodies, targeted therapies, and topoisomerase I inhibitors.
- Discuss nursing responsibilities and patient teaching required when administering cancer drugs.
- Describe precautions the nurse must take for self-protection when administering cancer drugs.

CHAPTER OVERVIEW

Cancer drugs, or *antineoplastics*, destroy cancer cells and normal tissue, especially rapidly dividing cells. This factor, along with the adverse effects and toxicity of antineoplastics, may limit their dosage or use. Therefore, combination therapy is usually used to kill as many cancerous cells as possible while avoiding toxic effects.

A&P highlights

- Proliferation: process of cell renewal and replacement
- In cancer, the proliferation process becomes unbalanced because normal control mechanisms can't halt the process.
- Differentiation: process by which cells diversify, acquire specific structural and functional characteristics, and mature
- In cancer, cells are poorly differentiated.
- Cells and tumors may be benign or malignant.
- Cells have altered biochemical properties, chromosomal instability, and the capacity to metastasize.
- Two types of antineoplastics: cell-cycle specific (act on cells undergoing division in the cell cycle) and cell-cycle nonspecific (act on cells during any phase of the cell cycle).
- Goal of cancer treatment is to kill cancer cells without destroying normal healthy cells by interfering with cancer-cell replication.

ANATOMY AND PHYSIOLOGY

⬤ **Anatomy of cancer**
  - Is disorder of cell differentiation and replication
  - Can affect any organ or body system

⬤ **Physiology**
  - Proliferation
    - Refers to the process of cell renewal and replacement
    - Is normally balanced
    - Is affected by cancer because normal control mechanisms can't halt proliferation and process becomes unbalanced
  - Differentiation
    - Refers to process by which cells diversify, acquire specific structural and functional characteristics, and mature
    - Is affected by cancer; the more undifferentiated the tumor cell, the more malignant the tumor

⬤ **Characteristics of cancer cells**
  - Have uncontrolled proliferation
  - Have altered biochemical properties (such as hormone secretion)
  - Chromosomal instability
    - Cell mutations—caused by alterations in deoxyribonucleic acid (DNA)
    - Genetic instability—causes new mutations with unique characteristics that are increasingly resistant to therapy
  - May metastasize (spread from the primary site to secondary sites); degree of cell malignancy correlates with its metastatic capacity

⬤ **Types of antineoplastic drugs**
  - Cell-cycle specific
    - Act on cells undergoing division in cell cycle (see *Chemotherapy's action in the cell cycle*)
    - Include antimetabolites and vinca plant alkaloids
    - Are effective against rapidly growing tumors
  - Cell-cycle nonspecific
    - Act on cells during any phase of cell cycle, whether undergoing division or in resting state
    - Include antitumor antibiotics, alkylating agents, hormones, and steroids
    - Are most effective against slow-growing tumors

Chemotherapy's action in the cell cycle

Some chemotherapeutic drugs are cell-cycle specific, impairing cellular growth by causing changes in the cell during specific phases of the cell cycle. Other drugs are cell-cycle nonspecific, affecting the cell at any phase during the cell cycle. The illustration below shows where the cell-cycle specific drugs work to disrupt cancer cell growth.

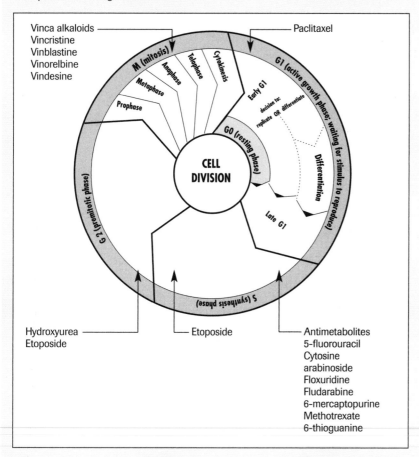

Vinca alkaloids
Vincristine
Vinblastine
Vinorelbine
Vindesine

Paclitaxel

M (mitosis)
Cytokinesis
Anaphase
Telophase
Metaphase
Prophase

G1 (active growth phase; waiting for stimulus to reproduce)
Early G1
decision to:
replicate OR differentiate
Differentiation

G0 (resting phase)

CELL DIVISION

G 2 (premitotic phase)

Late G1

S (synthesis phase)

Hydroxyurea
Etoposide

Etoposide

Antimetabolites
5-fluorouracil
Cytosine
arabinoside
Floxuridine
Fludarabine
6-mercaptopurine
Methotrexate
6-thioguanine

● **Cancer treatment**
- Tries to kill cancerous cells without destroying normal healthy cells by interfering with cancer-cell replication
- Involves combination therapy
  - Combines different classes of antineoplastics to maximize therapeutic response, leading to synergistic and additive qualities as well as various toxicities
  - Is used because single-agent therapy is usually unsuccessful in attaining long-term remission and increases risk of drug resistance
  - May involve combining antineoplastics with other treatments (surgery, radiation)

ALKYLATING DRUGS

- **Mechanism of action**
  - Affect the synthesis of DNA by causing cross-linking of DNA to inhibit cell reproduction (see *How alkylating drugs work*)
  - Cell-cycle nonspecific action; effective against rapidly growing tumors

- **Pharmacokinetics**
  - Absorption: Most drugs rapidly absorbed after oral administration
  - Distribution: Widely distributed
  - Metabolism: Metabolized in liver
  - Excretion: Excreted in urine

- **Drug examples**
  - Nitrogen mustards: chlorambucil (Leukeran), cyclophosphamide (Cytoxan, Neosar), estramustine (Emcyt), ifosfamide (Ifex), mechlorethamine (nitrogen mustard [Mustargen]), melphalan (Alkeran)
  - Alkyl sulfonates: busulfan (Busulfex, Myleran)
  - Nitrosoureas: carmustine (BiCNU, Gliadel), lomustine (CeeNU), streptozocin (Zanosar)
  - Triazenes: dacarbazine (DTIC [DTIC-Dome])
  - Ethylenimines: thiotepa (Thioplex)
  - Alkylating-like drugs: carboplatin (Paraplatin), cisplatin (Platinol-AQ)

- **Indications**
  - Treat many types of cancers, including but not limited to leukemia, brain tumors, multiple myeloma, Hodgkin's disease, non-Hodgkin's lymphoma, malignant melanoma, ovarian cancer, lung cancer, head and neck tumors, breast cancer, testicular tumors, prostatic cancer, osteosarcoma, and neuroblastoma; indications vary for each drug

- **Contraindications and precautions**
  - Contraindicated in pregnant patients and those with suppressed white or red blood cells and platelets or renal or liver failure
  - Busulfan contraindicated in patients with chronic myelogenous leukemia that has shown prior resistance to drug
  - Mechlorethamine contraindicated in patients with infectious disease
  - Used cautiously in patients with bone marrow depression, history of seizures, or hepatic impairment

- **Adverse reactions**
  - Fatigue, bone marrow suppression, nausea, vomiting, stomatitis, and alopecia (nitrogen mustards)
  - Bone marrow suppression, anemia, thrombocytopenia, pulmonary fibrosis, and seizures (alkyl sulfonates)
  - Nausea, vomiting, bone marrow suppression, and kidney toxicity and failure; carmustine may also cause liver and lung toxicity (nitrosoureas)

How alkylating drugs work

Alkylating drugs can attack deoxyribonucleic acid (DNA) in two ways, as shown in the illustrations below.

BIFUNCTIONAL ALKYLATION

Some drugs become inserted between two base pairs in the DNA chain, forming an irreversible bond between them. This is called bifunctional alkylation, which causes cytotoxic effects that can destroy or poison cells.

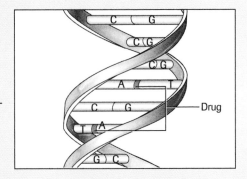

Drug

MONOFUNCTIONAL ALKYLATION

Other drugs react with just one part of a pair, separating it from its partner and eventually causing it and its attached sugar to break away from the DNA molecule. This is called monofunctional alkylation, which eventually may cause permanent cell damage.

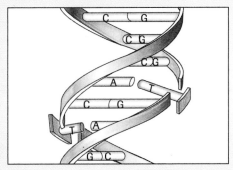

- Leukopenia, anemia, thrombocytopenia, pancytopenia, nausea, vomiting, stomatitis, hives, and pruritus (ethylenimines)
- Leukopenia, thrombocytopenia, nausea, vomiting, photosensitivity, flulike syndrome, and alopecia (triazenes)
- Bone marrow suppression, kidney toxicity, neurotoxicity, tinnitus, nausea, and vomiting (alkylating-like drugs)

● **Interactions**
- Use with other ototoxic and nephrotoxic drugs may cause additive ototoxicity and nephrotoxicity
- Cyclophosphamide may increase cardiac effects if taken with other cardiotoxic drugs
- Cimetidine taken with carmustine increases bone marrow toxicity
- Thiotepa taken with neuromuscular blockers may prolong muscle paralysis
- Aminoglycosides increase risk of nephrotoxicity of alkylating-like drugs

Adverse reactions

- Nausea and vomiting, stomatitis, bone marrow depression, pulmonary fibrosis, tinnitus, nephrotoxicity, alopecia, hemorrhagic cystitis, hepatotoxicity, skin reactions

Key nursing actions

- Ensure safe preparation and handling of antineoplastic drugs.
- Reduce pain with I.V. administration by altering the infusion rate, further diluting the drug, or warming the injection site to distend the vein and increase blood flow.
- When administering cisplatin, frequently assess for dizziness, tinnitus, hearing loss, incoordination, and numbness or tingling of extremities.
- Monitor for signs of hemorrhagic cystitis.
- Monitor for phlebitis with I.V. administration.
- Monitor for hemorrhagic cystitis (with cyclophosphamide or ifosfamide)
- Tell the patient to notify the practitioner immediately if fever, sore throat, unusual bleeding, or signs and symptoms of infection occur.

● Nursing responsibilities

- Prepare I.V. antineoplastic solutions in biologic cabinet to ensure safety; always wear gloves, gown, and mask when handling antineoplastic I.V. drugs
- Discard drug and any I.V. equipment used in specified containers according to facility policy
- Reduce pain with I.V. administration, as ordered, by altering the infusion rate, further diluting drug, or warming the injection site to distend the vein and increase blood flow
- Frequently assess for dizziness, tinnitus, hearing loss, incoordination, and numbness or tingling of extremities when administering cisplatin; such adverse effects may be irreversible
- Be aware that these drugs are given in short, high-dose, intermittent courses to maximize antineoplastic effects while allowing normal cells to recover
- Know that extravasation may cause tissue necrosis; if extravasation occurs, intervene as specified by facility protocol
- Monitor complete blood count (CBC), white blood cell count (WBC) differential, and platelet count; institute isolation precautions if the WBC count is low
- Assess for nausea and vomiting; give an antiemetic if needed
- Monitor for signs and symptoms of phlebitis with I.V. administration; many antineoplastics irritate the veins
- Monitor for signs of hemorrhagic cystitis (such as hematuria or dysuria) during cyclophosphamide or ifosfamide therapy
- Take bleeding precautions if thrombocytopenia occurs; avoid I.M. injections and venipunctures as much as possible
- Promote fluid intake (at least 2 qt [2 L] daily) to maintain adequate renal function
- Instruct the patient to notify the practitioner immediately if fever, sore throat, unusual bleeding, or signs and symptoms of infection occur
- Advise the patient to avoid crowds and those with infections to minimize the risk of infection
- Advise the patient to consult the practitioner before receiving any vaccinations
- Instruct the patient to use a soft toothbrush and an electric razor to decrease the risk of bleeding
- Instruct the patient to avoid alcohol (to decrease the risk of toxicity) and aspirin-containing products (to reduce the risk of bleeding)
- Warn the patient that drug may cause hair loss but that hair usually returns
- Know that many antineoplastics have teratogenic effects; explain the need for contraception during therapy, and discuss the effects of antineoplastics on fertility
- Instruct the patient to inspect the inside of the mouth for redness or ulcers and to rinse his mouth after meals if stomatitis occurs

ANTITUMOR ANTIBIOTICS

- **Mechanism of action**
  - Interfere with DNA and ribonucleic acid (RNA) synthesis
  - Cell-cycle nonspecific action
- **Pharmacokinetics**
  - Absorption: Administered I.V.
  - Distribution: Widely distributed
  - Metabolism: Metabolized in liver
  - Excretion: Excreted in urine
- **Drug examples**
  - Bleomycin (Blenoxane), dactinomycin (actinomycin D [Cosmegen]), daunorubicin (liposomal [DaunoXome]), daunorubicin, doxorubicin (Adriamycin), doxorubicin (liposomal [Doxil]), epirubicin (Ellence), idarubicin (Idamycin), mitomycin (Mutamycin), mitoxantrone (Novantrone), valrubicin (Valstar)
- **Indications**
  - Treat squamous cell carcinoma of the head and neck, lymphomas, Hodgkin's disease, embryonal cell carcinoma, bone carcinoma, Kaposi's sarcoma, and melanoma
  - Treat malignant pleural effusions and prevent recurrent pleural effusions (bleomycin)
- **Contraindications and precautions**
  - Contraindicated during pregnancy
  - Dactinomycin contraindicated in patients with chickenpox or herpes zoster
  - Doxorubicin contraindicated in patients with marked myelosuppression induced by previous antitumor drugs or radiotherapy or those who have had a lifetime cumulative dose of 550 mg/m^2 of doxorubicin or daunorubicin
  - Used cautiously in patients with liver or renal disease
- **Adverse reactions**
  - Alopecia, stomatitis, nausea, vomiting, anorexia, gonadal suppression, hyperuricemia, and phlebitis at I.V. site
  - Heart failure, myocardial toxicity, cardiomyopathy, electrocardiographic changes, and arrhythmias (daunorubicin, doxorubicin, epirubicin, and idarubicin)
  - Urinary tract infections, bladder pain, incontinence, and cystitis (valrubicin)
- **Interactions**
  - These drugs may decrease digoxin levels
  - Cardiotoxicity may increase if drugs are given with irradiation or cyclophosphamide

Key facts about antitumor antibiotics

- Interfere with DNA and ribonucleic acid synthesis
- Cell-cycle nonspecific
- Metabolized in liver
- Excreted in urine

When to use antitumor antibiotics

- Squamous cell carcinoma of the head and neck
- Lymphomas
- Hodgkin's disease
- Embryonal cell carcinoma
- Bone carcinoma
- Kaposi's sarcoma
- Melanoma
- Malignant pleural effusions

When NOT to use antitumor antibiotics

- Pregnancy
- Chickenpox
- Herpes zoster
- Myelosuppression induced by previous antitumor drugs or radiotherapy or a lifetime cumulative dose of 550 mg/m^2 of doxorubicin or daunorubicin

Adverse reactions

- Alopecia, stomatitis, nausea, vomiting, anorexia, gonadal suppression, hyperuricemia, phlebitis at the I.V. site, heart failure, myocardial toxicity, cardiomyopathy, electrocardiographic changes, arrhythmias, urinary tract infections, bladder pain, incontinence, cystitis

272 DRUGS AND CANCER

- Use with probenecid may increase the risk of hyperuricemia
- Concurrent use with vinca alkaloids may cause serious bronchospasms

● **Nursing responsibilities**
- Assess for signs and symptoms of heart failure (dyspnea, crackles, peripheral edema, and weight gain) when administering daunorubicin or idarubicin
- Assess for signs and symptoms of myocardial toxicity (dyspnea, arrhythmias, hypotension, and weight gain) when administering doxorubicin, epirubicin, or idarubicin.
- Monitor vital signs frequently during administration

ANTIMETABOLITES

● **Mechanism of action**
- Replace normal proteins required for DNA synthesis, thereby interfering with DNA and RNA synthesis
- Cell-cycle specific action

● **Pharmacokinetics**
- Absorption: Varies widely with drug
- Distribution: Varies widely with drug
- Metabolism: Metabolized in liver
- Excretion: Excreted in urine

● **Drug examples**
- Capecitabine (Xeloda), cytarabine (ARAC-DNR, cytosine arabinoside [Cytosar-U]), floxuridine (FUDR), fludarabine (Fludara), fluorouracil (5--FU [Adrucil]), hydroxyurea (Hydrea), mercaptopurine (6-MP [Purinethol]), methotrexate (Rheumatrex), pentostatin (Nipent), thioguanine (6-thioguanine, TG)

● **Indications**
- Treat acute myelogenous, acute lymphocytic, acute nonlymphocytic, and chronic myelogenous leukemia; non-Hodgkin's lymphoma; GI carcinomas; and breast and cervical carcinomas
- Treat painful sickle cell crises and reduce need for blood transfusions in patients with sickle cell anemia (hydroxyurea)

● **Contraindications and precautions**
- Contraindicated in pregnant patients and those with bone marrow suppression caused by previous chemotherapy or renal or liver toxicity
- Because cross-resistance to some drugs in this category occurs, patients with known resistance to mercaptopurine or thioguanine shouldn't receive further therapy with antimetabolites

● **Adverse reactions**
- Hepatotoxicity, GI disturbances, and myelosuppression

Key nursing actions

- When administering daunorubicin or idarubicin, assess for signs and symptoms of heart failure.
- When administering doxorubicin, epirubicin, or idarubicin, assess for signs and symptoms of myocardial toxicity

Key facts about antimetabolites

- Replace normal proteins required for DNA synthesis; interfere with DNA and RNA synthesis
- Cell-cycle specific
- Metabolized in liver
- Excreted in urine

When to use antimetabolites

- Acute myelogenous leukemia
- Acute lymphocytic leukemia
- Acute nonlymphocytic leukemia
- Chronic myelogenous leukemia
- Non-Hodgkin's lymphoma
- GI carcinomas
- Breast and cervical carcinomas
- Painful sickle cell crises

When NOT to use antimetabolites

- Pregnancy
- Bone marrow suppression
- Resistance to mercaptopurine or thioguanine

TIME-OUT FOR TEACHING

Teaching about antimetabolites

Include these topics in your teaching plan for the patient receiving an antimetabolite:

- medication regimen, including the drug's name, dosage, frequency, duration, and possible adverse effects
- signs and symptoms to discuss with the practitioner
- infection-control measures
- measures to combat common adverse reactions
- fluid requirements
- bleeding precautions
- energy conservation measures
- follow-up care, including laboratory tests and practitioner visits
- community resources for support, guidance, and education.

- Fatigue, paresthesia, abdominal pain, constipation, intestinal obstruction, hyperbilirubinemia, hand-and-foot syndrome, dermatitis, and fever (capecitabine)
- Alopecia, stomatitis, hyperuricemia, thrombophlebitis, and hepatotoxicity (cytarabine)
- Thromboembolic events, GI bleeding, renal failure, urinary tract infections, hepatotoxicity, myalgia, pneumonia, edema, fatigue, and alopecia (fludarabine)
- Alopecia, stomatitis, diarrhea, phototoxicity reactions, bone marrow suppression, and cerebellar dysfunction (fluorouracil)
- Hyperuricemia and hepatotoxicity (mercaptopurine)
- Alopecia, stomatitis, hyperuricemia, hepatotoxicity, pulmonary toxicity, seizures, and photosensitivity (methotrexate)

● **Interactions**

- Concurrent use of mercaptopurine or methotrexate with other hepatotoxic drugs causes additive hepatotoxicity
- Allopurinol decreases metabolism of mercaptopurine, increasing the risk of toxicity
- Chloramphenicol, oral hypoglycemics, phenytoin, probenecid, salicylates, and tetracyclines increase the risk of methotrexate toxicity

● **Nursing responsibilities**

- Assess for signs and symptoms of cerebellar dysfunction (dizziness, weakness, and ataxia) and stomatitis and diarrhea (which may necessitate drug discontinuation) when administering flourouracil; also monitor for bone marrow suppression
- Make sure the patient receives leucovorin (folinic acid or citrovorum factor ["leucovorin rescue"]) to prevent fatal toxicity when administering methotrexate in large doses
- Instruct the patient to use sunscreen and protective clothing to prevent photosensitivity reactions when administering fluorouracil or methotrexate (see *Teaching about antimetabolites*)

Key facts about hormonal drugs and drugs altering hormone response

- Suppress the immune system
- Block synthesis of RNA and new proteins
- Alter cell metabolism
- Metabolized in liver
- Excreted in urine, feces, or bile; some may be reabsorbed by intestines

When to use hormonal drugs and drugs altering hormone response

- Advanced breast cancer (postmenopausal and high-risk)
- Advanced prostate cancer
- Endometriosis and endometrial cancer
- Central precocious puberty
- Anemia related to uterine fibroids
- Anorexia, cachexia, or unexplained weight loss

When NOT to use hormonal drugs and drugs altering hormone response

- Estrogen-dependent neoplasia or thrombophlebitis
- Prostate cancer
- Male breast cancer
- Premenopause
- Genital cancer
- Abnormal vaginal bleeding

Mechanism of action

- Suppress the immune system and block synthesis of RNA and new proteins
- Alter cell metabolism by changing the hormonal environment of normal hormones in hormone sensitive tumors

Pharmacokinetics

- Absorption: Usually rapidly absorbed
- Distribution: Widely distributed
- Metabolism: Metabolized in liver
- Excretion: Excreted in urine, feces, or bile; some drug may be reabsorbed by intestines

Drug examples

- Aminoglutethimide (Cytadren), anastrozole (Arimidex), bicalutamide (Casodex), estramustine phosphate (Emcyt), exemestane (Aromasin), flutamide (Eulexin), fulvestrant (Faslodex), goserelin (Zoladex), letrozole (Femara), leuprolide (Lupron), megestrol (Megace), mitotane (Lysodren), nilutamide (Nilandron), prednisone (Deltasone), tamoxifen (Nolvadex), testolactone (Teslac), testosterone (Delatestryl), toremifene (Fareston), triptorelin (Trelstar Depot, Trelstar LA)

Indications

- Treat advanced breast cancer in postmenopausal women and advanced prostate cancer
- Palliative treatment in advanced cancers
- Treat endometriosis, central precocious puberty, and anemia related to uterine fibroids (leuprolide acetate)
- Treat endometrial cancer and anorexia, cachexia, or unexplained weight loss in patients with acquired immunodeficiency syndrome (AIDS) (megestrol acetate)
- Primary breast cancer prevention in high-risk patients (tamoxifen)

Contraindications and precautions

- Estrogens contraindicated in patients with estrogen-dependent neoplasia or thrombophlebitis
- Androgens contraindicated in patients with prostate cancer or male breast cancer and in premenopausal females
- Progesterones are contraindicated in patients with genital cancer or abnormal vaginal bleeding

Adverse reactions

- Headache, asthenia, nausea, pain, and hot flashes (anastrozole)

- Constipation, nausea, diarrhea, nocturia, hematuria, impotence, gynecomastia, peripheral edema, dyspnea, back pain, generalized pain, asthenia, pelvic pain, infection, and hot flashes (bicalutamide, flutamide, and nilutamide)
- Edema and hypercalcemia (tamoxifen and testosterone)
- Impotence and gynecomastia in males (testosterone)
- Depression, insomnia, anxiety, fatigue, pain, nausea, dyspnea, and hot flashes (exemestane)
- Breast tenderness, painful gynecomastia, edema, thromboembolic events, and skin irritations (estramustine)
- Headache, dizziness, nausea, vomiting, bone pain, asthenia, injection site pain, and cough (fulvestrant)
- Increased risk of thromboembolic events (tamoxifen and letrozole)
- Heart failure, arrhythmias, cataracts, dry eyes, thromboembolic events, hepatotoxicity, hypercalcemia, hot flashes, sweating, nausea, and vaginal bleeding or discharge (toremifene)

● **Interactions**
- Testosterone may alter the effects of insulin, oral anticoagulants, and oral hypoglycemics
- Drugs containing calcium may impair estramustine absorption
- Tamoxifen decreases effectiveness of estrogens
- Toremifene, testolactone, tamoxifen, and flutamide may increase warfarin's activity and increase the risk of bleeding

● **Nursing responsibilities**
- Warn the patient that she may experience severe bone pain when tamoxifen is administered because it's a sign of drug's effectiveness
- Reassure the patient that bone pain will resolve over time and may be controlled with analgesics

VINCA ALKALOIDS AND NATURAL PRODUCTS

● **Mechanism of action**
- Inhibit DNA or RNA synthesis and prevent mitosis, causing cell death
- Cell-cycle specific action

● **Pharmacokinetics**
- Absorption: Most drugs administered I.V.
- Distribution: Widely distributed
- Metabolism: Metabolized in liver
- Excretion: Excreted in urine

Adverse reactions

- Headache, asthenia, nausea, pain, hot flashes, constipation, diarrhea, nocturia, hematuria, impotence, gynecomastia, dyspnea, infection, edema, hypercalcemia, depression, insomnia, anxiety, fatigue, breast tenderness, thromboembolic events, skin irritations, dizziness, vomiting, cough, heart failure, arrhythmias, cataracts, dry eyes, hepatotoxicity, sweating, vaginal bleeding or discharge

Key nursing actions

- When administering tamoxifen, warn that it may cause severe bone pain.
- Reassure patient that such pain will resolve over time and may be controlled with analgesics.

Key facts about vinca alkaloids and natural products

- Inhibit DNA or RNA synthesis
- Prevent mitosis
- Cell-cycle specific
- Metabolized in liver
- Excreted in urine

When to use vinca alkaloids and natural products

- Testicular cancer
- Non-Hodgkin's lymphoma
- Breast cancer
- Lung cancer
- Head and neck cancer
- Neuroblastomas

When NOT to use vinca alkaloids and natural products

- Pregnancy
- Myelosuppression from previous chemotherapy or radiation
- Baseline neutrophil count below 1,500/mm^3
- AIDS or severe bacterial infection
- Pancreatitis
- History of hemorrhagic event

Adverse reactions

- Peripheral neuropathy, alopecia, stomatitis, anorexia, constipation, hyperuricemia, phlebitis at the I.V. infusion site, bradycardia, acute bronchospasms, myelosuppression

Key nursing actions

- Premedicate patients receiving paclitaxel with diphenhydramine, dexamethasone, and an H$_2$ antagonist.
- Always wear gloves when preparing drug.

Key facts about monoclonal antibodies

- Bind to target receptor or cancer cells and induce programmed cell death
- Metabolized in tissue
- Excreted in urine

● **Drug examples**
- Asparaginase (Elspar), docetaxel (Taxotere), etoposide (VePesid), paclitaxel (Taxol), pegaspargase (Oncaspar), teniposide (Vumon), vinblastine (Velban), vincristine (Oncovin), vinorelbine (Navelbine)

● **Indications**
- Treat testicular cancer, non-Hodgkin's lymphoma, breast cancer, lung cancer, head and neck cancer, and neuroblastomas

● **Contraindications and precautions**
- Contraindicated in pregnant patients, patients with myelosuppression from previous chemotherapy or radiation, patients with a baseline neutrophil count below 1,500/mm^3, and those with AIDS or severe bacterial infections
- Pegaspargase contraindicated in patients with pancreatitis and those who have suffered a hemorrhagic event while on L-asparaginase therapy
- Used cautiously in patients with liver impairment

● **Adverse reactions**
- Peripheral neuropathy, alopecia, stomatitis, anorexia, constipation, hyperuricemia, phlebitis at I.V. infusion site, bradycardia, acute bronchospasms, and myelosuppression

● **Interactions**
- Concurrent use of prednisone may enhance hyperglycemia, neurotoxicity, and myelosuppression
- Use with phenytoin may decrease phenytoin levels

● **Nursing responsibilities**
- Premedicate the patient receiving paclitaxel with diphenhydramine, dexamethasone, and a histamine-2 (H$_2$) antagonist to prevent hypersensitivity reactions
- Always wear gloves when preparing drug

MONOCLONAL ANTIBODIES

● **Mechanism of action**
- Bind to target receptor or cancer cells and cause tumor death by inducing programmed cell death
- Recruit other elements of the immune system to attack the cancer cell

● **Pharmacokinetics**
- Absorption: Usually administered I.V.; not given orally (large protein molecules prevent absorption)
- Distribution: Limited
- Metabolism: Metabolized in tissue; has long half-life
- Excretion: Excreted in urine

Drug examples
- Alemtuzumab (Campath), gemtuzumab (Mylotarg), ibritumomab (Zevalin), rituximab (Rituxan), trastuzumab (Herceptin)

Indications
- Treat non-Hodgkin's lymphoma (ibritumomab, rituximab)
- Treat metastatic breast cancer (trastuzumab)
- Treat chronic lymphocytic leukemia (alemtuzumab)
- Treat acute myeloid leukemia (gemtuzumab)

Contraindications and precautions
- Contraindicated in pregnant or breast-feeding patients and those with a previous hypersensitivity to drug or its components
- Used cautiously in patients with cardiac disease and bone marrow depression
- Gemtuzumab contraindicated in patients with known liver disease

Adverse reactions
- Fever, chills, shortness of breath, hypotension, anaphylaxis with infusion, malaise, headache, nausea, vomiting, diarrhea, anemia, and pain
- Serious cardiac toxicity, heart failure, and ventricular arrhythmias (trastuzumab)
- Myelosuppression and increased opportunistic infections (alemtuzumab)
- Tumor lysis syndrome, hyperuricemia, and liver toxicity (gemtuzumab)

Interactions
- Trastuzumab increases the risk of anthracycline cardiac toxicity
- Warfarin, aspirin, clopidogrel, ticlopidine, nonsteroidal anti-inflammatories, azathioprine, cyclosporine, and corticosteroids increase cytopenia when given with ibritumomab

Nursing responsibilities
- Administer trastuzumab in a dedicated line with no other solutions or additives
- Monitor for infusion reactions while drug is infusing and for 1 hour after infusion has completed; administering acetaminophen or diphenhydramine before infusion may help decrease the risk of transfusion reaction
- Monitor hemoglobin, hematocrit, and platelet count while the patient is taking drug
- Don't administer drug if the patient has a systemic infection
- Monitor liver function tests while the patient is taking gemtuzumab

TARGETED THERAPIES

Mechanism of action
- Target proteins associated with the growth patterns of specific cancers

---

When to use monoclonal antibodies
- Non-Hodgkin's lymphoma
- Metastatic breast cancer
- Chronic lymphocytic leukemia
- Acute myeloid leukemia

When NOT to use monoclonal antibodies
- Pregnant or breast-feeding patients
- Hypersensitivity
- Liver disease

Adverse reactions
- Fever, chills, hypotension, anaphylaxis with infusion, nausea, vomiting, diarrhea, anemia, serious cardiac toxicity, tumor lysis syndrome, liver toxicity

Key nursing actions
- Administer trastuzumab in a dedicated line with no other solutions or additives.
- Monitor for infusion reactions while the drug is infusing and for 1 hour after the infusion is complete.
- Don't administer if the patient has a systemic infection.

Key facts about targeted therapies
- Target proteins associated with the growth of specific cancers
- Metabolized in liver
- Excreted in feces

When to use targeted therapies

- Multiple myeloma
- Non-small-cell lung cancer
- Acute lymphocytic leukemia
- Chronic myeloid leukemia

When NOT to use targeted therapies

- Pregnant or breast-feeding patients
- Use caution with hepatic or renal dysfunction

Adverse reactions

- Fever, nausea, vomiting, diarrhea, abdominal pain, neutropenia, severe hepatotoxicity, interstitial lung disease, cerebral hemorrhage

Key nursing actions

- Weigh the patient daily.
- Monitor CBC closely.
- Administer with food if GI upset occurs.

Key facts about topoisomerase I inhibitors

- Inhibits topoisomerase I resulting in impaired DNA synthesis
- Metabolized in liver
- Excreted in urine and bile

- ● **Pharmacokinetics**
  - Absorption: Usually absorbed orally; bortezomib given I.V. because of poor oral absorption
  - Distribution: Widely distributed in tissue
  - Metabolism: Metabolized in liver
  - Excretion: Excreted in feces

- ● **Drug examples**
  - Bortezomib (Velcade), gefitinib (Iressa), imatinib (Gleevec)

- ● **Indications**
  - Treat multiple myeloma (bortezomib)
  - Treat non-small-cell lung cancer (gefitinib)
  - Treat chronic myeloid leukemia, acute lymphoid leukemia, GI stromal tumors (imatinib)

- ● **Contraindications and precautions**
  - Drugs must be used for specific tumors and cancers that contain targeted protein
  - Contraindicated in pregnant or breast-feeding patients
  - Used cautiously in patients with hepatic or renal dysfunction

- ● **Adverse reactions**
  - Malaise, insomnia, headache, abdominal pain, nausea, vomiting, diarrhea, anorexia, GI irritation, neutropenia, thrombocytopenia, cough, myalgia, fever, rash, and fatigue
  - Severe hepatotoxicity (bortezomib)
  - Abnormal eyelash growth, acne, and interstitial lung disease (gefitinib)
  - Cerebral hemorrhage, edema, epistaxis, and hypokalemia (imatinib)

- ● **Interactions**
  - Clarithromycin, erythromycin, itraconazole, and ketoconazole may increase targeted-therapy drug level of gefitinib or imatinib
  - Rifampin and phenytoin may decrease targeted-therapy drug levels of gefitinib and imatinib
  - H_2-receptor antagonist may decrease gefitinib level
  - Use with antiplatelets or anticoagulants may increase bleeding

- ● **Nursing responsibilities**
  - Weigh the patient daily
  - Monitor CBC closely
  - Give drug with food if the patient has GI upset
  - Monitor liver function test while the patient is receiving gefitinib

TOPOISOMERASE I INHIBITORS

- ● **Mechanism of action**
  - Inhibit the enzyme topoisomerase I, resulting in impaired DNA synthesis

- ● **Pharmacokinetics**
  - Absorption: Administered I.V.

- Distribution: Binds to albumin
- Metabolism: Metabolized in liver
- Excretion: Excreted in urine and bile

● **Drug examples**
  - Irinotecan (Camptosar), topotecan (Hycamtin)

● **Indications**
  - Treat solid tumors and hematologic malignancies

● **Contraindications and precautions**
  - Contraindicated in breast-feeding patients
  - Used cautiously in patients with bone marrow depression or diarrhea

● **Adverse reactions**
  - Abdominal pain and cramping, alopecia, anemia, anorexia, asthenia, myalgia, constipation, dyspnea, fever, headache, nausea, stomatitis, and vomiting
  - Diarrhea, insomnia, edema, rhinitis, dyspepsia, cough, and infection (irinotecan)
  - Significant myelosuppression, neutropenia, leucopenia, and thrombocytopenia (topotecan)

● **Interactions**
  - Ketoconazole increases the risk of toxicity when administered with irinotecan
  - Laxatives increase the chance of diarrhea with irinotecan
  - Prochlorperazine causes increased extrapyramidal toxicities when given with irinotecan
  - Fluorouracil and leucovorin may cause thromboembolic event when given with irinotecan

● **Nursing responsibilities**
  - Obtain baseline neutrophil and platelet counts and CBC
  - Don't administer diuretics with irinotecan when the patient is experiencing diarrhea or active vomiting
  - Monitor closely for diarrhea and subsequent dehydration

NCLEX CHECKS

It's never too soon to begin your NCLEX® preparation. Now that you've reviewed this chapter, carefully read each of the following questions and choose the best answer. Then compare your responses with the correct answers.

1. A client newly diagnosed with lung cancer is beginning chemotherapy. Which instruction is appropriate for the nurse to give this client?
- ☐ **1.** Increase daily fluid intake to 2 to 3 qt (2 to 3 L).
- ☐ **2.** Stay in direct sunlight as much as possible.
- ☐ **3.** Avoid brushing your teeth to prevent gum bleeding.
- ☐ **4.** Avoid eating for 6 hours after chemotherapy to prevent nausea.

When to use topoisomerase I inhibitors

- Solid tumors
- Hematologic malignancies

When NOT to use topoisomerase I inhibitors

- Breast-feeding patients
- Use caution in patients with bone marrow depression or diarrhea

Adverse reactions

- Abdominal pain, alopecia, anemia, constipation, fever, stomatitis, vomiting, infection, significant myelosuppression

Key nursing actions

- Obtain baseline neutrophil count, platelet count, and CBC.
- Monitor closely for diarrhea and dehydration.

TOP 5

Items to study for your next test on drugs and cancer

1. The rationale for using antineoplastics to treat cancer
2. Major adverse effects of antineoplastics
3. Nursing responsibilities when administering antineoplastics
4. Precautions the nurse must take for self-protection when administering antineoplastics
5. Appropriate teaching for the patient who is receiving an antineoplastic

2. A client taking antineoplastics develops leukopenia. Which nursing intervention has the highest priority?

☐ **1.** Assign the client to a private room.
☐ **2.** Use an electric shaver to help prevent cuts.
☐ **3.** Wear a gown and gloves when giving a bed bath.
☐ **4.** Dispose of the client's urine in a biohazard container.

3. A client asks about a drug to prevent breast cancer. Which agent is indicated for the primary prevention of breast cancer in females at high risk for developing breast cancer?

☐ **1.** Cyclophosphamide (Cytoxan)
☐ **2.** Ethinyl estradiol (Desogen)
☐ **3.** Methotrexate (Folex)
☐ **4.** Tamoxifen (Nolvadex)

4. A client receives the alkyl sulfonate busulfan (Myleran) for chronic myelogenous leukemia. The nurse assesses the client regularly for adverse drug reactions. Which adverse respiratory reaction is caused by long-term therapy?

☐ **1.** Asthma attacks
☐ **2.** Pulmonary fibrosis
☐ **3.** Pulmonary hypertension
☐ **4.** Chronic obstructive pulmonary disease (COPD)

5. A client is taking fluorouracil (Adrucil) for breast cancer. Stomatitis is a common adverse reaction to fluorouracil. The nurse should also assess for what other adverse reaction?

☐ **1.** Heart failure
☐ **2.** Pulmonary infiltrates
☐ **3.** Severe renal dysfunction
☐ **4.** Bone marrow suppression

6. A client who's receiving chemotherapy for breast cancer develops myelosuppression. Which instruction should the nurse include in the client's discharge teaching plan? Select all that apply.

☐ **1.** Avoid people who have recently received attenuated vaccines.
☐ **2.** Avoid activities that may cause bleeding.
☐ **3.** Wash hands frequently.
☐ **4.** Consume more fresh fruits and vegetables.
☐ **5.** Avoid crowded places such as shopping malls.
☐ **6.** Treat a sore throat with over-the-counter products.

7. A client is taking vinblastine (Velban) for ovarian cancer. The nurse should anticipate which complaint from the client?

☐ **1.** "I can't seem to sleep at night."
☐ **2.** "My heart keeps skipping beats."
☐ **3.** "The tips of my fingers have a tingling, numb feeling."
☐ **4.** "I'm having problems with regular bowel movements."

8. A client who's being treated with high-dose methotrexate (Folex) and folinic acid (Leucovorin) is seen in the clinic. Which laboratory test result indicates to the nurse that the client hasn't been taking folinic acid as directed?

- ☐ **1.** Platelet count of 150,000/mm³
- ☐ **2.** WBC count of 0.1/mm³
- ☐ **3.** Hemoglobin level of 16 mg/dl
- ☐ **4.** Hematocrit of 45%

9. A client takes megestrol (Megace) for advanced breast cancer. The nurse knows that the most common adverse reaction associated with megestrol is:

- ☐ **1.** dizziness.
- ☐ **2.** constipation.
- ☐ **3.** blurred vision.
- ☐ **4.** mild fluid retention.

10. A client has been taking doxorubicin (Adriamycin), fluorouracil (Adrucil), and cyclophosphamide (Cytoxan) for breast cancer. After six cycles, he reports dyspnea on exertion, pedal edema, and a cough. On physical examination, crackles and rhonchi are heard in both lung fields, and the client is afebrile. The nurse understands that the most likely explanation for these findings is:

- ☐ **1.** doxorubicin toxicity.
- ☐ **2.** tumor metastasis to the lung.
- ☐ **3.** chemotherapy-induced infection.
- ☐ **4.** fluorouracil pulmonary toxicity.

ANSWERS AND RATIONALES

1. CORRECT ANSWER: 1
The nurse should instruct the client to increase his daily fluid intake. Because many antineoplastics are nephrotoxic, increased fluid intake to 2 to 3 qt is recommended to decrease the risk of renal toxicity and prevent renal failure. Most chemotherapeutic agents cause photosensitivity, so avoiding exposure to sunlight is recommended. The client should be instructed to perform good oral care using a soft toothbrush. Avoiding food intake for 6 hours after treatment may increase nausea.

2. CORRECT ANSWER: 1
Leukopenia (low WBC count) is a common adverse reaction to many antineoplastics. Clients with leukopenia are more susceptible to infections, so a private room is necessary to reduce the risk of a nosocomial infection. Antineoplastics don't suppress the platelet count, so bleeding precautions aren't warranted and use of an electric shaver is unnecessary. Wearing a gown and gloves isn't necessary; however, practicing good hand-washing technique, using gloves when the risk of contact with any body fluids is probable, or wearing a face mask if a cough or obvious respiratory tract infection is present would be appropriate. The client's urine should be handled in the same manner as other body secretions.

3. CORRECT ANSWER: 4
Tamoxifen is indicated for primary breast cancer prevention in high-risk clients. How it works isn't fully clear, but it's an estrogen antagonist and may prevent tumor growth resulting from endogenous estrogen. Many breast cancers are estrogen-receptor positive; therefore, giving ethinyl estradiol would stimulate tumor growth. Cyclophosphamide and methotrexate are indicated for chemotherapy, not prevention.

4. CORRECT ANSWER: 2
Pulmonary fibrosis is an adverse reaction to long-term busulfan therapy; pulmonary tissue becomes fibrotic and interferes with normal oxygenation. Busulfan isn't known to cause COPD, pulmonary hypertension, or asthma attacks.

5. CORRECT ANSWER: 4
Bone marrow suppression, as evidenced by neutropenia and thrombocytopenia, is an adverse reaction to fluorouracil. Fluorouracil isn't known to cause pulmonary infiltrates, severe renal dysfunction, or heart failure.

6. CORRECT ANSWER: 1, 2, 3, 5
Chemotherapy can cause myelosuppression (reduced numbers of red blood cells, WBCs, and platelets). A client receiving chemotherapy needs to avoid people who have been vaccinated recently because he may contract the illness from the vaccination due to his immunocompromised status. Because platelet counts are reduced, the client also needs to avoid activities that could cause trauma and bleeding. The client should wash her hands frequently because hand washing is the best way to prevent the spread of infection. A client receiving chemotherapy should avoid crowded places, as well as people with colds during the flu season, because of the reduced ability to fight infection. Fresh fruits and vegetables should be avoided because they can harbor bacteria that can't be removed easily by washing. Signs and symptoms of infection, such as a sore throat, fever, and a cough, should be reported immediately to the physician.

7. CORRECT ANSWER: 3
Tingling and numbness of the extremities is a common adverse reaction to vinblastine because of its CNS effects. Irregular pulse, insomnia, and constipation aren't associated with this drug. Vinblastine usually produces diarrhea, not constipation.

8. CORRECT ANSWER: 2
High doses of methotrexate can cause fatal bone marrow toxicity; therefore, folinic acid is given at the same time to decrease this risk. A WBC count of $0.1/mm^3$ is indicative of bone marrow toxicity and suggests that the client hasn't been complying with the prescribed regimen. The platelet, hemoglobin, and hematocrit levels are all normal and not a concern.

9. CORRECT ANSWER: 4

Fluid retention is a common adverse reaction to megestrol and is usually dose-dependent. If it occurs, a dosage adjustment is recommended. If a dosage adjustment isn't possible, the client may need a sodium-restricted diet or diuretics. Megestrol acetate isn't known to cause blurred vision, constipation, or dizziness.

10. CORRECT ANSWER: 1

Doxorubicin toxicity commonly manifests as heart failure. It's more likely to occur toward the end of chemotherapy, when the total dose has approached 500 to 550 mg/m^2. Although it isn't possible to rule out metastasis, this presentation is more consistent with heart failure. If infection were present, the client would have other symptoms, such as fever and a productive cough. Fluorouracil doesn't cause pulmonary toxicity.

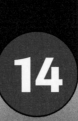

14

Drugs and the gastrointestinal system

PRETEST

1. Which class of drugs inhibits GI motility and gastric secretions?
- [ ] 1. Cholinergic blockers
- [ ] 2. Histamine-2 blockers
- [ ] 3. Proton pump inhibitors
- [ ] 4. 5-HT$_3$-receptor antagonists

CORRECT ANSWER: 1

2. Digestants work by:
- [ ] 1. binding to toxins in the GI tract.
- [ ] 2. creating a film on the intestine to help disperse gas pockets.
- [ ] 3. increasing the water content of stools.
- [ ] 4. reproducing the action of the substance they're replacing.

CORRECT ANSWER: 4

3. When teaching about potential adverse reactions, the nurse warns the client that blackening of the mouth, tongue, and stools can occur with which drug?
- [ ] 1. Aluminum hydroxide (Amphojel)
- [ ] 2. Bismuth subsalicylate (Pepto-Bismol)
- [ ] 3. Cimetidine (Tagamet)
- [ ] 4. Sucralfate (Carafate)

CORRECT ANSWER: 2

4. Which drug can be used only after a client signs a physician-client agreement?

☐ 1. Esomeprazole (Nexium)

☐ 2. Tegaserod (Zelnorm)

☐ 3. Alosetron (Lotronex)

☐ 4. Nizatidine (Axid)

CORRECT ANSWER: 3

5. How long before bedtime should a nurse administer sucralfate?

☐ 1. 1 hour

☐ 2. 45 minutes

☐ 3. 30 minutes

☐ 4. 15 minutes

CORRECT ANSWER: 1

LEARNING OBJECTIVES

After studying this chapter, you should be able to:

● Describe the major uses and mechanisms of action of the various types of drugs used to treat the GI system.

● List the major adverse effects of antiulceratives, adsorbents, antiflatulents, digestants, antiemetics, antidiarrheals, and laxatives.

● Identify important nursing responsibilities and teaching topics required for patients receiving different classes of GI system drugs.

CHAPTER OVERVIEW

Antiulceratives neutralize or block the release of hydrochloric acid and provide a barrier to the gastric mucosa. Aluminum hydroxide, used to neutralize hydrochloric acid, may also be used in renal failure to bind phosphate.

Adsorbents are used to bind to toxins in the GI tract to decrease systemic absorption. Antiflatulents foam in the GI tract, creating a film along the intestinal wall that helps disperse gas pockets. Digestants supplement or replace deficient digestive substances normally produced by the body, such as amylase and lipase.

Antiemetics are used to prevent or control nausea and vomiting secondary to pathologic conditions, drugs, toxins, radiation, or motion sickness. These drugs may be administered orally, I.M., rectally, or transdermally.

Antidiarrheals are used to control or treat acute or nonspecific diarrhea. Laxatives are used to treat constipation or to clean the bowel before surgery or diagnostic studies. Bulk-forming laxatives may help incorporate water into stools and are occasionally used to treat diarrhea. Lactulose may also be used to decrease ammonia levels in hepatic encephalopathy.

5-HT$_3$-receptor antagonists decrease GI motility and the perception of pain in patients with irritable bowel disease. 5-HT$_4$-receptor agonists stimulate the release of serotonin in the GI tract, which helps normalize peristalsis and relieves the pain and discomfort associated with irritable bowel disease and chronic constipation.

ANATOMY AND PHYSIOLOGY

- **Anatomy**
  - GI system
    - Is a continuous tube open at both ends
    - Consists of oral cavity, pharynx, esophagus, stomach, and small and large intestines
    - Is surrounded by peritoneum
  - Small intestine structures: duodenum, jejunum, ileum
  - Large intestine structures: cecum, vermiform appendix, colon (ascending, transverse, descending, and sigmoid), rectum, anus
  - Accessory organs: gastrin glands, liver, gallbladder, pancreas
- **Physiology**
  - Digestion
    - Begins in oral cavity, where food and liquid are propelled through esophagus, into stomach, and through small and large intestine
    - Propelled via mechanisms of peristalsis (rhythmic contraction of smooth muscle) and segmenting contractions (alternating contraction and relaxation of adjacent intestinal segments)
      - Esophageal sphincter—keeps swallowed foods and gastric juices in stomach; failure to close or remain closed causes gastroesophageal reflux disease (GERD)

A&P highlights

- The GI system consists of the oral cavity, pharynx, esophagus, stomach, and small and large intestines.
- Accessory organs include gastrin glands, the liver, the gallbladder, and the pancreas.
- Digestion begins in the oral cavity.
- Food and liquid are propelled through the GI tract via peristalsis and segmenting contractions.
- A normally functioning esophageal sphincter keeps swallowed foods and gastric juices in the stomach.
- GI hormones regulate gastric secretions and motility.
- Gastric acid secretion is prompted by the sight, smell, or anticipation of food.
- After food is in the stomach, gastrin stimulates secretion of gastric acids from the parietal cells.
- Gastric acid also activates pepsinogen to form pepsin, which digests proteins.
- The major nutrients in the body are carbohydrates, proteins, and lipids; they are digested in the GI tract by enzymes and are then absorbed by the small intestines.
- Digested carbohydrates are converted to glucose, which supplies energy.
- Proteins are absorbed as amino acids, which are converted to protein or glucose or catabolized for energy.
- Lipids are stored in adipose tissue for later use as energy.

- Peristalsis—propels fecal material into rectum and causes the defecation reflex; if abnormal, can lead to constipation, diarrhea, or both (as in irritable bowel syndrome)
  - Aided by GI hormones (gastrin, gastric inhibitory peptides, secretin, and cholecystokinin), which regulate gastric secretions and motility
    - Gastric acid secretion—prompted by sight, smell, or anticipation of food
    - Gastrin—released in response to food in stomach and duodenum and stimulates secretion of gastric acids from parietal cells
    - Gastric acid—activates the gastric enzyme precursor pepsinogen to form pepsin, which digests proteins by breaking peptide bonds
- Nutrients
  - Include carbohydrates, proteins, and lipids
    - Are digested in GI tract by enzymes that hydrolyze them into smaller units
    - Are absorbed from small intestine
  - Digested carbohydrates
    - Are converted to glucose, which supplies the body and cells with energy
    - Are catabolized in three phases: glycolysis, citric acid cycle, and electron transport system
  - Ingested proteins
    - Are absorbed as amino acids
    - Must be converted to protein or glucose or catabolized for energy, which occurs by deamination and transamination
  - Lipids
    - Are stored in adipose (fat) tissue
    - Are hydrolyzed when the body needs energy

● **Function of the GI system**
- Obtains and processes almost all of the body's nutrient intake and needs (including energy and building materials required for daily activities, growth, and repair)
  - Stomach—serves as a temporary storage area for food, which remains there until it's partially digested
  - Small intestine—completes digestion and absorbs most of the nutrients, water, and electrolytes in foods
  - Large intestine absorbs water and minerals and eliminates digestive waste products; intestinal bacteria also release intestinal gases and synthesize vitamin K and some B vitamins, which are absorbed in colon
  - Peritoneum—lines walls of the abdominal cavity; holds intestines and other GI organs in place with peritoneal folds (mesenteries)
- Involves accessory organs, which produce or store secretions used in digestion
  - Liver

Functions of GI structures

- The stomach is a temporary storage and digestion area for food.
- The small intestines complete the digestion of food; they're also the site of nutrient, water, and electrolyte absorption.
- The large intestines absorb water and minerals and eliminate digestive waste products; intestinal bacteria in the large intestines release intestinal gases and synthesize vitamin K and some B vitamins.
- The peritoneum lines the walls of the abdominal cavity; the folds of the peritoneum hold the intestines and other GI organs in place.

Functions of accessory GI organs

- The liver produces bile, blood proteins, lipoproteins, and proteins involved with blood coagulation. It also stores fat, glycogen, iron, and vitamins A, B_{12}, D, E, and K; detoxifies and excretes wastes and toxins; and excretes cholesterol.
- The gallbladder stores and concentrates bile.
- The exocrine pancreas secretes digestive enzymes.
- The endocrine pancreas secretes hormones.

- Has digestive, metabolic, and regulatory functions
- Produces bile (chief digestive function); bile acts as a fat emulsifier in small intestine
- Produces blood proteins, such as albumin and globulin, lipoproteins, and proteins involved with blood coagulation
- Stores small reserve of fat, glycogen, iron, and vitamins (A, B_{12}, D, E, and K)
- Detoxifies or excretes many wastes and toxins; it also excretes cholesterol
- Gallbladder—stores and concentrates bile secreted by liver
- Exocrine pancreas—contains cells that secrete digestive enzymes into the duodenum via the pancreatic duct; pancreatic fluid contains amylase to digest starch; trypsin, chymotrypsin, and carboxypeptidase to digest proteins; lipase to digest certain lipids; cholesterol esterase to digest cholesterol esters; and ribonuclease and deoxyribonuclease to digest nucleic acids
- Endocrine pancreas—secretes hormones (such as glucagon, insulin, and somatostatin) directly into bloodstream
  - Glucagon, epinephrine, growth hormone, cortisol, and thyroxine increase the blood glucose level
  - Insulin decreases blood glucose level

ANTIULCERATIVES

ANTACIDS

Key facts about antacids

- Neutralize gastric acid, thereby increasing the pH in the GI tract
- Metabolism action unknown
- Excreted in feces and breast milk

- **Mechanism of action**
  - Neutralize gastric acid, thereby increasing pH in the GI tract
- **Pharmacokinetics**
  - Absorption: Minimally absorbed
  - Distribution: Distributed throughout GI tract
  - Metabolism: Unknown
  - Excretion: Excreted in feces; some may be excreted in breast milk
- **Drug examples**
  - Aluminum hydroxide (AlternaGEL, Amphojel), aluminum hydroxide and magnesium hydroxide (Gaviscon, Gelusil, Maalox, Mylanta), calcium carbonate (Tums), magaldrate (aluminum-magnesium complex [Riopan]), magnesium hydroxide (Mag-Ox, Milk of Magnesia)

When to use antacids

- Indigestion
- Reflux esophagitis
- Peptic ulcers
- Renal failure

- **Indications**
  - Treat indigestion, reflux esophagitis, and peptic ulcers
  - Bind dietary phosphate in renal failure (calcium carbonate)

Contraindications and precautions
- Contraindicated in abdominal pain of unknown origin, heart failure, hypertension, and gastric outlet destruction
- Used cautiously in pregnant patients or those with renal failure

Adverse reactions
- Constipation, diarrhea, electrolyte imbalances, and serum aluminum accumulation

Interactions
- Antacids decrease absorption of quinolones, iron, isoniazid, ketoconazole, phenytoin, and digoxin if administered within 2 hours of each other
- Antacids cause premature dissolution of enteric-coated tablets

Nursing responsibilities
- Know that antacids containing both aluminum and magnesium hydroxide balance the constipating effects of aluminum with the laxative effects of magnesium
- Instruct the patient to shake the suspension well, or, if taking chewable tablets, to chew them thoroughly and then drink half a glass of water to promote passage to stomach
- Give antacids at least 1 hour apart from enteric-coated tablets
- Teach the patient who has heart failure or hypertension or who must restrict sodium intake to check antacid labels for sodium content and to use only low-sodium preparations
- Instruct the patient not to take antacids for more than 2 weeks or for recurring problems without consulting a practitioner (see *Teaching about antacids*)
- Flush with enough water to make sure the drug reaches the stomach and the tube is clear if administering through a nasogastric (NG) tube
- Assess the patient for epigastric or abdominal pain, frank bleeding, and occult bleeding

TIME-OUT FOR TEACHING
Teaching about antacids

Include these topics in your teaching plan for the patient receiving an antacid:
- medication regimen, including the drug's name, dose, frequency, duration, and possible adverse effects
- signs and symptoms to discuss with the practitioner

- possible dietary interactions
- measures to promote bowel elimination
- avoidance of over-the-counter self-medication
- follow-up care.

- Teach the patient to avoid gastric irritants (alcohol, smoking, products containing aspirin, caffeine, nonsteroidal anti-inflammatory drugs [NSAIDs], and foods that cause GI irritation); these may counteract drug effects and worsen the ulcer

Histamine-2 RECEPTOR ANTAGONISTS

● **Mechanism of action**
- Inhibit gastric acid secretion by inhibiting the action of histamine at histamine-2 (H_2) receptors in gastric parietal cells

● **Pharmacokinetics**
- Absorption: Most drugs absorbed rapidly and completely
- Distribution: Widely distributed throughout body; cimetidine crosses placental barrier and appears in breast milk
- Metabolism: Metabolized by the liver
- Excretion: Primarily excreted in bile

● **Drug examples**
- Cimetidine (Tagamet, Tagamet HB), famotidine (Pepcid, Pepcid AC), nizatidine (Axid), ranitidine (Zantac)

● **Indications**
- Long-term treatment of pathologic GI hypersecretory conditions (Zollinger-Ellison syndrome)
- Promote healing of duodenal and gastric ulcers
- Decrease gastric acid production and prevent stress ulcers in severely ill patients and those with reflux esophagitis or upper GI bleeding
- Treat heartburn, acid indigestion, and sour stomach (over-the-counter preparations)

● **Contraindications and precautions**
- Contraindicated in breast-feeding patients and those with known hypersensitivity
- Used cautiously in pregnant patients, those with impaired renal or hepatic function, and elderly patients (because of increased risk of central nervous system [CNS] effects, such as dizziness and confusion)

● **Adverse reactions**
- Headache, dizziness, confusion, mild diarrhea, and rash

● **Interactions**
- Cimetidine may cause increased serum levels and consequent toxicity of benzodiazapenes, calcium channel blockers, tricyclic antidepressants, procainamide, lidocaine, oral anticoagulants, phenytoin, propranolol, quinidine, and theophylline
- Antacids may inhibit absorption of H_2-receptor antagonists
- Cimetidine administered with carmustine increases the risk of bone marrow toxicity

---

Key facts about H_2-receptor antagonists

- Inhibit gastric acid secretion by inhibiting the action of histamine at H_2 receptors in gastric parietal cells
- Metabolized by the liver
- Primarily excreted in bile

When to use H_2-receptor antagonists

- Active duodenal ulcers
- Gastric hypersecretory states
- Prophylaxis for stress ulcer
- Heartburn
- Acid indigestion
- Sour stomach

When NOT to use H_2-receptor antagonists

- Breast-feeding
- Hypersensitivity to H_2-receptor antagonists

Adverse reactions

- Headache, mild diarrhea, dizziness, confusion

Nursing responsibilities

- Teach the patient that smoking worsens ulcer disorders and counteracts the effects of H_2-receptor antagonists
- Don't give an antacid within 1 hour of administering drug; may decrease absorption of drug
- Caution the patient about possible dizziness; recommend avoidance of hazardous activities that require alertness
- Assess for epigastric or abdominal pain, frank bleeding, and occult bleeding
- Teach the patient to avoid gastric irritants (smoking, alcohol, products containing aspirin, caffeine, NSAIDs, and foods that cause GI irritation), which may counteract drug effects and worsen the ulcer

PROTON PUMP INHIBITORS

Mechanism of action

- Block gastric acid secretions by inhibiting acid pump in gastric parietal cells

Pharmacokinetics

- Absorption: Rapidly absorbed in small intestines
- Distribution: Highly protein-bound
- Metabolism: Extensively metabolized in liver
- Excretion: Eliminated by kidneys

Drug examples

- Esomeprazole (Nexium), lansoprazole (Prevacid), omeprazole (Prilosec, Prilosec OTC), pantoprazole (Protonix), rabeprazole (Aciphex)

Indications

- Treat erosive esophagitis and GERD
- Treat duodenal ulcer
- Short-term treatment of active gastric ulcer
- Long-term treatment of hypersecretory conditions
- Eradicate *Helicobacter pylori* infection (esomeprazole, lansoprazole, omeprazole, and rabeprazole)
- Prevent and treat NSAID-related gastric ulcers (lansoprazole)

Contraindications and precautions

- Contraindicated in patients with known hypersensitivity
- Used cautiously in pregnant and breast-feeding patients

Adverse reactions

- Abdominal pain, nausea, vomiting, and diarrhea

Interactions

- May interfere with metabolism of diazepam, phenytoin, and warfarin, increasing their half-lives and plasma levels

Key nursing actions

- Don't give an antacid within 1 hour of administering H_2-receptor antagonists.
- Assess the patient for epigastric or abdominal pain, frank bleeding, and occult bleeding.
- Teach the patient to avoid gastric irritants, such as smoking, alcohol, aspirin-containing products, caffeine, NSAIDs, and foods that cause GI irritation.

Key facts about proton pump inhibitors

- Block gastric acid secretions by inhibiting the acid pump in the gastric parietal cells
- Extensively metabolized in liver
- Eliminated by kidneys

When to use proton pump inhibitors

- Erosive esophagitis
- GERD
- Duodenal ulcer
- Gastric ulcer
- Hypersecretory conditions
- *H. pylori* infection
- NSAID-related gastric ulcers

When NOT to use proton pump inhibitors

- Hypersensitivity to proton pump inhibitors
- Pregnancy
- Breast-feeding

Adverse reactions

- Diarrhea, abdominal pain, nausea, vomiting

Key nursing actions

- Administer 1 hour before meals.
- Teach the patient to swallow capsules whole.
- Teach the patient to avoid gastric irritants, such as smoking, alcohol, aspirin-containing products, caffeine, NSAIDs, and foods that cause GI irritation.

Key facts about local-acting drugs

- Protect the gastric mucosa by coating the ulcer crater
- Metabolism is unknown
- Excreted in feces

When to use local-acting drugs

- Gastric, duodenal, and stress ulcers

When NOT to use local-acting drugs

- Hypersensitivity
- Pregnancy
- Breast-feeding
- Chronic renal failure

Adverse reactions

- Constipation

Key nursing actions

- Administer at least 1 hour before meals and at bedtime.
- Give at least 2 hours apart from cimetidine, digoxin, phenytoin, tetracyclines, theophylline, or warfarin.

- May interfere with absorption of drugs that depend on gastric pH for absorption (such as ketoconazole, ampicillin, and iron)

● **Nursing responsibilities**
  - Monitor for diarrhea and abdominal pain
  - Instruct the patient to swallow capsules whole and not to chew or crush them
  - Administer 1 hour before meals
  - Instruct the patient to avoid gastric irritants (smoking, alcohol, products containing aspirin, caffeine, NSAIDs, and foods that cause GI irritation), which may counteract drug effects and worsen the ulcer

LOCAL-ACTING DRUGS

● **Mechanism of action**
  - Protect gastric mucosa by coating the ulcer crater

● **Pharmacokinetics**
  - Absorption: Only 3% to 5% of drug is absorbed after oral administration
  - Distribution: Acts locally at ulcer site
  - Metabolism: Unknown
  - Excretion: Excreted in feces

● **Drug examples**
  - Sucralfate (Carafate)

● **Indications**
  - Short-term treatment and prevention of gastric, duodenal, and stress ulcers

● **Contraindications and precautions**
  - Contraindicated in patients with known hypersensitivity
  - Used cautiously in pregnant or breast-feeding patients and those with chronic renal failure

● **Adverse reactions**
  - Constipation

● **Interactions**
  - Binds with other drugs in GI tract; may decrease absorption of cimetidine, phenytoin, tetracyclines, warfarin, and theophylline
  - Antacids increase gastric pH and may decrease drug effectiveness
  - Sucralfate decreases absorption of lansoprazole; separate doses of drugs by giving lansoprazole 30 minutes before sucralfate

● **Nursing responsibilities**
  - Give at least 2 hours apart from cimetidine, digoxin, phenytoin, tetracyclines, theophylline, or warfarin
  - Don't administer with an antacid; separate administration times by at least 30 minutes
  - Administer drug at least 1 hour before meals and at bedtime for maximum effectiveness

- Assess for epigastric or abdominal pain, frank bleeding, occult bleeding, and constipation
- Instruct the patient to avoid gastric irritants (smoking, alcohol, products containing aspirin, caffeine, NSAIDs, and foods that cause GI irritation), which may counteract drug effects and worsen the ulcer
- Know that sucralfate is poorly water-soluble; administering drug through an NG tube requires special preparation by a pharmacist

CHOLINERGIC BLOCKERS

- **Mechanism of action**
  - Inhibit GI motility and gastric secretions
- **Pharmacokinetics**
  - Absorption: Poorly absorbed from GI tract (about 10% to 25%)
  - Distribution: Rapidly distributed
  - Metabolism: Unknown
  - Excretion: Unknown
- **Drug examples**
  - Glycopyrrolate (Robinul), mepenzolate (Cantil), methscopolamine (Pamine), propantheline (Pro-Banthine)
- **Indications**
  - Adjunctive therapy for peptic ulcer disease
- **Contraindications and precautions**
  - Contraindicated in children and breast-feeding patients and in those with angle-closure glaucoma, uncontrolled tachycardia, urinary or GI tract obstruction, hypersensitivity, severe ulcerative colitis, myasthenia gravis, tachycardia caused by cardiac insufficiency or thyrotoxicosis, acute or severe hemorrhage, or unstable cardiovascular status
- **Adverse reactions**
  - Tachycardia, dry mouth, constipation, urine retention, and urinary hesitancy
- **Interactions**
  - Use with similar-acting drugs causes additive anticholinergic effects
  - Antacids may decrease absorption of anticholinergic antiulceratives
- **Nursing responsibilities**
  - Assess for epigastric or abdominal pain, frank bleeding, and occult bleeding
  - Instruct the patient to avoid gastric irritants (smoking, alcohol, aspirin-containing products, caffeine, NSAIDs, and foods that cause GI irritation); may counteract drug effects and worsen the ulcer

Key facts about cholinergic blockers

- Inhibit GI motility and gastric secretions
- Metabolism and excretion are unknown

When to use cholinergic blockers

- Peptic ulcer disease

When NOT to use cholinergic blockers

- Uncontrolled tachycardia
- Urinary or GI tract obstruction
- Hypersensitivity
- Severe ulcerative colitis
- Myasthenia gravis
- Tachycardia caused by cardiac insufficiency or thyrotoxicosis
- Acute or severe hemorrhage
- Unstable cardiovascular status
- Children
- Breast-feeding

Adverse reactions

- Tachycardia, dry mouth, constipation, urine retention, urinary hesitancy

Key nursing actions

- Assess the patient for epigastric or abdominal pain, frank bleeding, occult bleeding, and constipation.
- Teach the patient to avoid gastric irritants.

Key facts about antiulceratives

- Reduce GI motility and gastric secretions, replace gastric prostaglandins, and enhance natural local protective mechanisms
- Metabolism and excretion unknown

When to use antiulceratives

- *H. pylori* ulcers
- Gastric ulcer prevention related to NSAID use
- Duodenal ulcers

When NOT to use antiulceratives

- Hypersensitivity
- Pregnancy
- Breast-feeding
- Chronic renal failure
- Liver impairment
- Allergy to prostaglandins

Adverse reactions

- Darkened tongue or stools, diarrhea, abdominal pain, flatulence, dyspepsia, infertility, nausea, vomiting, vaginal spotting, uterine cramping, miscarriage

Key nursing actions

- Watch for diarrhea.
- Know that women of childbearing age should be assessed for pregnancy before receiving misoprostol.
- Assess the patient for epigastric or abdominal pain, frank bleeding, and occult bleeding.
- Teach the patient to avoid gastric irritants, such as smoking, alcohol, aspirin-containing products, caffeine, NSAIDs, and foods that cause GI irritation.

MISCELLANEOUS ANTIULCERATIVES

- **Mechanism of action**
  - Bismuth subsalicylate: Reduces GI motility and gastric secretions
  - Misoprostol: Replaces gastric prostaglandins and enhances natural local protective mechanisms

- **Pharmacokinetics**
  - Absorption: Misoprostol is extensively and rapidly absorbed
  - Distribution: Unknown
  - Metabolism: Unknown
  - Excretion: Unknown

- **Drug examples**
  - Bismuth (Pepto-Bismol), misoprostol (Cytotec)

- **Indications**
  - Adjunct to antibiotic therapy to eradicate *Helicobacter pylori* (bismuth subsalicylate)
  - Prevent gastric ulcers resulting from use of NSAIDs or treat duodenal ulcers not responding to other medication regimens (misoprostol)

- **Contraindications and precautions**
  - Contraindicated in patients with known hypersensitivity
  - Used cautiously in pregnant or breast-feeding patients and those with chronic renal failure or liver impairment
  - Misoprostol contraindicated in pregnant or breast-feeding patients and those allergic to prostaglandins

- **Adverse reactions**
  - Darkened tongue or stools (bismuth)
  - Diarrhea (most common), abdominal pain, flatulence, dyspepsia, infertility, nausea and vomiting, vaginal spotting, uterine cramping, and miscarriage (misoprostol)

- **Interactions**
  - Bismuth increases action of warfarin and oral hypoglycemic agonists
  - Bismuth and misoprostol decrease absorption of tetracyclines

- **Nursing responsibilities**
  - Administer misoprostol with food or after meals and at bedtime to decrease the risk of diarrhea
  - Observe for diarrhea
  - Know that females of childbearing age should be assessed for pregnancy before receiving misoprostol
    - Begin therapy on second or third day of menses following a negative pregnancy test
    - Encourage contraceptive use throughout therapy

- Assess for epigastric or abdominal pain, frank bleeding, and occult bleeding
- Instruct the patient to avoid gastric irritants (smoking, alcohol, aspirin-containing products, caffeine, NSAIDs, and foods that cause GI irritation); may counteract drug effects or worsen the ulcer

ADSORBENTS, ANTIFLATULENTS, AND DIGESTANTS

● Mechanism of action
- Adsorbents: Attract and bind to toxins in GI tract, thereby preventing absorption
- Antiflatulents: Cause foaming action in GI tract, creating a film on intestines that helps to disperse mucus-enclosed gas pockets and to prevent their formation
- Digestants: Resembles action of deficient substance (bile acid, which increases output of bile in the liver, or pancreatic enzymes) normally produced by body

● Pharmacokinetics
- Absorption: Not absorbed into body; acts locally in GI tract and excreted whole
- Distribution: Not distributed
- Metabolism: Not metabolized
- Excretion: Excreted unchanged in feces

● Drug examples
- Adsorbents: Activated charcoal
- Antiflatulents: Simethicone (Flatulex, Gas-X, Maalox Anti-Gas, Mylanta Gas, Mylicon, Phazyme)
- Digestants: Dehydrocholic acid, pancreatic enzymes (pancreatin, pancrelipase [Pancrease], lipase, protease, amylase)

● Indications
- Antidote for oral ingestion of toxins that can lead to poisoning or overdose (activated charcoal)
- Treat conditions involving excessive air or gas in stomach or intestines, such as gastric bloating, diverticular disease, or spastic or irritable colon (simethicone)
- Treat constipation and promote bile flow (dehydrocholic acid)
- Supplement deficient natural pancreatic enzymes, such as occurs in patients with pancreatitis or cystic fibrosis (pancreatic enzymes)

● Contraindications and precautions
- Activated charcoal contraindicated in patients with acute poisoning from mineral acids, alkalines, cyanide, ethanol, methanol, iron, inorganic acids, or organic solvents

---

Key facts about adsorbents, antiflatulents, and digestants

- Adsorbents: Attract and bind to toxins in the GI tract to prevent absorption
- Antiflatulents: Foaming action in GI tract creates a film on intestines that helps disperse gas pockets
- Digestants: Resemble action of deficient substance that's normally produced in the body

When to use adsorbents, antiflatulents, and digestants

- Oral ingestion of toxins
- Gastric bloating or diverticular disease
- Constipation
- Deficient production of natural pancreatic enzymes (such as in cystic fibrosis)

When NOT to use adsorbents, antiflatulents, and digestants

- Acute poisoning from alkalines, cyanide, ethanol, iron, or organic solvents

Adverse reactions

- Blackened stools, constipation, abdominal cramping, diarrhea, nausea

Key nursing actions

- Know that a patient who has recently eaten will require an increased amount of charcoal.
- Be aware that several doses of charcoal may be needed to treat severe poisoning.
- Don't mix activated charcoal with dairy products.

Key facts about antiemetics

- Mechanisms vary; some act on CNS to prevent nausea and vomiting, some reduce motion sickness, some increase the rate of gastric emptying and enhance gastroesophageal sphincter tone
- Extensively metabolized by liver
- Excreted in urine and feces

Adverse reactions

- Blackened stools and constipation (activated charcoal)
- Abdominal cramping, biliary colic, diarrhea, and nausea (digestive enzymes)

Interactions

- Activated charcoal decreases absorption of oral medications
- Antacids reduce effects of pancreatic enzymes
- Pancreatic enzymes decrease absorption of folic acid and iron

Nursing responsibilities

- Know that a patient who has recently eaten requires an increased amount of activated charcoal
- Be aware that multiple doses of activated charcoal may be needed to treat severe poisoning involving certain drugs (acetaminophen, digoxin, phenobarbital, phenytoin, theophylline, carbamazepine, dapsone, and quinidine)
- Don't mix activated charcoal with dairy products because activated charcoal decreases the drug's ability to absorb toxins
- Shake simethicone well before administration to thoroughly mix drug
- Administer drug at appropriate time
  - Simethicone: After meals and at bedtime
  - Pancreatic enzymes: With meals
  - Dehydrocholic acid: After meals

ANTIEMETICS

Mechanism of action

- Aprepitant, dronabinol, granisetron, ondansetron, palonosetron, phenothiazines, and trimethobenzamide: Act on CNS to prevent nausea and vomiting
- Dimenhydrinate, meclizine, and scopolamine: Reduce motion sickness by inhibiting impulses from inner ear to the vestibular pathway
- Metoclopramide: Increases the rate of gastric emptying and enhances gastroesophageal sphincter tone

Pharmacokinetics

- Absorption: Usually well absorbed from GI tract
- Distribution: Widely distributed
- Metabolism: Extensively metabolized by liver
- Excretion: Excreted in urine and feces

Drug examples

- Aprepitant (Emend), dimenhydrinate (Dramamine), dronabinol ([Marinol]), droperidol (Inapsine), granisetron (Kytril), meclizine (Antivert, Bonine), metoclopramide (Reglan), ondansetron (Zofran), palonosetron (Aloxi), phenothiazines (chlorpromazine [Thorazine], perphenazine

[Trilafon], prochlorperazine [Compazine], promethazine [Phenergan], scopolamine (Scopace), thiethylperazine [Torecan]), trimethobenzamide (Tigan)

● **Indications**
- Manage nausea and vomiting associated with chemotherapy (aprepitant, palonosetron, ondansetron, granisetron, and dronabinol)
- Treat motion sickness (dimenhydrinate, meclizine)
- Promote gastric emptying in patients receiving tube feedings and those with diabetic gastroparesis (metoclopramide)
- Prevent vomiting during surgery (droperidol)

● **Contraindications and precautions**
- Metoclopramide contraindicated in suspected GI obstruction; used cautiously and at reduced dose in patients with renal impairment
- Phenothiazines contraindicated in angle-closure glaucoma, bone marrow depression, and severe liver or heart disease
- Dimenhydrinate contraindicated in patients hypersensitive to drug or its components; I.V. form contains benzyl alcohol, which has been associated with fatal "gasping syndrome" in neonates

● **Adverse reactions**
- Hypotension, constipation, blurred vision, dryness of eyes and mouth, extrapyramidal reactions, and photosensitivity reactions (phenothiazines)
- Hypotension, pain at I.M. injection site, and rectal irritation (with suppositories) (trimethobenzamide)
- Drowsiness (antiemetics)

● **Interactions**
- Use with antihistamines, other CNS depressants (including opioids), or sedative-hypnotics causes additive CNS depression
- Use of phenothiazines with other hypotensive drugs causes additive hypotension
- Use of phenothiazines or meclizine with anticholinergic drugs causes additive anticholinergic effects
- Metoclopramide affects GI motility, possibly altering GI absorption of other drugs (such as salicylates, diazepam, levodopa, lithium, tetracycline, and digoxin)

● **Nursing responsibilities**
- Decrease initial dose of metoclopramide by 50% of usual recommended dose if creatinine clearance is less than 40 ml/minute
- Instruct the patient to change position slowly when administering phenothiazines (to minimize orthostatic hypotension) and to wear sunscreen and protective clothing (to prevent photosensitivity reactions) (see *Teaching about antiemetics,* page 298)
- Assess for nausea and vomiting and fluid and electrolyte imbalances
- Caution the patient to avoid activities requiring alertness until drug response is known

When to use antiemetics

- Nausea and vomiting associated with chemotherapy
- Motion sickness
- Tube feedings
- Diabetic gastroparesis

When NOT to use antiemetics

- Suspected GI obstruction
- Angle-closure glaucoma
- Bone marrow depression
- Severe liver or heart disease
- Hypersensitivity

Adverse reactions

- Hypotension, constipation, blurred vision, dryness of the eyes and mouth, extrapyramidal reactions, photosensitivity reactions, hypotension, pain at I.M. injection site, rectal irritation, drowsiness

Key nursing actions

- Assess the patient for nausea and vomiting and fluid and electrolyte imbalances.
- Instruct the patient not to consume alcohol when taking an antiemetic.
- Teach the patient to take oral antiemetics 1 hour before exposure to conditions causing motion sickness.

Topics for patient discussion

- Medication regimen, including proper timing of and technique for administration
- Signs and symptoms to discuss with the practitioner
- Safety measures
- Measures to alleviate anticholinergic effects and problems with bowel elimination
- Importance of changing position slowly and wearing sunscreen and protective clothing as appropriate
- Ways to reduce dry mouth
- Follow-up care

Key facts about antidiarrheals

- Reduce fluid content of stool
- Decrease the volume of gastric and intestinal secretions
- Metabolized by liver
- Excreted by kidneys or in feces

TIME-OUT FOR TEACHING

Teaching about antiemetics

Include these topics in your teaching plan for the patient receiving an antiemetic:

- medication regimen, including the drug's name, dosage, frequency, duration, and possible adverse effects
- signs and symptoms to discuss with the practitioner

- proper timing of and technique for administration
- safety measures
- measures to alleviate anticholinergic effects and problems with bowel elimination
- follow-up care, including practitioner visits.

- Inform the patient that frequent mouth rinses, good oral hygiene, and sugarless gum or candy may reduce dry mouth
- Instruct the patient not to consume alcohol when taking an antiemetic to prevent additive CNS depression
- Advise the patient to take oral antiemetics 1 hour before exposure to conditions causing motion sickness

ANTIDIARRHEALS AND LAXATIVES

ANTIDIARRHEALS

Mechanism of action

- Camphorated opium tincture, difenoxin, diphenoxylate, and loperamide: Slow intestinal motility, ultimately reducing water absorption from stools
- Bismuth, kaolin and pectin mixture, and polycarbophil: Reduce fluid content of stools
- Octreotide: Decreases volume of gastric and intestinal secretions and diarrhea secondary to vasoactive intestinal tumors (such as carcinoid tumors)

Pharmacokinetics

- Absorption: Opium preparations are absorbed systemically; others are absorbed readily from GI tract, except for loperamide
- Distribution: Varies with drug
- Metabolism: Metabolized by liver
- Excretion: Opium preparations are excreted by kidneys; others are excreted primarily in feces

Drug examples

- Bismuth (Pepto-Bismol), camphorated opium tincture (Paregoric), difenoxin (with atropine [Motofen]), diphenoxylate (with atropine [Lomotil]), kaolin and pectin mixture (Kapectolin), loperamide (Imodium), octreotide (Sandostatin), polycarbophil (FiberCon)

● **Indications**
  • Control and relieve symptoms of acute or chronic nonspecific diarrhea

● **Contraindications and precautions**
  • Contraindicated in patients with abdominal pain of unknown cause, especially if accompanied by fever

● **Adverse reactions**
  • Constipation, drowsiness (camphorated opium tincture, difenoxin, diphenoxylate, and loperamide), nausea, abdominal pain, pain at injection site, and gallstones (octreotide)

● **Interactions**
  • Use of camphorated opium tincture, difenoxin, diphenoxylate, or loperamide with other CNS depressants causes additive CNS depression
  • Use of difenoxin, diphenoxylate, or loperamide with similar-acting drugs causes additive anticholinergic effects
  • Concurrent use of kaolin with digoxin may decrease digoxin absorption

● **Nursing responsibilities**
  • Assess skin turgor and monitor fluid and electrolyte balance for evidence of dehydration resulting from diarrhea
  • Assess for abdominal pain and distention, nausea and vomiting, and frank or occult bleeding; auscultate for bowel sounds; and evaluate stools for frequency and consistency
  • Know that high-dose, long-term use of difenoxin or diphenoxylate may cause dependence (atropine has been added to these preparations to discourage abuse)
  • Don't confuse camphorated opium tincture with deodorized tincture of opium, which is 25 times more potent
  • Caution the patient to avoid activities requiring alertness until drug response is known; also instruct him to avoid alcohol and CNS depressants when administering camphorated opium tincture, difenoxin, diphenoxylate, or loperamide
  • Instruct the patient to notify the practitioner if diarrhea persists or fever occurs

LAXATIVES

● **Mechanism of action**
  • Bulk-forming laxatives: Increase water content of stools, forming a viscous solution that promotes peristalsis and improves elimination rate
  • Lubricant laxatives: Increase water retention in stools, prevent water absorption from stools, and lubricate and soften intestinal contents
  • Hyperosmotic laxatives: Increase water content of stools and soften stools; lactulose also inhibits diffusion of ammonia from the colon into the blood, reducing serum ammonia levels in patients with liver dysfunction

When to use laxatives

- Constipation
- Radiologic and endoscopic procedures
- Chronic watery diarrhea
- Hepatic encephalopathy

When NOT to use laxatives

- Persistent or severe abdominal pain of unknown cause

Adverse reactions

- Nausea, vomiting, abdominal cramping, esophageal or intestinal obstruction, lipid pneumonia, nutritional deficiencies, cramps, distention, flatulence, belching, dehydration, electrolyte imbalance, loss of colonic motility, dependence

- Saline cathartic laxatives: Draw water into bowel, increasing the bulk of intestinal contents and stimulating peristalsis
- Stimulant laxatives: Stimulate peristalsis and inhibit water and electrolyte reabsorption from intestine
- Stool softeners: Allow more fluid and fat to penetrate feces, producing a softer fecal mass

Pharmacokinetics
- Absorption: Minimally absorbed
- Distribution: Distributed in intestines
- Metabolism: Metabolized by intestinal microflora
- Excretion: Excreted in feces

Drug examples
- Bulk-forming laxatives: Methylcellulose (Citrucel), polycarbophil (Fiber-Con), psyllium (Fiberall, Konsyl, Metamucil, Perdiem)
- Lubricant laxatives: Mineral oil (Fleet Mineral Oil Enema, Kondremul)
- Hyperosmotic laxatives: Lactulose (Cephulac, Chronulac)
- Saline cathartic laxatives: Magnesium citrate, magnesium hydroxide (Milk of Magnesia), magnesium sulfate, polyethylene glycol and electrolytes (GoLYTELY, HalfLytely, MiraLax), sodium phosphates (sodium phosphate and sodium biphosphate [Fleet Phospho-soda])
- Stimulant laxatives: Bisacodyl (Dulcolax), cascara sagrada, castor oil, glycerin suppositories, senna (Senokot)
- Stool softeners: Docusate calcium (Surfak), docusate potassium, docusate sodium (Colace, Peri-Colace)

Indications
- Treat or prevent constipation and prepare bowel for radiologic or endoscopic procedures
- Manage chronic watery diarrhea (methylcellulose and psyllium)
- Adjunctive treatment in managing hepatic encephalopathy (lactulose)

Contraindications and precautions
- Contraindicated in patients with persistent or severe abdominal pain of unknown cause, especially when accompanied by fever

Adverse reactions
- Nausea, vomiting, and abdominal cramping
- Esophageal obstruction or intestinal obstruction (bulk-forming laxatives)
- Lipid pneumonia and nutritional deficiencies (lubricant laxatives)
- Cramps, distention, flatulence, and belching (osmotic laxatives)
- Dehydration and electrolyte imbalances (saline cathartic laxatives)
- Possible permanent loss of colonic motility, laxative dependence, and electrolyte imbalances with long-term use or abuse of laxatives

Interactions
- Laxatives reduce intestinal transit time and may decrease absorption of orally administered drugs

TIME-OUT FOR TEACHING
Teaching about laxatives

Include these topics in your teaching plan for the patient receiving a laxative:

- medication regimen, including the drug's name, dosage, frequency, duration, and possible adverse effects
- signs and symptoms to discuss with the practitioner

- proper timing of and technique for administration
- nonpharmacologic bowel elimination measures, including diet and exercise
- dietary fibers and fluids
- follow-up care, including practitioner visits.

● Nursing responsibilities
- Assess for abdominal pain and distention, nausea and vomiting, and frank or occult bleeding; auscultate for bowel sounds; and evaluate stools for frequency and consistency
- Monitor for fluid and electrolyte imbalances
- Mix bulk-forming laxatives in a full glass of water or juice; give an additional glass of fluid after administering
- Assess the patient's mental status, including level of consciousness and orientation when administering laxatives as adjunctive drugs for hepatic encephalopathy
- Dilute sodium phosphates with water before giving, and monitor for electrolyte disturbances
- Inform the patient that most laxatives are for short-term use only and that long-term use may cause electrolyte imbalances and laxative dependence by causing a permanent loss of colonic motility; encourage use of other methods to regulate bowel, such as increasing dietary bulk and fluid intake and engaging in exercise (see *Teaching about laxatives*)

5-HT₃-RECEPTOR ANTAGONISTS

● Mechanism of action
- Block 5-HT₃ (serotonin) receptors in GI tract, thereby increasing colonic transit time and decreasing GI motility; may also decrease perception of pain and discomfort in GI tract

● Pharmacokinetics
- Absorption: Orally absorbed
- Distribution: Widely distributed
- Metabolism: Metabolized in the liver
- Excretion: Excreted in urine and bile

● Drug examples
- Alosetron (Lotronex)

When to use 5-HT₃-receptor antagonists

- Diarrhea-predominant IBS

When NOT to use 5-HT₃-receptor antagonists

- Constipation
- Hypersensitivity to alosetron
- Abnormal GI anatomy
- History of Crohn's disease, ulcerative colitis, or diverticulitis

Adverse reactions

- Potentially fatal GI complications, anxiety, tremors, headache, sweating, abdominal pain, nausea, constipation, fatigue

Key nursing actions

- Explain and have patient sign practitioner-patient agreement.
- Monitor for adverse reactions.

● **Indications**
- Treatment of severe diarrhea-predominant irritable bowel syndrome (IBS) in females
- Not intended for females with anatomic or biochemical GI tract abnormalities; also not intended as first-line drug

● **Contraindications and precautions**
- Serious adverse reactions have occurred in patients taking the drug; the drug may by prescribed only by practitioners registered in the prescribing program with the manufacturer; patients must sign a practitioner-patient agreement before taking the drug
- Contraindicated in patients who are currently constipated or have a history of constipation, patients with previous hypersensitivity reaction to alosetron, and those with any abnormal anatomy of the GI tract or a history of Crohn's disease, ulcerative colitis, or diverticulitis

● **Adverse reactions**
- Anxiety, tremors, headache, sweating, abdominal pain, nausea, constipation, and fatigue
- Serious, potentially fatal GI complications, including ischemic colitis and serious complications of constipation (such as obstruction, perforation, and toxic megacolon) (alosetron)

● **Interactions**
- Use with other drugs that decrease GI motility may worsen constipation

● **Nursing responsibilities**
- Explain to the patient that she must sign and follow the practitioner-patient agreement while taking alosetron
- Monitor for adverse reactions
- Teach the patient the signs and symptoms of possible serious adverse effects, including constipation, ischemic colitis, intestinal obstruction, and perforation

NCLEX CHECKS

It's never too soon to begin your NCLEX® preparation. Now that you've reviewed this chapter, carefully read each of the following questions and choose the best answer. Then compare your responses with the correct answers.

1. A client is using aluminum hydroxide (AlternaGEL) as an antacid. The nurse should warn the client about which adverse reaction?

☐ **1.** Black stools
☐ **2.** Constipation
☐ **3.** Acid rebound
☐ **4.** Reduced iron absorption

2. As part of the treatment regimen for a client with a peptic ulcer, the physician orders cimetidine (Tagamet), 300 mg P.O., before meals and at bedtime. The best response to the order is to:
- ☐ **1.** give the drug as ordered.
- ☐ **2.** change the drug times to be given with meals.
- ☐ **3.** withhold the drug and check the dosage with the physician.
- ☐ **4.** withhold the drug and ask the physician to change the dosage to twice daily.

3. A 48-year-old client takes large doses of a nonsteroidal anti-inflammatory drug (NSAID) for rheumatoid arthritis. Misoprostol (Cytotec) is ordered to prevent NSAID-induced ulcers. Which common dose-related adverse reaction to misoprostol does the nurse need to discuss with the client?
- ☐ **1.** Diarrhea
- ☐ **2.** Dyspepsia
- ☐ **3.** Headache
- ☐ **4.** Tinnitus

4. A nurse gave metoclopramide (Reglan) to a postoperative client 1 hour ago. Which assessment finding best indicates the drug's effectiveness?
- ☐ **1.** Increased peristalsis and decreased nausea
- ☐ **2.** Decreased drowsiness
- ☐ **3.** Decreased disorientation
- ☐ **4.** Increased gastric secretions as measured through the nasogastric tube

5. A client complains of severe nausea and vomiting caused by radiotherapy for metastatic breast cancer. Which antiemetic would the nurse expect to be most effective?
- ☐ **1.** Chlorpromazine (Thorazine)
- ☐ **2.** Meclizine (Antivert)
- ☐ **3.** Ondansetron (Zofran)
- ☐ **4.** Trimethobenzamide (Tigan)

6. A child with cystic fibrosis is taking pancrelipase (Pancrease) with each meal. The nurse is reviewing discharge instructions with the child and his parents. Which statement indicates that the parents understand the primary reason for giving this drug?
- ☐ **1.** "My child's appetite should increase while taking this drug."
- ☐ **2.** "There should be less fat in my child's stools with this drug."
- ☐ **3.** "This drug will help prevent mouth ulcers."
- ☐ **4.** "This drug will cause my child to gain weight quickly."

TOP 4

Items to study for your next test on drugs and the gastrointestinal system

1. Mechanisms of action of the various types of antiulceratives, antiemetics, emetics, antidiarrheals, and laxatives
2. Major adverse effects of antiulceratives, antiemetics, emetics, antidiarrheals, and laxatives
3. Nursing responsibilities when administering antiulceratives, antiemetics, emetics, antidiarrheals, and laxatives
4. Teaching for the patient receiving antiulceratives, antiemetics, emetics, antidiarrheals, or laxatives

7. A nurse advises a client not to take a stimulant laxative for an extended period. Which condition could result from long-term use of a stimulant laxative?

- ☐ **1.** Hepatotoxicity
- ☐ **2.** Small-intestine blockage
- ☐ **3.** Permanent loss of colonic motility
- ☐ **4.** Withdrawal reactions when the laxative is stopped

8. A client returns from the operating room after receiving extensive abdominal surgery. He has 1,000 ml of lactated Ringer's solution infusing via a central line. The physician orders the I.V. fluid to be infused at 125 ml/hour plus the total output of the previous hour. The drop factor of the tubing is 15 gtt/minute, and the output for the previous hour was 75 ml via indwelling urinary catheter, 50 ml via nasogastric tube, and 10 ml via Jackson-Pratt tube. For how many drops per minute should the nurse set the I.V. flow rate to deliver the correct amount of fluid? Record your answer as a whole number.

_____ gtt/minute

9. A client wants to know why his antacid contains simethicone. The nurse tells him that the rationale for adding simethicone to antacid products is to:

- ☐ **1.** reduce GI motility.
- ☐ **2.** reduce gas in the GI tract.
- ☐ **3.** improve the acid-neutralizing capacity of the product.
- ☐ **4.** protect the esophagus during reflux of gastric contents.

10. A physician orders propantheline bromide (Pro-Banthine), 15 mg P.O. q.i.d., for a client with neurogenic bladder. What should the nurse include in the teaching plan for this medication?

- ☐ **1.** Increase the amount of dietary fat to help with absorption of the drug.
- ☐ **2.** Take the drug 30 minutes before meals and at bedtime.
- ☐ **3.** Take the drug 30 minutes after meals and at bedtime.
- ☐ **4.** The drug needs to be taken 1 hour before or 2 hours after meals.

ANSWERS AND RATIONALES

1. CORRECT ANSWER: 2
Aluminum can cause constipation. It doesn't change stool color, it neutralizes acid without rebound, and it has little impact on iron absorption unless taken in excessive amounts.

2. CORRECT ANSWER: 1
The nurse should give the drug as ordered. Cimetidine, which inhibits gastric acid secretions, works best when the stomach is empty, so giving it before meals and at bedtime is appropriate. The dosage is correct. Changing the times is inappropriate and would require a physician's order. Withholding the drug and seeking a dosage change would interfere with the drug's maximum effectiveness.

3. CORRECT ANSWER: 1

Diarrhea is the most common adverse reaction to misoprostol. The client can minimize the reaction by taking the drug after meals and at bedtime and by avoiding antacids containing magnesium. He should contact his physician if the diarrhea becomes severe. Dyspepsia, headache, and tinnitus aren't common adverse reactions to misoprostol.

4. CORRECT ANSWER: 1

The antiemetic metoclopramide helps increase peristalsis and gastric emptying in postoperative clients. It doesn't affect the production of gastric secretions or orientation. It may cause, not decrease, drowsiness.

5. CORRECT ANSWER: 3

Ondansetron is used specifically to manage nausea and vomiting caused by radiotherapy. Trimethobenzamide is indicated for general mild-to-moderate nausea and vomiting, whereas chlorpromazine is used for severe nausea and vomiting. Meclizine is used to treat motion sickness.

6. CORRECT ANSWER: 2

The main reason for giving pancrelipase is that it substitutes for the pancreatic enzymes that are typically lacking in a client with cystic fibrosis. The drug helps the client to digest fats better, so the stools contain less fat. Although pancrelipase may increase the client's appetite and cause him to gain weight, these aren't the primary reasons for administering the drug. Mouth ulcers are a common adverse effect of the drug.

7. CORRECT ANSWER: 3

Prolonged use or abuse of stimulant laxatives may lead to permanent loss of colonic motility or laxative dependence as a result of chronic stimulation of smooth-muscle activity. In general, these drugs aren't hepatotoxic, don't significantly affect the small intestines, and aren't associated with withdrawal reactions.

8. CORRECT ANSWER: 65

First, calculate the volume to be infused (in milliliters):

75 ml + 50 ml + 10 ml = 135 ml total output for the previous hour

135 ml + 125 ml ordered as a constant flow =
260 ml to be infused over the next hour.

Next, use the formula:

Volume to be infused/Total minutes to be infused × Drop factor =
Drops per minute.

In this case, 260 ml divided by 60 minutes × 15 gtt/minute = 65 gtt/minute.

9. CORRECT ANSWER: 2

Simethicone, an antiflatulent, reduces gas by reducing the surface tension of gas bubbles so they coalesce and become easier to eliminate. It doesn't act as a protectant or affect GI motility, and it has no acid-neutralizing capacity.

10. CORRECT ANSWER: 2

Propantheline bromide should be taken 30 minutes before meals and at bedtime. There's no need to increase dietary fat intake, and the drug doesn't need to be taken on an empty stomach.

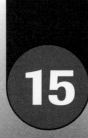

15

Drugs and the reproductive system

PRETEST

1. Which class of drugs reverses catabolic or tissue-depleting processes?
- ☐ 1. Anabolic steroids
- ☐ 2. Erectile dysfunction drugs
- ☐ 3. Estrogen replacement drugs
- ☐ 4. Androgens

CORRECT ANSWER: 1

2. A postpartum client is typically started on oxytocin (Pitocin) to:
- ☐ 1. increase milk production.
- ☐ 2. decrease vaginal tone.
- ☐ 3. increase uterine contractions.
- ☐ 4. decrease urine output.

CORRECT ANSWER: 3

3. Prolactin secretion inhibitors may produce which adverse reaction?
- ☐ 1. Anorexia
- ☐ 2. Rash
- ☐ 3. Bradycardia
- ☐ 4. Orthostatic hypotension

CORRECT ANSWER: 4

4. A nurse should advise a client taking erectile dysfunction drugs that these medications shouldn't be taken with:

☐ 1. grapefruit juice.

☐ 2. bananas.

☐ 3. orange juice.

☐ 4. spinach.

CORRECT ANSWER: 1

5. A client taking estrogen hormonal therapy should be instructed to immediately report:

☐ 1. weight gain.

☐ 2. severe mental depression.

☐ 3. diminished dysmenorrhea.

☐ 4. increased vaginal lubrication.

CORRECT ANSWER: 2

LEARNING OBJECTIVES

After studying this chapter, you should be able to:

- List the major classes and uses of reproductive system drugs.
- Describe the mechanisms of action of androgens, androgen hormone inhibitors, anabolic steroids, hormonal contraceptives, estrogens, progestins, prolactin secretion inhibitors, fertility drugs, abortifacients, obstetric drugs, and erectile dysfunction drugs.
- Name common adverse effects of reproductive system drugs.
- Identify important nursing responsibilities and patient teaching needs related to the administration of reproductive system drugs.

CHAPTER OVERVIEW

Androgens are used to provide replacement therapy for hormonal deficiencies in men and to create an environment unfavorable for tissue or tumor growth. Finasteride specifically decreases prostate size and improves urine flow in patients with benign prostatic hyperplasia (BPH).

Estrogens and progestins are used for contraception, treatment of hormone-sensitive tissue or tumors, restoration of hormone balance during menopause, and treatment of osteoporosis. Lactation suppressants, fertility drugs, oxytocics, and labor suppressants are used during the childbearing cycle.

ANATOMY AND PHYSIOLOGY

- **Anatomy**
  - Male reproductive system: Scrotum, testes, duct system, accessory reproductive glands, penis
  - Female reproductive system: Ovaries, fallopian tubes, uterus, vagina, external genitalia, mammary glands

- **Physiology**
  - Hormones and puberty
    - Hypothalamus begins to release gonadotropin-releasing hormones (follicle-stimulating hormone [FSH] and luteinizing hormone [LH])
    - Release of gonadotropin-releasing hormones stimulates gonads to release sex hormones (testosterone in males, estrogen and progesterone in females)
    - Sex hormones induce sexual development and body changes characteristic of sexual maturity
    - Puberty is marked by production of mature spermatozoa in males and onset of menarche in females
  - Male hormones
    - Male testicular function is regulated by FSH and LH
    - FSH maintains normal spermiogenesis (production of sperm)
    - LH maintains normal spermiogenesis and promotes testosterone secretion
    - Testosterone is responsible for sexual drive, development of secondary sex characteristics, and growth
  - Female reproductive hormones
    - LH and FSH promote follicle maturation and ovarian secretion of estrogen and progesterone
    - Estrogen is responsible for secondary sex characteristics and stimulates
      - Endometrial growth during first half of menstrual cycle
      - Cervical secretion of mucus that facilitates passage of sperm into uterus and fallopian tubes
      - Bone growth

A&P highlights

- Male reproductive system includes scrotum, testes, duct system, accessory reproductive glands, and penis.
- Female reproductive system includes ovaries, fallopian tubes, uterus, vagina, external genitalia, and mammary glands.
- During puberty, the hypothalamus releases FSH and LH, and these hormones stimulate gonads to release sex hormones.
- Male testicular function is regulated by FSH and LH.
- In females, LH and FSH promote follicle maturation and ovarian secretion of estrogen and progesterone.
- Estrogen is responsible for secondary sex characteristics in females.

Key facts about the menstrual cycle

- Menstrual cycle beginning is dated from the first day of the menstrual flow.
- Ovulation occurs around the middle of the cycle.
- Preovulatory stage varies.
- Postovulatory phase is usually constant and lasts for about 14 days.

Key facts about childbirth

- Labor is the process by which the fetus is expelled from the uterus.
- Oxytocin receptors, uterine stretch, and fetal stimulation of oxytocin and estrogen contribute to the onset of labor.
- Labor is maintained by cervical dilation.

Key facts about lactation

- Milk produced by mammary glands in the breasts
- Regulated by estrogen, progesterone, prolactin, and oxytocin

– Progesterone prepares the endometrium for implantation of fertilized ovum during second half of menstrual cycle; also causes breast development
– LH and FSH have a reciprocal relationship with ovarian hormones (estrogen and progesterone)
  · High estrogen level inhibits FSH output (which stabilizes estrogen levels) and stimulates LH release (which in turn increases progesterone output)
  · High progesterone level inhibits LH output

• Menstrual cycle
  – Beginning of menstrual cycle is dated from first day of menstrual flow
  – Ovulation occurs around midpoint of cycle, which is divided into preovulatory (follicular) and postovulatory (luteal) phases
  – Preovulatory (follicular) phase varies among individuals
    · Pituitary gland releases FSH, which stimulates a group of ovarian follicles to grow
    · One follicle typically grows faster and reaches maturity; the others atrophy
    · Soon after FSH levels increase, LH levels rise; together, these hormones promote estrogen secretion by the ovarian follicle
    · LH surge lasts about 24 hours and causes the mature follicle to rupture, leading to ovulation
  – Postovulatory (luteal) phase is usually constant; lasts about 14 days
    · Phase is characterized by conversion of ruptured follicle into the corpus luteum, which produces estrogen and progesterone
    · Corpus luteum reaches maturity 8 to 9 days after ovulation and begins to degenerate if pregnancy hasn't occurred
    · Decline in corpus luteum activity, which reduces estrogen and progesterone output, results in menstruation
    · Eventually, when estrogen and progesterone levels have fallen, FSH and LH are released again and a new menstrual cycle begins

• Childbirth
  – Labor is the process by which a fetus is expelled from the uterus by uterine contractions
  – Several factors contribute to onset of labor
    · Oxytocin receptors on uterine muscle fibers
    · Uterine stretch that stimulates oxytocin secretion
    · Fetal stimulation of oxytocin and estrogen with decreased progesterone secretion
  – Labor process is sustained by cervical dilation, which increases oxytocin secretion

• Lactation
  – Milk is produced by mammary glands in the breasts
  – Process is regulated by four major hormones
    · Estrogen and progesterone (stimulate proliferation of breast tissue)
    · Prolactin (causes milk production when stimulated by estrogen and progesterone)

- Oxytocin (helps expel milk during breast-feeding)
  - Prolactin levels affect reestablishment of menstrual cycle
    - High prolactin level inhibits FSH and LH release immediately postpartum
    - If breast-feeding doesn't occur, prolactin level declines, FSH and LH levels rise, and cyclic release soon follows
    - Amount of prolactin released in response to breast-feeding gradually decreases normally, and ovulation and menstrual cycle resume
- Hormones and aging
  - With age, production and release of reproductive hormones slowly decline
  - Decreased testosterone secretion in males leads to a decrease in sex drive and spermatogenesis
  - As females age, ovarian follicles gradually degenerate and don't produce any more mature egg cells; by age 45, few follicles remain
  - Aging ovaries no longer produce sufficient hormones to stimulate cyclic changes in endometrium, and menstruation ceases (menopause)

Function
- Produces offspring
- Has endocrine functions
- Contributes to the development of and is an integral part of individual's self-concept

ANDROGENS

Mechanism of action
- Simulate action of endogenous hormones to replace deficient hormones or treat hormone-sensitive disorders
- Stimulate production of red blood cells (RBCs) by enhancing production of erythropoietic stimulating factor

Pharmacokinetics
- Absorption
  - Oral testosterone: GI tract
  - I.M. injections of esters in oil: Slowly absorbed; can be given at 2- to 4-week intervals
  - Topical testosterone: Absorbed by skin; effects continue for 24 hours after application
- Distribution: Varies with drug
- Metabolism: Varies with drug
- Excretion: Varies with drug

Drug examples
- Danazol (Danocrine), fluoxymesterone, methyltestosterone (Methitest, Testred, Virilon), testolactone (Teslac), testosterone (Androderm, Andro-Gel, Delatestryl, Depo-Testosterone, Testoderm, Testopel)

When to use androgens

- Hypogonadism
- Delayed puberty
- Postpartum breast engorgement
- Androgen-sensitive inoperable metastatic breast cancer (palliative care)
- Endometriosis
- Fibrocystic breast disease
- Hereditary angioedema
- Advanced disseminated breast carcinoma (palliative care)

When NOT to use androgens

- Cardiac disease
- Hepatic disease
- Renal disease
- Prostate or breast cancer
- Hypersensitivity
- Pregnancy

Adverse reactions

- Nausea, vomiting, diarrhea, sodium and water retention, edema, weight gain, mood swings, changes in libido, impotence, precocious puberty, priapism, premature epiphyseal closure, breast tenderness, impotence, sterility, hirsutism, reduced breast size, hoarseness

Key nursing actions

- Know that most androgens are Schedule III controlled substances.
- Testosterone must be administered I.M. only.
- Warn women that androgen therapy may cause hoarseness, deeper voice, facial hair, acne, and menstrual irregularities.
- Advise male adolescents receiving androgens for delayed puberty to have bone development checked every 6 months.

Indications

- Treat hypogonadism, delayed puberty, and postpartum breast engorgement; also palliative treatment for androgen-sensitive inoperable metastatic (skeletal) breast cancer in females 1 to 5 years postmenopause (testosterone and methyltestosterone)
- Treat endometriosis; palliative treatment for fibrocystic breast disease; and prophylaxis for hereditary angioedema (danazol)
- Treat androgen deficiencies and inoperable breast cancer that's androgen-responsive (fluoxymesterone)
- Adjunctive therapy in the palliative treatment of advanced disseminated breast carcinoma in postmenopausal females when hormonal therapy is indicated and in premenopausal females with disseminated breast carcinoma whose ovarian function has been terminated (testolactone)

Contraindications and precautions

- Contraindicated in patients with serious cardiac, hepatic, or renal diseases; those hypersensitive to drug or its components; males with known or suspected prostate or breast cancer; and pregnant patients (pregnant patients should also avoid skin contact with AndroGel)
- Testosterone transdermal systems and gels contraindicated in female patients

Adverse reactions

- Nausea, vomiting, diarrhea, sodium and water retention, edema, weight gain, mood swings, changes in libido, and impotence
- In boys: Precocious puberty, priapism, and premature epiphyseal closure
- In men: Breast tenderness, impotence, and sterility
- In women: Hirsutism, reduced breast size, and hoarseness

Interactions

- Use with other hepatotoxic drugs increases risk of hepatotoxicity
- Androgens may decrease serum glucose levels, thereby reducing insulin requirements
- Androgens may increase effects of anticoagulants

Nursing responsibilities

- Know that most androgens, including all anabolic steroids (such as testolactone), are Schedule III controlled substances
- Use deep I.M. injections for parenteral forms, preferably into a large muscle mass
- Give fluoxymesterone with food to reduce abdominal discomfort
- Assess for weight gain and edema
- Monitor blood pressure, weight, electrolyte and lipid levels, and liver function test results
- Instruct the female patient to use a nonhormonal contraceptive (barrier method) during therapy
- Advise the female patient taking danazol to expect amenorrhea

- Warn the female patient that androgen therapy may cause hoarseness, deeper voice, facial hair, acne, and menstrual irregularities; advise her to notify the practitioner if these effects occur
- Advise the male adolescent receiving androgens for delayed puberty to have bone development checked every 6 months

ANDROGEN HORMONE INHIBITORS

- **Mechanism of action**
  - Inhibit steroid 5alpha-reductase, an enzyme that converts testosterone into dihydrotestosterone (DHT)
  - Decrease high levels of DHT in males with an enlarged prostate or balding scalp

- **Pharmacokinetics**
  - Absorption: Well absorbed orally
  - Distribution: Highly protein-bound
  - Metabolism: Metabolized in liver
  - Excretion: Excreted in bile and feces

- **Drug examples**
  - Dutasteride (Avodart), finasteride (Propecia, Proscar)

- **Indications**
  - Treat BPH
  - Treat androgenic alopecia (male-pattern baldness)

- **Contraindications and precautions**
  - Contraindicated in females, children, and those hypersensitive to drug
  - Used cautiously in patients with hepatic impairment
  - Pregnant patients shouldn't handle or come in contact with crushed or broken tablets

- **Adverse reactions**
  - Generally mild and transient reactions, including erectile dysfunction, decreased libido, breast tenderness and enlargement, testicular pain, and hypersensitivity reactions (lip swelling and rash)
  - Possible hepatic impairment

- **Interactions**
  - Increased serum levels when used with ketoconazole, ritonavir, verapamil, diltiazem, cimetidine, or ciprofloxacin

- **Nursing responsibilities**
  - Warn the male patient that females who are or may become pregnant shouldn't come in contact with crushed or broken tablets because of the risk to the male fetus
  - Warn the male patient that he may have a decreased volume of ejaculate during treatment; impotence and decreased libido may also occur
  - Explain that treatment for alopecia is long-term; discontinuing drug will cause balding to resume

Key facts about androgen hormone inhibitors

- Finasteride inhibits steroid 5alpha-reductase.
- Finasteride leads to a decrease in high levels of DHT found in some men.
- They undergo hepatic metabolism.
- They're excreted in bile and feces.

When to use androgen hormone inhibitors

- BPH
- Androgenic alopecia

When NOT to use androgen hormone inhibitors

- Hypersensitivity
- Women
- Children
- Pregnancy

Adverse reactions

- Erectile dysfunction, decreased libido, breast tenderness and enlargement, testicular pain, hypersensitivity reactions

Key nursing actions

- Warn that women who are or may become pregnant shouldn't come in contact with crushed or broken tablets because of the risk to the male fetus.
- Know that men treated for BPH still must be evaluated for prostate cancer before and during therapy.

- Be aware that male patients treated for BPH still must be evaluated for prostate cancer before and during therapy because drug doesn't protect against prostate cancer; decreases prostate-specific antigen levels, even in the presence of prostate cancer

ANABOLIC STEROIDS

- ### Mechanism of action
  - Promote body tissue-building processes and reverse catabolic or tissue-depleting processes (such as anemias, trauma, surgery, arthritis, and osteoporosis)
  - Inhibit release of testosterone through the inhibition of pituitary LH
  - May suppress spermatogenesis through feedback inhibition of pituitary FSH when given in large doses

- ### Pharmacokinetics
  - Unknown

- ### Drug examples
  - Nandrolone decanoate (Deca-Durabolin), oxandrolone (Oxandrin), oxymetholone (Anadrol-50), stanozolol (Winstrol)

- ### Indications
  - Treat anemias (oxymetholone)
  - Adjunctive therapy to promote weight gain after weight loss from catabolic disorders, such as surgery, severe trauma, anemia, arthritis, chronic infections, and osteoporosis (oxandrolone)
  - Prophylactic treatment to decrease frequency and severity of attacks from hereditary angioedema (stanozolol)
  - Treat renal insufficiency–induced anemia (nandrolone decanoate)

- ### Contraindications and precautions
  - Contraindicated in pregnant patients; those hypersensitive to drug; male patients with prostate or breast carcinoma; and female patients with breast carcinoma and hypercalcemia, nephrosis, or nephrotic phase of nephritis
  - Shouldn't be used to enhance physical appearance or athletic performance
  - Classified as Schedule III controlled substances because of their potential for abuse, especially among athletes

- ### Adverse reactions
  - Virilization (most common); acne (mostly in females and prepubertal males), insomnia, edema from sodium retention, ankle swelling, nausea, vomiting, and diarrhea
  - In young children: Possible direct effect on testes, causing serious growth and developmental disturbances (drug suppresses gonadotropic functions of the pituitary); possible stunting of linear growth

Key facts about anabolic steroids

- Promote body tissue-building processes
- Reverse catabolic or tissue-depleting processes
- May suppress spermatogenesis (in large doses)
- Metabolism and excretion are unknown

When to use anabolic steroids

- Anemia, including renal insufficiency-induced anemia
- Promote weight gain
- Hereditary angioedema

When NOT to use anabolic steroids

- Hypersensitivity
- Prostate carcinoma
- Breast carcinoma
- Hypercalcemia
- Nephrosis
- Pregnancy

- In postpubertal males: Acne, inhibition of testicular function with oligospermia, gynecomastia, testicular atrophy, chronic priapism, epididymitis, bladder irritability, change in libido, and impotence
- In females: Irreversible hirsutism, acne, hoarseness or deepening of the voice, clitoral enlargement, change in libido, and menstrual irregularities
- In elderly patients: Increased risk of BPH and prostatic carcinoma
- Drug use has been associated with peliosis hepatitis (blood-filled cysts in liver and spleen) and liver cell tumors, which may cause liver failure or malignant and fatal tumors
- Drug use has been linked to blood lipid changes, which may increase cholesterol and low-density lipoprotein levels and the risk of atherosclerosis

Interactions
- Anabolic steroids increase effects of anticoagulants
- May increase the hypoglycemic effects of sulfonylureas when used together

Nursing responsibilities
- Warn the athletic patient that use of anabolic steroids to improve physical appearance or athletic performance is contraindicated; adverse effects may be serious and irreversible
- Warn the female patient that virilization may occur while on drug therapy; advise her to discontinue drug and contact the practitioner if amenorrhea, menstrual irregularities, hoarseness, hirsutism, or acne occurs
- Monitor glucose levels in the diabetic patient carefully; glucose tolerance may be altered
- Monitor liver function test results

HORMONAL CONTRACEPTIVES

Mechanism of action
- Suppress production and release of gonadotropins, thereby inhibiting ovulation

Pharmacokinetics
- Absorption: Orally or transdermally absorbed (Ortho Evra)
- Distribution: Widely distributed
- Metabolism: Metabolized renally
- Excretion: Excreted in urine and feces

Drug examples
- Various concentrations of hormones may be available for the trade names listed below
  - Ethinyl estradiol and desogestrel (Apri, Cyclessa, Desogen, Kariva, Mircette, Ortho-Cept)
  - Ethinyl estradiol and drospirenone (Yasmin)
  - Ethinyl estradiol and ethynodiol diacetate (Demulen 1/35 and 1/50, Zovia 1/35E and 1/50E)

– Ethinyl estradiol and levonorgestrel (Alesse, Aviane, Enpresse, Levlen, Levlite, Nordette, Portia, Seasonale, Tri-Levlen, Triphasil)
– Ethinyl estradiol and norethindrone (Brevicon; Estrostep 21; Estrostep Fe; Modicon; Loestrin 21 1/20 and 21 1.5/30; Microgestin Fe 1/20 and 1.5/30; Norinyl (1+35); Ovcon-35 and -50; Ortho-Novum 1/35, 10/11, and 7/7/7; Tri-Norinyl)
– Ethinyl estradiol and norgestimate (Necon, Norinyl, Ortho-Novum, Ortho Tri-Cyclen, Ortho Tri-Cyclen Lo)
– Ethinyl estradiol and norgestrel (Cryselle, Lo/Ovral, Low-Ogestrel, Ogestrel)
– Mestranol and norethindrone (Necon 1/50, Norinyl 1 + 50, Ortho-Novum 1/50, Ovcon-50)

● Indications
- Prevent pregnancy in females
- Treat moderate acne in females older than age 15 (Ortho Tri-Cyclen)

● Contraindications and precautions
- Contraindicated in patients who are pregnant, trying to become pregnant, or breast-feeding; patients who have delivered within previous 4 weeks; and those with a history of thrombophlebitis or thromboembolic disorders, deep vein thrombosis (DVT), stroke, coronary artery disease (CAD), known carcinoma of the breast, any estrogen-dependent neoplasm, abnormal genital bleeding, or cholestatic jaundice during pregnancy
- Used cautiously in patients who smoke; patients with fibrocystic breast disease or an abnormal mammogram; and those with a history of migraines, high blood pressure, or diabetes

● Adverse reactions
- Potentially serious reactions: Arterial thrombosis, thrombophlebitis, pulmonary embolism, myocardial infarction, cerebral hemorrhage or thrombosis, hypertension, gallbladder disease, and hepatic adenomas
- Stomach upset, vomiting, bloating, diarrhea, weight fluctuations, acne, unusual hair growth, breast tenderness or enlargement, difficulty wearing contact lenses, and changes in libido
- Possible bleeding or spotting between menses

● Interactions
- Use with antibiotics, oxcarbazepine, phenobarbital, phenytoin, topiramate, or modafinil may decrease effectiveness of these drugs; patient should be instructed to use barrier contraceptive when drugs are taken together
- Use with atorvastatin may increase serum estrogen levels
- Increased risk of cyclosporine or theophylline toxicity when taken with hormonal contraceptives
- Use with prednisone increases therapeutic and possibly toxic drug effects
- Serum drug levels may be affected by various herbal medications

When to use hormonal contraceptives
- Pregnancy prevention
- Acne

When NOT to use hormonal contraceptives
- Pregnancy or breast-feeding
- History of thrombophlebitis or thromboembolism, DVT, stroke, CAD, breast cancer, or estrogen-dependent neoplasm

Adverse reactions
- Arterial thrombosis, thrombophlebitis, pulmonary embolism, myocardial infarction, cerebral hemorrhage or thrombosis, hypertension, gallbladder disease, hepatic adenomas

● **Nursing responsibilities**
- Instruct the patient to take the drug at the same time every day
- Advise the patient how to take her pills (21-, 28-, or 91-day packet)
- Teach the patient how to make up for missed doses
  - If she misses one dose: Take missed dose as soon as she remembers, or take two tablets the next day
  - If she misses two doses: Take two tablets each day for the next 2 days, then resume regular drug schedule
  - If she misses three or more tablets: Begin a new cycle of pills 7 days after start of next menses, and use additional (barrier) method of birth control
- Stress to the patient that hormonal contraceptives don't protect against human immunodeficiency virus and other sexually transmitted diseases (STDs)
- Teach the patient about possible drug interactions, life-threatening reactions, and when additional form of contraception is needed
- Advise the patient to call the practitioner immediately if she misses two consecutive periods; she may be pregnant

ESTROGENS, PROGESTINS, AND PROLACTIN SECRETION INHIBITORS

ESTROGENS AND PROGESTINS

● **Mechanism of action**
- Simulate endogenous hormones to restore hormonal balance and treat hormone-sensitive tumors

● **Pharmacokinetics**
- Absorption: Well absorbed from GI tract
- Distribution: Largely protein-bound; distributed into virtually all body tissues
- Metabolism: Metabolized in liver; skin metabolizes transdermal systems to a small extent
- Excretion: Some estrogens are excreted in bile, reabsorbed from intestines, and returned to liver; water-soluble estrogens are excreted in urine, and tubular reabsorption is minimal

● **Drug examples**
- Conjugated estrogenic substances (Premarin), drospirenone and estradiol, estradiol (Delestrogen, Depo-Estradiol, Estrace, Estraderm), medroxyprogesterone (Provera), megestrol (Megace), norethindrone/mestranol (Norinyl, Ortho-Novum), progesterone

● **Indications**
- Provide contraception; treat hormonal deficiencies, breast cancer, endometriosis, and (during menopause) hot flashes and atrophic vaginitis; and restore positive calcium balance in postmenopausal osteoporosis (estrogens)

Key nursing actions

- Instruct the patient to take the drug at the same time every day.
- Provide patient teaching (administration schedule, missed dose, drug interactions, adverse effects).

Key facts about estrogens and progestins

- Simulate endogenous hormones to restore hormonal balance and treat hormone-sensitive tumors
- Metabolized in liver and skin
- Varied excretion

When to use estrogens and progestins

- Contraception
- Hormonal deficiencies
- Breast cancer
- Endometriosis
- Menopausal hot flashes and atrophic vaginitis
- Calcium restoration
- Menstrual cycle regulation or restoration
- Endometrial or renal cancer
- Premenstrual syndrome

When NOT to use estrogens and progestins

- Embolism
- Thrombophlebitis
- Breast cancer
- History of stroke
- Unexplained abnormal genital bleeding
- Pregnancy
- Cardiovascular disease prevention

Adverse reactions

- Nausea, vomiting, diarrhea, weight gain, edema, rash, headache, insomnia, hypertension, thromboembolic disorders, endometrial and breast cancer, gall bladder disease, thromboembolic disease, hepatic adenoma, massive elevations in triglyceride levels that lead to pancreatitis, depression

Key nursing actions

- Assess for edema; monitor blood pressure, weight, and cholesterol and triglyceride levels.
- Warn the patients not to smoke while taking these drugs because smoking increases the risk of thromboembolism.
- Instruct the patient to immediately notify the practitioner if she experiences groin, calf, or chest pain; shortness of breath; or abdominal bleeding.

- Provide contraception; regulate or restore the menstrual cycle; and treat endometrial or renal cancer, endometriosis, and premenstrual syndrome (progestins)

● **Contraindications and precautions**
- Contraindicated in patients with cardiovascular disease, embolism, thrombophlebitis, breast cancer, history of stroke, unexplained abnormal genital bleeding, and known or suspected pregnancy
- Used cautiously in patients with asthma, epilepsy, migraine, or heart or kidney disease
- Estrogens and progestins shouldn't be used to prevent cardiovascular disease

● **Adverse reactions**
- Nausea, vomiting, diarrhea, anorexia, malaise, weight gain, edema, rash, headache, insomnia, hypertension, and thromboembolic disorders (including deep vein thrombosis and pulmonary embolism)
- Increased risk of endometrial and breast cancer, gall bladder disease requiring surgery (in postmenopausal patients), thromboembolic disease, hepatic adenoma, and massive elevations in triglyceride levels that lead to pancreatitis (in patients with a family history of lipoprotein metabolism) (estrogens)
- Estrogens may increase the risk of depression

● **Interactions**
- Penicillins, sulfonamides, and tetracyclines alter normal GI flora, decreasing effects of estrogen
- Estrogens decrease effects of barbiturates, anticonvulsants, antidiabetics, and oral anticoagulants
- Estrogens may increase effects and risk of toxicity of corticosteroids
- Hydantoins may decrease effects of estrogens and cause breakthrough bleeding, spotting, and pregnancy

● **Nursing responsibilities**
- Assess for edema; monitor blood pressure, weight, and cholesterol and triglyceride levels
- Teach the patient the appropriate administration technique (oral, intravaginal, or transdermal use)
- Explain the importance of complying with therapy (see *Teaching about estrogen replacement therapy*)
- Warn the patient not to smoke while taking these drugs; smoking increases the risk of thromboembolism (especially in females older than age 35)
- Advise the patient to receive routine breast, pelvic, and blood pressure examinations and Papanicolaou tests to detect adverse effects
- Advise the patient who suspects she's pregnant to notify her practitioner immediately

TIME-OUT FOR TEACHING

Teaching about estrogen replacement therapy

Include these topics in your teaching plan for the patient receiving estrogen replacement therapy:
- medication regimen, including the drug's name, dosage, frequency, duration, and possible adverse effects
- signs and symptoms to discuss with the practitioner, including headache, shortness of breath, chest pain, breast lumps, and calf tenderness or swelling
- proper administration technique
- cyclic nature of therapy
- breast self-examination
- follow-up care, including breast and pelvic examinations, Papanicolaou tests, and practitioner visits.

- Urge the patient to immediately notify the practitioner if she experiences pain in the groin or calves, sharp chest pain or sudden shortness of breath, abnormal bleeding, sudden severe headaches, dizziness, fainting, vision or speech disturbances, weakness in arms or legs, severe abdominal pain, yellowing of skin or eyes, or severe depression

PROLACTIN SECRETION INHIBITORS

● **Mechanism of action**
- Decrease serum prolactin level in hyperprolactinemia by mimicking the action of prolactin inhibitory factor, which decreases release of prolactin and galactorrhea

● **Pharmacokinetics**
- Absorption: Bromocriptine is poorly (about 28%) absorbed in GI tract; bioavailability of cabergoline is unknown
- Distribution: Bromocriptine is highly (90% to 96%) protein-bound to albumin; cabergoline not highly protein-bound
- Metabolism: Completely metabolized by liver
- Excretion: Primarily excreted in feces with minor excretion in urine

● **Drug examples**
- Bromocriptine (Parlodel), cabergoline (Dostinex)

● **Indications**
- Inhibit prolactin secretion in idiopathic or pituitary adenoma–induced hyperprolactinemia
- Treat hyperprolactinemia-associated dysfunctions, including amenorrhea with or without galactorrhea, infertility, and hypogonadism (bromocriptine)
- Treat acromegaly and Parkinson's disease (bromocriptine)

Key facts about prolactin secretion inhibitors

- Decrease the serum prolactin level
- Metabolized in liver
- Excreted primarily in feces

When to use prolactin secretion inhibitors

- Idiopathic or pituitary adenoma–induced hyperprolactinemia
- Hyperprolactinemia-associated dysfunctions
- Acromegaly
- Parkinson's disease

When NOT to use prolactin secretion inhibitors

- Hypersensitivity
- Uncontrolled hypertension
- Severe ischemic heart disease
- Peripheral vascular disease

Adverse reactions

- Orthostatic and symptomatic hypotension, nausea, headache, dizziness, vertigo, fatigue, light-headedness, vomiting, abdominal cramps, nasal congestion, constipation, diarrhea, psychosis, hypotension, pulmonary infiltrates, pleural effusion, pleural thickening

Key nursing actions

- Know that for patients being treated for amenorrhea and galactorrhea, bromocriptine suppresses galactorrhea and reinitiates normal ovulatory menstrual cycles; some may respond in a few days, whereas others may take up to 8 months.
- Know that dizziness and fainting may occur.

Key facts about fertility drugs

- Stimulate ovarian function by increasing levels of pituitary gonadotropins
- Metabolism unknown
- Excreted in feces

● **Contraindications and precautions**
- Contraindicated in patients with hypersensitivity to ergot alkaloids
- Cabergoline contraindicated in patients with uncontrolled hypertension
- Bromocriptine contraindicated in patients with severe ischemic heart disease or peripheral vascular disease

● **Adverse reactions**
- Orthostatic and symptomatic hypotension
- Various adverse reactions (usually ranging from mild to moderate), including nausea, headache, dizziness, vertigo, fatigue, light-headedness, vomiting, abdominal cramps, nasal congestion, constipation, diarrhea, psychosis, and hypotension; long-term treatment may cause pulmonary infiltrates, pleural effusion, and pleural thickening (bromocriptine)
- Headache, nausea, and vomiting (cabergoline)

● **Interactions**
- Erythromycin may increase bromocriptine levels
- Sympathomimetics exacerbate adverse effects of bromocriptine
- Phenothiazines decrease efficacy of bromocriptine and cabergoline
- Cabergoline has additive hypotensive effects when given with antihypertensive medications

● **Nursing responsibilities**
- Know that for patients being treated for amenorrhea and galactorrhea, bromocriptine suppresses galactorrhea and reinitiates normal ovulatory menstrual cycles, usually in 6 to 8 weeks; however, some patients may respond in as little as a few days, whereas others may take up to 8 months
- Perform pituitary evaluation before start of treatment because bromocriptine has been associated with pituitary tumors
- Give bromocriptine with food
- Know that dizziness and fainting may occur, particularly following the first dose or if the patient stands up too quickly
  - Instruct the patient to take the first dose lying down
  - Advise the patient to avoid sudden position changes, such as rising immediately from a sitting position

FERTILITY DRUGS (OVULATION STIMULANTS)

● **Mechanism of action**
- Stimulate ovarian function by increasing levels of pituitary gonadotropins, thereby stimulating the maturation and endocrine activity of ovarian follicles and subsequent development and function of the corpus luteum

● **Pharmacokinetics**
- Absorption: Well-absorbed, except for follitropins, which have absorption-rate limitations; absorption rate following I.M. and subcutaneous (subQ) administration is slower than excretion rate

- Distribution: Unknown
- Metabolism: Unknown
- Excretion: Excreted in feces

Drug examples

- Choriogonadotropin alfa (Ovidrel), clomiphene citrate (Clomid, Milophene, Serophene), follitropin alfa (Gonal-F), follitropin beta (Follistim), human chorionic gonadotropin (hCG [Chorex-5, Choron 10, Gonic, Pregnyl, Profasi]), human menopausal gonadotropin (Pergonal), menotropins (Pergonal, Repronex), urofollitropin (Bravelle, Fertinex)

Indications

- Treat infertility secondary to anovulation (through stimulation of endocrine gland)
- Follicle stimulation in patients undergoing in vitro fertilization or other assisted reproductive technology
- Concomitant treatment to stimulate spermatogenesis in males with primary or secondary hypogonadotropic hypogonadism (menotropins [Pergonal only] with hCG)
- Treat infertility in females with polycystic ovary syndrome (urofollitropin)
- Treat prepubertal cryptorchidism and hypogonadism in males and induce ovulation in females (chorionic gonadotropin)

Contraindications and precautions

- hCG contraindicated in pregnant patients and those with precocious puberty, prostatic carcinoma or other androgen-dependent neoplasm, or prior allergic reaction to hCG; used cautiously in patients with epilepsy, migraines, asthma, or cardiac or renal disease (androgens may cause fluid retention)
- Menotropins contraindicated in female patients who are pregnant or who have high gonadotropin levels indicating primary ovarian failure, overt thyroid dysfunction, any cause of infertility other than anovulation, abnormal bleeding, ovarian cysts or enlargement not due to polycystic ovary syndrome, or organic intracranial lesion (such as pituitary tumor); also contraindicated in male patients with normal gonadotropin levels, elevated gonadotropin levels indicating primary testicular failure, or infertility disorders other than hypogonadotropic hypogonadism
- Follitropins contraindicated in pregnant patients and those with high FSH levels indicating primary ovarian failure, uncontrolled thyroid or adrenal dysfunction, infertility not due to anovulation, abnormal vaginal bleeding, ovarian cysts or enlargement not due to polycystic ovary syndrome, or tumors of the breast, ovary, uterus, hypothalamus, or pituitary gland
- Clomiphene contraindicated in pregnant patients or those with liver disease or a history of liver dysfunction, abnormal bleeding, organic intracranial lesion, ovarian cysts, or uncontrolled thyroid or adrenal dysfunction

When to use fertility drugs

- Infertility
- Follicle stimulation
- Spermatogenesis stimulation (with primary or secondary hypogonadotropic hypogonadism)
- Prepubertal cryptorchidism and hypogonadism
- Ovulation inducement

When NOT to use fertility drugs

- Pregnancy
- Precocious puberty
- Prostatic carcinoma or other androgen-dependent neoplasm
- Allergies to hCG
- High gonadotropin levels (women)
- Normal or elevated gonadotropin levels (men)
- High levels of FSH
- Liver disease
- History of liver dysfunction
- Abnormal bleeding
- Organic intracranial lesion
- Ovarian cysts
- Uncontrolled thyroid or adrenal dysfunction

Adverse reactions

- Cyst formation, hot flashes, dizziness, light-headedness, nausea, vomiting, abnormal uterine bleeding, pulmonary and vascular complications, adnexal torsion, breast pain, gynecomastia, mastitis

Key nursing actions

- Instruct in infertility measures and the importance of complying with therapy.
- Warn of the risk of ovarian hyperstimulation syndrome and multiple births.

Key facts about abortifacients

- Compete with progesterone at progesterone receptor sites
- Result in termination of pregnancy
- Primarily metabolized in liver
- Primarily excreted in feces

When to use abortifacients

- Pregnancy termination
- Uterine content evacuation
- Nonmetastatic gestational trophoblastic disease management

When NOT to use abortifacients

- Ectopic pregnancy
- Adnexal mass
- IUD
- Chronic adrenal failure
- Hemorrhagic disorders
- Concurrent anticoagulation therapy
- Inherited porphyrias
- Hypersensitivity
- Acute pelvic inflammatory disease
- Active cardiac, pulmonary, hepatic, or renal disease

- ● **Adverse reactions**
  - Hot flashes, dizziness, light-headedness, nausea, vomiting, bloating, and abnormal uterine bleeding
  - Possible multiple births, ovarian enlargement, and cyst formation
  - Pulmonary and vascular complications and adnexal torsion as a complication of ovarian enlargement (follitropins)
  - In males, may cause breast pain, gynecomastia, mastitis, nausea, and abnormal liver enzyme levels (menotropins)

- ● **Interactions**
  - None significant

- ● **Nursing responsibilities**
  - Instruct the patient in infertility measures and the importance of complying with therapy
  - Offer emotional support
  - Encourage compliance with follow-up diagnostic testing to evaluate drug effectiveness
  - Warn the patient about the risk of ovarian hyperstimulation syndrome and multiple births with treatment

ABORTIFACIENTS

- ● **Mechanism of action**
  - Compete with progesterone at progesterone receptor sites, resulting in inactivity of progesterone and termination of pregnancy

- ● **Pharmacokinetics**
  - Absorption: Rapidly absorbed following oral administration
  - Distribution: Highly protein-bound
  - Metabolism: Primarily metabolized in liver
  - Excretion: Primarily excreted in feces

- ● **Drug examples**
  - Mifepristone (Mifeprex, RU-486), prostaglandins, carboprost tromethamine (Hemabate), dinoprostone (prostaglandin E_2 [Prostin E2]), misoprostol (Cytotec)

- ● **Indications**
  - Termination of pregnancy
  - Uterine content evacuation and management of nonmetastatic gestational trophoblastic disease (benign hydatidiform mole) (dinoprostone)

- ● **Contraindications and precautions**
  - Mifepristone contraindicated in patients with intrauterine devices (IUDs), ectopic pregnancy, adnexal mass, chronic adrenal failure, concurrent long-term corticosteroid therapy, hemorrhagic disorders, concurrent anticoagulation therapy, allergy to drug or other prostaglandins, or inherited porphyrias

- Prostaglandins contraindicated in patients with hypersensitivity to drug, acute pelvic inflammatory disease, or active cardiac, pulmonary, hepatic, or renal disease

● **Adverse reactions**
- Nausea, vomiting, diarrhea, headache, abdominal pain, and heavy uterine bleeding

● **Interactions**
- Use with oxytocics may enhance oxytocic effects

● **Nursing responsibilities**
- Inform the patient that treatment with abortifacients requires three office visits
- Warn the patient that surgical intervention may be needed in cases of incomplete abortion or severe bleeding; other measures may be required to ensure complete abortion
- Explain to the patient that she may experience bleeding or spotting for 9 to 16 days or up to 30 days after treatment; urge her to seek medical treatment if she experiences persistent, moderate to heavy vaginal bleeding
- Teach the patient about the use of an appropriate contraceptive method after treatment is completed

OBSTETRIC DRUGS

OXYTOCIC DRUGS

● **Mechanism of action**
- Enhance uterine motility by directly stimulating uterine and smooth-muscle contraction

● **Pharmacokinetics**
- Absorption: Immediate
- Distribution: Unknown
- Metabolism: Unknown
- Excretion: Eliminated through kidneys, liver, and mammary glands

● **Drug examples**
- Ergonovine maleate (Ergotrate Maleate), methylergonovine maleate (Methergine), oxytocin (Pitocin, Syntocinon), dinoprostone (prostaglandin E_2 [Prostin E2])

● **Indications**
- Manage postpartum hemorrhage
- Promote labor, initiate milk letdown reflex, induce therapeutic abortion, and test uteroplacental respiratory reserve (unlabeled use) (oxytocin)

Adverse reactions

- Nausea, vomiting, diarrhea, headache

Key nursing actions

- Warn the patient that surgical intervention may be needed in cases of incomplete abortion or severe bleeding.
- Explain that she may experience bleeding or spotting for 9 to 16 days after treatment.

Key facts about oxytocic drugs

- Enhance uterine mobility by stimulating uterine and smooth-muscle contraction
- Metabolism unknown
- Excreted through kidneys, liver, and mammary glands

When to use oxytocic drugs

- Postpartum hemorrhage
- Labor promotion
- Milk letdown reflex initiation
- Therapeutic abortion
- Uteroplacental respiratory reserve test

When NOT to use oxytocic drugs

- Obstetric emergencies
- Maternal hypertension
- Significant cephalopelvic disproportions
- Unfavorable fetal positions
- Fetal distress
- Drug hypersensitivity

Adverse reactions

- Nausea, vomiting, bradycardia, hypertension, anaphylaxis

Of oxytocin
- Fetal: bradycardia, hypoxia, intracranial hemorrhage
- Maternal: tetanic contractions, arrhythmias

Key nursing actions

- Oxytocin is given by I.V. infusion only when inducing labor.
- I.V. infusion of oxytocin requires continuous monitoring and observations.
- Monitor the fetal heart rate.

Key facts about labor suppressants

- Relax uterine muscles
- Decrease uterine contractions
- Metabolism unknown
- Excreted primarily in urine

When to use labor suppressants

- Premature labor prevention

● Contraindications and precautions
- Contraindicated in obstetric emergencies, maternal hypertension, and gestational hypertension
- Contraindicated in patients with significant cephalopelvic disproportions, unfavorable fetal positions, fetal distress, or hypersensitivity to drug

● Adverse reactions
- Nausea, vomiting, bradycardia, hypertension, anaphylaxis, and severe water intoxication
- Oxytocin: May cause separate effects for fetus and mother
    - Fetal: Bradycardia, hypoxia, and intracranial hemorrhage
    - Maternal: Tetanic contractions and arrhythmias

● Interactions
- Use of dopamine or other vasoconstrictors with ergonovine or methylergonovine may increase peripheral vasoconstriction
- Use of ergonovine or methylergonovine with a vasoconstrictor or regional anesthetic may cause severe hypertension

● Nursing responsibilities
- Be aware that oxytocin is given by I.V. infusion only when used to induce labor; I.V. infusion of oxytocin requires continuous monitoring and observation and a practitioner must be immediately available
- Monitor blood pressure, pulse rate, urine output, uterine contractions, and vaginal bleeding
- Monitor fetal heart rate
- Know that hypocalcemia may decrease the patient's response to ergonovine maleate; administer I.V. calcium salts, if necessary

LABOR SUPPRESSANTS (UTERINE RELAXANTS)

● Mechanism of action
- Relax uterine muscles and decrease uterine contractions
- Exert beta-adrenergic agonist effects on uterine smooth muscles, thereby inhibiting uterine contractions

● Pharmacokinetics
- Absorption: Administered I.V.
- Distribution: 100% bioavailable and 32% protein-bound; drug crosses placental barrier
- Metabolism: Unknown
- Excretion: Primarily excreted in urine

● Drug examples
- Terbutaline (Brethine)

● Indications
- Prevent premature labor from 29 to 36 weeks of gestation

Contraindications and precautions
- Contraindicated in patients with ruptured membranes, abruptio placentae, hypertension, preeclampsia, fetal distress, or pregnancy of less than 20 weeks

Adverse reactions
- Causes separate adverse effects for mother and fetus
  - Maternal: Widening pulse pressure, hypotension, tachycardia, and electrolyte imbalances
  - Fetal: Increased heart rate, hypotension, and hypocalcemia
- Possible transient cerebral ischemia, chorioamnionitis, and intrauterine growth retardation; drug should be used only if benefits outweigh risks

Interactions
- Use with beta-adrenergic blockers interferes with terbutaline's uterine-inhibiting action
- Use with corticosteroids may cause pulmonary edema

Nursing responsibilities
- Place the patient in a left lateral recumbent position to promote venous return to heart and decrease hypotension
- Monitor the patient and fetus closely for adverse effects
- Know that the patient initially will receive the drug by I.V. route but will be switched to oral administration when stable

GONADOTROPIN-RELEASING HORMONES

Mechanism of action
- Initially: Stimulate release of pituitary gonadotropins (LH and FSH), resulting in increased steroidogenesis (gonadotropin-releasing hormone [GnRH] agonistic action)
- With repeated doses: Inhibit stimulatory effects on pituitary gland, leading to decreased secretion of gonadal steroids after about 4 weeks of therapy

Pharmacokinetics
- Absorption:
  - Leuprolide: Rapidly absorbed after subQ administration; unknown for I.M.
  - Gonadorelin: Well-absorbed after I.V. administration
  - Goserelin: Slowly absorbed
- Distribution: Highly protein-bound
- Metabolism: Unknown
- Excretion: Excreted in urine and feces

Drug examples
- Gonadorelin (Lutrepulse), goserelin (Zoladex), leuprolide (Lupron), nafarelin acetate (Synarel)

When NOT to use labor suppressants

- Ruptured membranes
- Abruptio placentae
- Hypertension
- Preeclampsia
- Fetal distress
- Pregnancy of less than 20 weeks

Adverse reactions

- Maternal: transient cerebral ischemia, chorioamnionitis, intrauterine growth retardation; widening pulse pressure, hypotension, tachycardia, electrolyte imbalances; fetal: increased heart rate, hypotension, hypocalcemia

Key nursing actions

- Place in left lateral recumbent position to promote venous return to the heart and decrease hypotension.
- Monitor patient and fetus closely.

Key facts about gonadotropin-releasing hormones

- GnRH agonists that at first stimulate release of pituitary gonadotropins, LH and FSH
- Result is steroidogenesis increase
- Repeated doses inhibit stimulatory effect on pituitary gland
- Metabolism unknown
- Excreted in urine and feces

When to use gonadotropin-releasing hormones

- Endometriosis
- Central precocious puberty
- Advanced prostatic cancer
- Primary hypothalamic amenorrhea

When NOT to use gonadotropin-releasing hormones

- Drug hypersensitivity
- Undiagnosed abnormal vaginal bleeding
- Pregnancy
- Breast-feeding

Adverse reactions

- Hot flashes, headache, nausea, vomiting, constipation, emotional lability, vaginitis, decreased libido

Key nursing actions

- Monitor hydration status to prevent fluid loss from vomiting.
- Closely monitor cardiac status during goserelin therapy.

Key facts about erectile dysfunction drugs

- Inhibit breakdown of cGMP, which increases cGMP levels and causes prolonged smooth-muscle relaxation
- Metabolized in liver and lungs
- Excreted in urine and feces

When to use erectile dysfunction drugs

- Erectile dysfunction

● **Indications**
- Treat endometriosis (leuprolide and nafarelin)
- Treat central precocious puberty (nafarelin)
- Palliative treatment for advanced prostate cancer (goserelin and leuprolide)
- Treat primary hypothalamic amenorrhea (gonadorelin)

● **Contraindications and precautions**
- Contraindicated in pregnant and breast-feeding patients, patients hypersensitive to GnRH agonists, and those with undiagnosed abnormal vaginal bleeding
- Repeated uses aren't recommended for patients who have major risk factors for decreased bone mineral content, such as occurs with alcoholism, drug or tobacco use, or a strong family history of osteoporosis

● **Adverse reactions**
- Hot flashes, headache, nausea, vomiting, constipation, emotional lability, vaginitis, and decreased libido

● **Interactions**
- None reported

● **Nursing responsibilities**
- Administer drug by the appropriate route
- Monitor hydration status to prevent fluid loss from vomiting
- Monitor cardiac status closely during goserelin therapy; drug has been associated with cardiac complications, including heart failure and arrhythmias

ERECTILE DYSFUNCTION DRUGS

● **Mechanism of action**
- Inhibit breakdown of cyclic guanosine monophosphate (cGMP) by phosphodiesterase, which leads to increased cGMP levels and prolonged smooth-muscle relaxation, thereby promoting blood flow into the corpus cavernosum

● **Pharmacokinetics**
- Absorption: Orally absorbed; alprostadil absorbed via I.V. or intracavernous route
- Distribution: Widely distributed; highly protein-bound
- Metabolism: Hepatically metabolized; alprostadil metabolized in lungs
- Excretion: Excreted in urine and feces; alprostadil excreted solely in urine

● **Drug examples**
- Alprostadil (Caverject, Caverject Impulse), sildenafil (Viagra), tadalafil (Cialis), vardenafil (Levitra)

● **Indications**
- Treat erectile dysfunction

- **Contraindications and precautions**
  - Not intended for use in females
  - Shouldn't be used by patients taking nitrates
  - Used cautiously in patients with hepatic or renal dysfunction or known cardiac disease, patients taking alpha-blocker therapy for BPH, or those with a prolonged QT interval (rare prolongation of QT has occurred)

- **Adverse reactions**
  - Headache, dizziness, flushing, dyspepsia, and vision changes
  - Possible prolonged erections (lasting longer than 4 hours), which may result in irreversible damage to erectile tissue
  - Alprostadil: Penile pain

- **Interactions**
  - Use with nitrates may cause severe hypotension and potentially serious cardiac events
  - Increased drug levels may occur with use of cimetidine, amlodipine, erythromycin, or protease inhibitors
  - Absorption is decreased when taken with grapefruit juice

- **Nursing responsibilities**
  - Inform the patient that the drug doesn't protect against pregnancy or transmission of STDs
  - Advise the patient that the drug won't work without sexual stimulation
  - Instruct the patient to seek medical attention if erection lasts longer than 4 hours
  - Warn the patient taking HIV medications about the risk of adverse effects, including hypotension and priapism
  - Advise the patient that the drug must be taken 30 minutes to 4 hours before anticipated sexual activity
  - Inform the patient about the need to tell all health care providers that he's taking an erectile dysfunction drug

NCLEX CHECKS

It's never too soon to begin your NCLEX® preparation. Now that you've reviewed this chapter, carefully read each of the following questions and choose the best answer. Then compare your responses with the correct answers.

1. A client asks, "Why is the physician prescribing danazol (Danocrine) for my endometriosis?" The nurse's best answer would be that the drug:

☐ **1.** increases the activity of the ovaries.

☐ **2.** increases the production of estrogen.

☐ **3.** causes the body to release an LH surge.

☐ **4.** decreases the secretion of FSH and LH.

2. A client with metastatic breast cancer is ordered testosterone, an androgenic steroid. Although androgenic and anabolic steroids produce similar effects, which rationale correctly describes how they differ?

- [ ] **1.** Androgenic steroids produce masculinizing effects; anabolic steroids build muscle mass.
- [ ] **2.** Androgenic steroids promote a positive nitrogen balance; anabolic steroids stimulate cellular protein synthesis.
- [ ] **3.** Androgenic steroids promote tissue growth; anabolic steroids stimulate the development of male sex characteristics.
- [ ] **4.** Androgenic steroids promote the development of female sex characteristics; anabolic steroids suppress their development.

3. A nurse is administering estrogen therapy to a postmenopausal client. Which adverse reaction should the nurse specifically mention in her teaching plan for this drug?

- [ ] **1.** Renal calculi
- [ ] **2.** Uterine atony
- [ ] **3.** Deep vein thrombosis
- [ ] **4.** Narrowing of the visual fields

4. A pregnant client experiences fetal demise during the 30th week of gestation. She asks the nurse why she's being given a prostaglandin E_2 suppository at this time. The nurse appropriately responds by stating that prostaglandin suppositories:

- [ ] **1.** cause labor to start.
- [ ] **2.** prevent postpartum infections in cases like this.
- [ ] **3.** help relieve pain when the baby is delivered.
- [ ] **4.** allow the client to relax and decrease her anxiety.

5. A client is taking a hormonal contraceptive. The nurse must instruct her about the possibility of decreased effectiveness of hormonal contraceptives if she's also taking:

- [ ] **1.** an anticoagulant.
- [ ] **2.** a benzodiazepine.
- [ ] **3.** a corticosteroid.
- [ ] **4.** a tetracycline.

6. While monitoring a client who's receiving oxytocin (Pitocin) to induce labor, the nurse should be prepared for which possible maternal adverse reactions? Select all that apply.

- [ ] **1.** Hypertension
- [ ] **2.** Jaundice
- [ ] **3.** Dehydration
- [ ] **4.** Fluid overload
- [ ] **5.** Uterine tetany
- [ ] **6.** Bradycardia

7. A sexually active client is ordered tetracycline for treatment of acne. Because the client is currently taking ethinyl estradiol and norethindrone (Ortho-Novum), the nurse informs her that:

- ☐ **1.** diabetes can be caused by this combination of medications.
- ☐ **2.** both medications must be taken as ordered and spaced 2 hours apart.
- ☐ **3.** this drug combination places the client at increased risk for stroke.
- ☐ **4.** an alternate method of birth control must be used during tetracycline therapy.

8. A client develops abnormal uterine bleeding caused by a hormonal imbalance. Before giving conjugated estrogenic substances, 25 mg. I.M., as ordered, the nurse obtains a thorough medical history. Which condition revealed during the history is of special concern to the nurse?

- ☐ **1.** Diabetes mellitus
- ☐ **2.** Epilepsy
- ☐ **3.** Gallbladder disease
- ☐ **4.** Pregnancy

9. A client taking ethinyl estradiol and norgestrel (Lo/Ovral) calls the women's health clinic because she missed taking her pills for 2 days and doesn't know how to proceed. Which instruction should the nurse provide in addition to the use of an alternative birth control method for the rest of the month?

- ☐ **1.** "Take three pills tonight, and then resume the rest of your pack tomorrow."
- ☐ **2.** "Stop taking your pills this month, and begin a new pack after your period."
- ☐ **3.** "Take two pills tonight, two pills tomorrow night, and then resume the rest of your pack."
- ☐ **4.** "Just resume the pack with tonight's pill, and continue as scheduled."

10. Which complication may be potentially life-threatening in a client who's receiving terbutaline (Brethine) for preterm labor?

- ☐ **1.** Diabetic ketoacidosis
- ☐ **2.** Hyperemesis gravidarum
- ☐ **3.** Pulmonary edema
- ☐ **4.** Sickle cell anemia

ANSWERS AND RATIONALES

1. Correct answer: 4
Danazol is an antigonadotropin that suppresses the production of LH and FSH, reducing engorgement in ectopic endometrial tissue and its accompanying pain. The drug decreases ovarian activity and estrogen production, and it reduces LH.

2. CORRECT ANSWER: 1

Androgenic steroids produce masculinizing effects; anabolic steroids build muscle mass. Androgenic steroids don't promote the development of female sex characteristics, a positive nitrogen balance, or tissue growth. Anabolic steroids don't suppress female sex characteristics, stimulate cellular protein synthesis, or stimulate the development of male sex characteristics.

3. CORRECT ANSWER: 3

Estrogen therapy increases clotting tendencies. The nurse should warn the client to call her physician if she experiences leg pain, redness, or swelling because she may have developed deep vein thrombosis. A client who smokes should also be warned to avoid smoking during drug therapy because smoking increases the risk of blood clots. Estrogen therapy doesn't cause narrowing of the visual fields, uterine atony, or renal calculi.

4. CORRECT ANSWER: 1

Prostaglandin vaginal suppositories or gels are used to induce labor in cases of second- or third-trimester fetal demise. They stimulate smooth muscle and cause the uterus to contract. They're also sometimes used before induction of normal pregnancies. Prostaglandin has no analgesic, anxiolytic, or antimicrobial effects.

5. CORRECT ANSWER: 4

Tetracycline, ampicillin, and penicillin V cause alterations in the normal flora of the GI tract that can lead to a decreased efficacy of the contraceptive agent and result in pregnancy. Use of a hormonal contraceptive with any of the other drugs listed can cause an increase or decrease in the drug's (anticoagulant, benzodiazepine, or corticosteroid) level, but it won't affect the level or efficacy of the hormonal contraceptive.

6. CORRECT ANSWER: 1, 4, 5

Adverse reactions to oxytocin in the mother include hypertension, fluid overload, and uterine tetany. The antidiuretic effect of oxytocin increases renal reabsorption of water, leading to fluid overload—not dehydration. Jaundice and bradycardia are adverse reactions that may occur in the neonate. Tachycardia, not bradycardia, is reported as a maternal adverse reaction.

7. CORRECT ANSWER: 4

Tetracycline interferes with the effectiveness of such hormonal contraceptives as ethinyl estradiol and norethindrone; an alternative method of birth control must be used. Hormonal contraceptive use already places the client at risk for stroke; the client's new drug combination doesn't further compound this risk. Diabetes isn't caused by this drug combination. Taking both medications 2 hours apart doesn't increase the effectiveness of the hormonal contraceptive.

8. CORRECT ANSWER: 4

Estrogens are contraindicated for use during pregnancy because they may result in congenital fetal defects. Caution is required for clients with epilepsy, gallbladder disease, and diabetes mellitus.

9. CORRECT ANSWER: 3

When a client misses two consecutive doses of oral contraceptives, the nurse should advise her to take two tablets the first night, two tablets the next night, and then resume the pack as scheduled. There's no need to stop taking the pills; however, an alternative method of birth control should be used for the rest of the month. The other options aren't appropriate for this product.

10. CORRECT ANSWER: 3

The most common adverse reaction associated with the use of terbutaline is pulmonary edema. Unless the client has diabetes, it isn't necessary to observe for diabetic ketoacidosis. Hyperemesis gravidarum doesn't result from terbutaline use. Sickle cell anemia is an inherited genetic condition and doesn't develop spontaneously.

16

Drugs and the integumentary system

PRETEST

1. Which type of dermatologic agent helps the skin retain water?
- [ ] 1. Antipruritic
- [ ] 2. Emollient
- [ ] 3. Keratolytic
- [ ] 4. Antiviral

CORRECT ANSWER: 2

2. A nurse should expect which agent to be ordered for a client with a viral skin infection?
- [ ] 1. Acyclovir (Zovirax)
- [ ] 2. Bacitracin
- [ ] 3. Hydrocortisone (Acticort)
- [ ] 4. Silver sulfadiazine (Silvadene)

CORRECT ANSWER: 1

3. Which adverse reaction is common to all dermatologic agents?
- [ ] 1. Tachycardia
- [ ] 2. Constipation
- [ ] 3. Skin irritation
- [ ] 4. Photosensitivity

CORRECT ANSWER: 3

4. Which class of drugs kills or inhibits the growth of fungi?

☐ 1. Antifungals
☐ 2. Antivirals
☐ 3. Antipruritics
☐ 4. Antiparasitics

CORRECT ANSWER: 1

5. Which test parameters should be monitored in a client taking isotretinoin (Accutane)?

☐ 1. Serum creatinine level and red blood cell count
☐ 2. Serum glucose level and white blood cell count
☐ 3. Serum lipid levels and hepatic function test results
☐ 4. Thyroid function test results and ophthalmic examinations

CORRECT ANSWER: 3

LEARNING OBJECTIVES

After studying this chapter, you should be able to:

● Describe the general uses and mechanism of action of various topical drugs.
● List common adverse reactions to topical drugs.
● Identify important nursing responsibilities and patient teaching requirements related to the administration of topical drugs.

CHAPTER OVERVIEW

Topical drugs are lotions and ointments that are applied directly to the skin. Used to treat various dermatologic conditions, they include emollients, keratolytics, antibacterial drugs, antifungals, antivirals, antiparasitics, anti-inflammatories, debriding drugs, antipruritics, and acne products.

ANATOMY AND PHYSIOLOGY

A&P highlights

- The integumentary system consists of the skin and its derivatives, such as hair, nails, and sweat, sebaceous, and ceruminous glands.
- The epidermis is the skin's surface layer and the body's outermost protective covering.
- The dermis lies just below the epidermis and constitutes the bulk of the skin.
- Beneath the dermis is subcutaneous tissue that attaches the skin to underlying structures.
- Chemically, acidic skin secretions inhibit bacteria from multiplying on the body's surface.
- Keratinized cells of the epidermis, hair, and nails provide a barrier to invading organisms.
- Macrophage-like Langerhans' cells attack bacteria and viruses.
- The skin maintains body temperature at about 98.6° F (37° C) via thermoregulation.
- When the body is hot, sweat glands produce perspiration and blood vessels dilate.
- When the body is cold, blood vessels constrict to prevent heat loss.

● **Anatomy of the integumentary system**
- Consists of skin and its derivatives (hair, nails, the sudoriferous [sweat] glands, sebaceous [oil] glands, and ceruminous glands)
- Skin
  - Is the body's largest and most visible organ
  - Contains blood vessels, nerves, sweat glands, oil glands, sensory receptors, and cells in every square inch
- Skin layers
  - Epidermis
    - Surface layer of skin
    - Body's outermost protective covering
  - Dermis
    - Lies just below epidermis
    - Constitutes bulk of skin
  - Subcutaneous tissue
    - Located beneath dermis
    - Also called *hypodermis* or *superficial fascia*
    - Is loose connective tissue that attaches skin to underlying structures

● **Physiology**
- Protective mechanisms of skin
  - Chemically, acidic skin secretions inhibit bacteria from multiplying on body's surface
  - Physically, keratinized cells of the epidermis, hair, and nails provide barrier to invading organisms
  - Biologically, skin contains macrophage-like Langerhans' cells that attack bacteria and viruses
  - When exposed to ultraviolet light, skin converts cholesterol to vitamin D
- Thermoregulation
  - In this homeostatic process, skin maintains body's temperature at about 98.6° F (37° C)
  - Process is regulated by a negative feedback mechanism
    - Skin receptors sense temperature stimulus (heat or cold) and then send impulses to control center of brain

· Brain transmits impulses to effector organs (sweat glands and blood vessels)
· Effector organs respond accordingly to brain's message
  - When body is hot, sweat glands produce perspiration and blood vessels dilate; evaporation of sweat from surface dissipates heat; vasodilation brings more warm blood to skin, where it's cooled
  - When the body is cold, blood vessels constrict to prevent heat loss
- Nutrition and hormones influence hair growth and distribution and affect sebaceous gland secretions

● **Function**
- Skin has six major functions
  - Protects body chemically, physically, and biologically
  - Excretes waste products from body
  - Helps regulate body temperature
  - Provides cutaneous sensation
  - Promotes vitamin D synthesis
  - Acts as reservoir for blood
- Hair protects body from heat loss and ultraviolet rays, shields the eyes, and helps keep dust out of upper respiratory tract
- Nails protect ends of fingers and toes
- Sudoriferous glands help maintain normal body temperature
- Sebaceous glands secrete sebum that softens and lubricates hair and skin, impedes water loss from skin, and acts as bactericide
- Ceruminous glands line external ear canal; secretions combine with those of sebaceous gland to form cerumen (earwax)

TOPICAL DRUGS

● **Mechanism of action**
- Emollients: Allow skin to retain water
- Keratolytics: Break down protein in keratin, causing loss of the skin's stratum corneum layer
- Antibacterial drugs: Kill (bactericidal action) or inhibit growth of (bacteriostatic action) susceptible bacteria
- Antifungals: Kill or inhibit growth of susceptible fungi
- Antivirals: Kill or inhibit growth of susceptible viruses
- Antiparasitics: Kill parasitic arthropods
- Anti-inflammatories: Decrease inflammation and itching and cause vasoconstriction
- Debriding and wound-healing agents: Digest necrotic collagenous tissue, thereby removing substances necessary for bacterial growth and allowing better access to the site for antibodies, leukocytes, and anti-infectives
- Antipruritics: Relieve itching of skin and mucous membranes

---

Functions of skin

- Protects the body
- Excretes waste products
- Helps regulate body temperature
- Provides cutaneous sensations
- Promotes vitamin D synthesis
- Acts as a reservoir for blood

Key facts about topical drugs

- Allow skin to retain water
- Break down protein in keratin, causing a loss of the stratum corneum skin layer
- Bactericidal or bacteriostatic
- Kill or inhibit growth of fungi and viruses
- Kill parasitic arthropods
- Decrease inflammation and itching and cause vasoconstriction
- Digest necrotic collagenous tissue
- Relieve itching
- Clean and dry skin and reduce the size and activity of sebaceous glands
- Metabolism varies by drug
- Excretion varies by drug

• Acne products: Clean and dry skin (cleaner and antiseptic drugs), reduce bacteria that cause infection (antibiotics), and reduce size and activity of sebaceous glands (isotretinoin)

● **Pharmacokinetics**
• Absorption: Varies with drug
  – Some topical drugs are systemically absorbed through skin
  – Some are minimally absorbed or not absorbed at all
• Distribution: Varies with drug
• Metabolism: Varies with drug
• Excretion: Varies with drug; may be excreted in urine and feces

● **Drug examples**
• Emollients: Lanolin, mineral oil
• Keratolytics and antipsoriatics: Coal tar preparations (Fototar, Oxipor VHC, Polytar, PsoriGel), resorcinol, salicylic acid (Clearasil, PROPApH Astringent, Sal-Acid, Stridex Pads)
• Antibacterial drugs: Bacitracin; gentamicin sulfate (Garamycin); mafenide acetate (Sulfamylon); neomycin sulfate (Mycifradin); neomycin sulfate, polymyxin B, and bacitracin combination (Neosporin); neomycin sulfate, gramicidin, and polymyxin B combination; silver sulfadiazine (Silvadene)
• Antifungals: Clotrimazole (Lotrimin, Mycelex), griseofulvin (Grifulvin), ketoconazole (Nizoral), miconazole nitrate (Monistat-Derm, Micatin), nystatin (Mycostatin), terbinafine (Lamisil)
• Antivirals: Acyclovir (Zovirax), famciclovir (Famvir), penciclovir (Denavir)
• Antiparasitics: Crotamiton (Eurax), lindane, malathion (Ovide), permethrin (Acticin, Elimite, Nix), pyrethrin (RID)
• Anti-inflammatories: Betamethasone valerate (Valisone), coal tar (Balnetar, Fototar), dexamethasone (Decadron), hydrocortisone (Cort-Dome), triamcinolone (Aristocort, Kenalog)
• Debriding and wound-healing drugs: Becaplermin (Regranex), chlorophyll derivatives (Chloresium), dextranomer (Debrisan), trypsin (Granulex)
• Antipruritics: Calamine lotion, cyproheptadine, diphenhydramine (Benadryl), oatmeal (Aveeno)
• Acne products: Antibiotics (clindamycin [Cleocin T], erythromycin [Eryderm], tetracycline), cleaners and antiseptic drugs (azelaic acid [Azelex], benzoyl peroxide, isotretinoin [Accutane]), tretinoin [Retin-A]

● **Indications**
• Lubricate and moisturize skin to treat dryness and itching (emollients)
• Treat superficial fungal infections, psoriasis, seborrheic dermatitis, corns, and calluses (keratolytics and antipsoriatics)
• Fight bacterial skin infections (antibacterials)
• Treat burn wounds (mafenide and silver sulfadiazine)
• Treat fungal skin infections (antifungals)

When to use topical drugs

• Dryness and itching
• Psoriasis
• Seborrheic dermatitis
• Corns
• Calluses
• Bacterial and fungal skin infections
• Burns
• Types 1 and 2 herpes simplex virus infections
• Scabies
• Pediculosis
• Dermatitis
• Allergic skin reactions
• Pressure ulcers
• Venous and peripheral vascular ulcers
• Infected traumatic or surgical wounds
• Pruritus
• Acne vulgaris

- Treat Types 1 and 2 herpes simplex virus infections (antivirals)
- Treat scabies (mites), pediculosis (lice), and their eggs (antiparasitics)
- Treat dermatitis and allergic skin reactions (anti-inflammatories)
- Treat and clean pressure ulcers, venous and peripheral vascular ulcers, burns, infected traumatic or surgical wounds, and other skin injuries (debriding drugs)
- Treat pruritus (antipruritics)
- Treat acne vulgaris (acne products)

● **Contraindications and precautions**
- Contraindicated in patients with hypersensitivity to drug or its components
- Mafenide, silver sulfadiazine, isotretinoin, and tretinoin contraindicated in pregnant and breast-feeding patients

● **Adverse reactions**
- Skin irritation may occur with any topical drug, especially acne products
- Metabolic acidosis, hemolytic anemia, and bone marrow suppression (mafenide)
- Leukopenia (silver sulfadiazine)
- Systemic adverse effects with absorption of large quantities (behavioral changes, fluid and electrolyte imbalances, impaired wound healing, and suppressed immune response) (anti-inflammatories)
- Nosebleeds; burning, redness, or itching of eyes; and scaling, redness, burning, or pain of lips (acne products)
- Photosensitivity reactions (isotretinoin and tretinoin)

● **Interactions**
- No significant drug interactions have been reported
- Increased use of acne products may increase skin irritation

● **Nursing responsibilities**
- Assess the skin lesion and remove remains of previously applied medication before applying drug
- Use sterile technique when applying drug to an open lesion
- Provide psychological support to the patient with a skin disorder as appropriate
- Teach the patient how to apply the drug
- Advise the patient that topical drugs are for external use only and to avoid contact with the eyes
- Warn against breast-feeding while using mafenide or silver sulfadiazine
- Assess respiratory status and blood pH level for signs of metabolic acidosis if the patient is using mafenide
- Advise family members of the patient infected with parasites about the need to be treated with antiparasitics to control spread of infestation
- Follow these guidelines when applying acne products
  - Clean the affected area before applying drug

When NOT to use topical drugs

- Hypersensitivity
- Pregnancy
- Breast-feeding

Adverse reactions

- Skin irritation; metabolic acidosis; hemolytic anemia; bone marrow suppression; leukopenia; behavioral changes; fluid and electrolyte imbalances; impaired wound healing; suppressed immune response; nosebleeds; burning, redness, or itching of the eyes; scaling, redness, burning, or pain of the lips; photosensitivity reactions

Key nursing actions

- Before applying a topical drug, assess skin and remove remains of previously applied medication.
- Use sterile technique when applying medications to open lesions.
- As appropriate, provide psychological support.

Topics for patient discussion

- Medication regimen, including proper administration
- Signs and symptoms to discuss with the practitioner
- Skin care measures
- Normal skin reactions
- Follow-up care

TIME-OUT FOR TEACHING

Teaching about acne products

Include these topics in your teaching plan for the patient receiving an acne product:
- medication regimen, including the drug's name, dosage, frequency, duration, and possible adverse effects
- signs and symptoms to discuss with the practitioner
- proper administration technique
- skin care measures
- normal skin reactions
- follow-up care, including practitioner visits.

– Advise the patient using isotretinoin or tretinoin to apply sunscreen and wear protective clothing to prevent photosensitivity reactions

– Advise the female patient using isotretinoin or tretinoin to use contraception while taking drug; severe fetal abnormalities may occur

– Instruct any patient using isotretinoin or tretinoin to avoid donating blood during and for 30 days after therapy (to prevent pregnant women from receiving the blood)

• Teach the patient using topical tetracycline to be careful to cover the entire affected area (see *Teaching about acne products*)

NCLEX CHECKS

It's never too soon to begin your NCLEX® preparation. Now that you've reviewed this chapter, carefully read each of the following questions and choose the best answer. Then compare your responses with the correct answers.

1. A nurse is caring for a client with third-degree burns of the upper torso. The treatment plan includes applying mafenide (Sulfamylon) 10% cream to the burn twice daily. After three applications of the cream, the nurse notes a significant increase in the client's respiratory rate. Arterial blood gas analysis shows the following values: pH, 7.30; partial pressure of arterial carbon dioxide ($PaCO_2$), 35 mm Hg; partial pressure of arterial oxygen, 90 mg Hg; and bicarbonate (HCO_3^-), 10 mEq/L. Based on these findings, which acid-base disturbance has occurred as a result of mafenide therapy?

- ☐ **1.** Metabolic acidosis
- ☐ **2.** Metabolic alkalosis
- ☐ **3.** Respiratory acidosis
- ☐ **4.** Respiratory alkalosis

2. A client has had athlete's foot for 12 weeks that hasn't responded to clotrimazole (Lotrimin). Which drug should the nurse anticipate administering as ordered?

- ☐ **1.** Aluminum acetate (Domeboro) soaks
- ☐ **2.** Hydrocortisone cream (Cort-Dome)
- ☐ **3.** Miconazole cream (Micatin)
- ☐ **4.** Neomycin ointment (Neosporin)

TOP 4

Items to study for your next test on drugs and the integumentary system

1. Mechanisms of action of the various topical drugs
2. Common adverse effects of topical drugs
3. Nursing responsibilities when administering topical drugs
4. Teaching for the patient receiving a topical drug

3. While obtaining a history from the parents of a 4-year-old child, the nurse discovers the child has been recently treated with permethrin (Nix). Which nursing action is appropriate in response to this information?

- [ ] **1.** Carefully check the child's hair and scalp.
- [ ] **2.** Obtain a stool specimen for ova and parasites.
- [ ] **3.** Assess the child for age-appropriate cognitive ability and motor development.
- [ ] **4.** Put on a mask and sterile gown to keep the child from getting a respiratory infection.

4. A client has a viral infection. The nurse would expect the physician to order which dermatologic agent?

- [ ] **1.** Acyclovir (Zovirax)
- [ ] **2.** Bacitracin
- [ ] **3.** Hydrocortisone (Cort-Dome)
- [ ] **4.** Silver sulfadiazine (Silvadene)

5. When applying a dermatologic agent, what's the first and last thing the nurse should do?

- [ ] **1.** Wash the hands.
- [ ] **2.** Check the medication label.
- [ ] **3.** Keep the medication in a cool place.
- [ ] **4.** Wash the affected area with soap and water.

6. A client is admitted to the burn unit with third-degree burns of his left leg. Silver sulfadiazine (Silvadene) 1% cream is applied to the burn twice daily. What abnormal laboratory findings can result from therapy with silver sulfadiazine?

- [ ] **1.** Decreased blood pH
- [ ] **2.** Decreased sodium level
- [ ] **3.** Increased blood glucose level
- [ ] **4.** Decreased WBC count

7. A client using isotretinoin (Accutane) may experience which adverse reactions? Select all that apply.

- [ ] **1.** Birth defects
- [ ] **2.** Nausea and vomiting
- [ ] **3.** Photosensitivity reaction
- [ ] **4.** Vaginal yeast infection
- [ ] **5.** Gram-negative folliculitis
- [ ] **6.** Nosebleeds

8. A client has just started topical tretinoin (Retin-A) 0.025% cream for acne. Within 3 weeks of starting the drug, he reports that his acne is getting worse. What should the nurse tell the client?

- [ ] **1.** The cream is too potent.
- [ ] **2.** The worsened acne is caused by an allergy to the cream, and he should stop using it.
- [ ] **3.** Benzoyl peroxide cream needs to be added to the therapy.
- [ ] **4.** An acne flare-up early in therapy doesn't indicate drug failure.

9. Which antibacterial agent is commonly used to prevent infections of burns?

☐ **1.** Ketoconazole (Nizoral)
☐ **2.** Gentamicin (Garamycin)
☐ **3.** Silver sulfadiazine (Silvadene)
☐ **4.** Terbinafine (Lamisil)

10. When applying hydrocortisone (Cort-Dome) topically, a nurse shouldn't use an occlusive dressing because:

☐ **1.** the tissue will become denuded.
☐ **2.** skin lesions do better if kept dry.
☐ **3.** systemic absorption can be increased.
☐ **4.** the risk of infection is increased by moisture.

ANSWERS AND RATIONALES

1. CORRECT ANSWER: 1
Mafenide is a carbonic anhydrase inhibitor that slows the production of the enzyme that breaks down carbonic acid. Thus, it increases carbonic acid levels in the body and causes metabolic acidosis. The increased respiratory rate is a compensatory mechanism to try to reduce the $PaCO_2$ level. The less-than-normal pH and HCO_3^- levels are consistent with metabolic acidosis.

2. CORRECT ANSWER: 3
Miconazole, a broad-spectrum antifungal, should be more effective against the organism causing this problem than clotrimazole. Hydrocortisone isn't indicated as the sole agent for fungal infections because it doesn't kill the organism and may compromise the immune response. Soaks with aluminum acetate, an astringent, may help with the itching but won't effectively treat the fungus. Neomycin is an antibacterial and therefore won't be effective against this fungal infection.

3. CORRECT ANSWER: 1
Permethrin is a topical agent that's used to treat head lice and scabies in children and adults. A careful examination of the client's hair and scalp is indicated. The drug has no effect on intestinal parasites. Assessing the child for mental ability and motor development level is an appropriate action, but it isn't related to the drug's effects. It isn't necessary to use a mask and sterile gown with this client.

4. CORRECT ANSWER: 1
Acyclovir is an antiviral dermatologic agent. Bacitracin and silver sulfadiazine are antibacterial agents. Hydrocortisone is an anti-inflammatory.

5. CORRECT ANSWER: 1
Although standard precautions require gloves when touching broken or excoriated skin, hand washing is still imperative before and after applying medication to the skin. The medication label should be checked before the procedure begins. It's important to keep the medication in a cool area, but that isn't an action

at these points. Soap and water are usually detrimental to the skin being treated, and washing the area after applying the agent would wash away the drug.

6. CORRECT ANSWER: 4

Leukopenia (a decrease in WBC count) commonly occurs with the initiation of silver sulfadiazine therapy. The WBC count usually returns to normal after the first few days of therapy. Acid-base disturbances and changes in blood pH aren't associated with silver sulfadiazine therapy. The drug doesn't interfere with blood glucose or sodium levels.

7. CORRECT ANSWER: 1, 3, 6

Birth defects can result with use of even small amounts of isotretinoin. In fact, female clients who use isotretinoin are commonly prescribed hormonal contraceptives. Photosensitivity reactions and nosebleeds are also adverse reactions to isotretinoin. Diarrhea and gram-negative folliculitis are associated with clindamycin (Cleocin T) use. Yeast infections are associated with tetracycline use.

8. CORRECT ANSWER: 4

The client is experiencing a flare-up of his acne. This reaction commonly occurs during the first few weeks of tretinoin therapy. Clients usually respond to the drug after this phase. The client has been started on the lowest potency of tretinoin cream, so potency isn't an issue. An acne flare-up isn't an allergic reaction. The client shouldn't use another irritating product, such as benzoyl peroxide, because it will only increase skin irritation.

9. CORRECT ANSWER: 3

Silver sulfadiazine, a bacteriostatic cream, is applied to burns to prevent infection by occluding open areas that act as a direct portal for infection. The skin is the body's largest organ and the first defense against infection. Ketoconazole and terbinafine are antifungal agents. Gentamicin is an antibacterial drug used to treat gram-negative aerobic infections.

10. CORRECT ANSWER: 3

An occlusive dressing shouldn't be used if hydrocortisone or another anti-inflammatory agent is applied; such a dressing may increase systemic absorption. Although moisture may denude the tissue, the drug's systemic effect is the greater concern. If skin lesions responded better when dry, a topical agent wouldn't be used. Anti-inflammatory agents shouldn't be applied to areas at risk for infection.

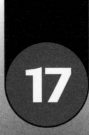

Drugs and the sensory system

PRETEST

1. Beta-adrenergic blockers help control open-angle glaucoma by:
- ☐ 1. causing miosis.
- ☐ 2. causing mydriasis.
- ☐ 3. increasing aqueous humor drainage.
- ☐ 4. decreasing aqueous humor production.

CORRECT ANSWER: 4

2. To prevent vertigo from eardrop instillation, a client should:
- ☐ 1. wash the hands before instillation.
- ☐ 2. lie down to receive eardrops.
- ☐ 3. make sure the drops are room temperature.
- ☐ 4. shake excess medication out of the ears.

CORRECT ANSWER: 3

3. What's a contraindication to eardrop administration?
- ☐ 1. Perforated eardrum
- ☐ 2. Sensory hearing loss
- ☐ 3. Cochlear implant
- ☐ 4. Otitis media

CORRECT ANSWER: 1

4. Which adverse reaction is most commonly associated with atropine eyedrops?

☐ 1. Abdominal pain
☐ 2. Bradycardia
☐ 3. Headache
☐ 4. Tachycardia

CORRECT ANSWER: 4

5. The correct way for a nurse to straighten the ear canal before instilling eardrops in an adult is to:

☐ 1. pull the pinna of the ear up and back.
☐ 2. pull the pinna of the ear down and back.
☐ 3. pull the pinna of the ear up and forward.
☐ 4. pull the pinna of the ear down and forward.

CORRECT ANSWER: 1

LEARNING OBJECTIVES

After studying this chapter, you should be able to:

● Name the mechanisms of action of ophthalmic and otic drugs.
● Explain the rationales for using anti-infectives, anti-inflammatories, anesthetics, lubricants, miotics, beta-adrenergic blockers, mydriatics, and cycloplegics to treat eye disorders.
● List common adverse effects of ophthalmic and otic drugs.
● Identify nursing responsibilities and patient teaching requirements related to administering ophthalmic and otic drugs.

A&P highlights

- The sensory system includes vision, hearing, equilibrium, smell, taste, touch, pressure, temperature, and pain.
- The eyes are complex, sensory organs for vision composed of three layers of tissues and a lens.
- The accessory structures of the eye include the eyebrows, eyelids, eyelashes, conjunctivae, lacrimal glands, and eye muscles.
- The eyebrows, eyelids, and eyelashes keep debris from entering the eye.
- The conjunctivae line the inner surface of the eyelids and sclerae.
- The lacrimal glands discharge fluid secretions to moisten the conjunctivae.
- Eye muscles allow eye movement.
- The external ear consists of the auricle and the external auditory canal.
- The middle ear is a mucosa-lined structure that contains three small bones: the malleus, stapes, and incus.
- The inner ear consists of the vestibule, semicircular canals, and cochlea.
- When stimulated, the eye receptors collect light waves and transmit them as nerve impulses along the visual pathways to the brain, which translates them into images.
- The eye with normal refractive powers can form clear images of an object 20 feet away.
- When stimulated, the ear receptors gather sound waves and transmit them as nerve impulses to the brain; the brain interprets these impulses as hearing.

CHAPTER OVERVIEW

Ophthalmic drugs, which are applied onto the conjunctival sac, may be anti-infective, anti-inflammatory, anesthetic, lubricating, topical, systemic, miotic, beta-adrenergic blocking, mydriatic, cycloplegic, antiallergic, or diuretic.

Otic drugs (also called *aural medications*) help to treat infection and inflammation of the ear, remove excess cerumen, and provide anesthesia. Antihistamines and decongestants may help to clear obstruction of a eustachian tube. Locally instilled otic medications may be administered to treat pain associated with infection or to reduce excess cerumen.

ANATOMY AND PHYSIOLOGY

- **Anatomy**
  - Sensory system
    - Special senses: Vision, hearing, equilibrium, smell, and taste
    - General senses: Touch, pressure, temperature, and pain
  - Eyes
    - Are paired, complex spherical structures composed of a lens and three layers of tissue: the cornea and sclera, middle choroid coat, and an inner retina, which contains receptor cells (rods and cones)
    - Anterior and posterior chambers
      - Are located in the space between the cornea and lens
      - Contain aqueous humor, a clear, watery fluid that flows into Schlemm canal; if imbalanced, can lead to buildup of intraocular pressure (IOP); vision impairment and loss may occur if pressure is transmitted to vitreous humor in posterior cavity, thereby damaging the retina
    - Accessory structures of the eye
      - Eyebrows, eyelids, and eyelashes—keep debris from entering eye
      - Conjunctivae—thin vascular membranes lining the inner surface of eyelids and sclerae
      - Lacrimal glands—discharge fluid secretions to moisten conjunctivae
      - Eye muscles—paired; work together to perform eye movement
  - Ears
    - Paired structures composed of three major parts: external (outer) ear, middle ear, and inner ear
    - External ear—consists of auricle (pinna) and external auditory canal
    - Middle ear (tympanic cavity)—mucosa-lined and contains three small bones
      - Malleus (hammer)—attached to the tympanic membrane
      - Stapes (stirrup)—attached to the oval window
      - Incus (anvil)
        - Is located between the malleus and stapes

- Articulates with malleus and stapes when vibrations are transmitted from eardrum to fluid of inner ear and excite receptor nerve endings in the inner ear
  – Inner ear (osseus canal)—consists of the vestibule, semicircular canals, and cochlea

Physiology
- Eyes
  – Stimulated eye receptors collect light waves and transmit them as nerve impulses along visual pathways to brain, which translates them into images
  – Image forms on retina when light stimulates rods and cones
  – Eye with normal refractive powers can form clear images of objects 20′ (6 m) away
  – Eyes must make many changes (accommodation, papillary constriction, eye convergence) to adapt and form clear images of objects closer than 20′ (near vision)
  – Binocular vision contributes to depth perception (ability to judge relative distances of objects)
- Ears
  – Stimulated ear receptors gather sound waves and transmit them as nerve impulses to brain; brain interprets these impulses as hearing
  – Equilibrium is controlled by semicircular canals of inner ear

Function
- Eye is responsible for vision
  – Rods are photoreceptors that provide vision when it's dark
  – Cones provide colored vision when it's light
- Ear is responsible for hearing and maintaining balance
  – External ear collects sound
  – Middle ear conducts sound
  – Inner ear structures transmit sound waves and maintain equilibrium

OPHTHALMIC DRUGS

Mechanism of action
- Anti-infectives: Kill or inhibit growth of susceptible bacteria, fungi, and viruses
- Anti-inflammatories: Control inflammation, thereby reducing vision loss and scarring
- Anesthetics: Produce corneal anesthesia
- Lubricants: Replace tears or add moisture to the eye
- Miotics: Reduce IOP by constricting the pupil, contracting ciliary muscles, opening anterior chamber angle, and increasing outflow of aqueous humor
  – Miotic cholinergic agonists: Reduce IOP by mimicking action of acetylcholine

Functions of eye structures
- Rods are photoreceptors that provide vision when it's dark.
- Cones provide colored vision when it's light.

Functions of ear structures
- External ear collects sound.
- Middle ear conducts sound.
- Inner ear contains structures that transmit sound waves and maintain equilibrium.

Key facts about ophthalmic drugs
- Kill or inhibit growth of susceptible bacteria, fungi, and viruses
- Control inflammation, thereby reducing vision loss and scarring
- Produce corneal anesthesia
- Replace tears or add moisture to the eye
- Reduce intraocular pressure
- Dilate and paralyze the pupil
- Diminish allergic response
- Reduce aqueous humor production
- Metabolism varies by drug
- Excretion varies by drug

– Miotic acetylcholinesterase inhibitors: Reduce IOP by inhibiting action of cholinesterase
- Beta-adrenergic blockers: Reduce IOP by decreasing sympathetic impulses to the eye and decreasing aqueous humor production without affecting accommodation or pupil size
- Mydriatics and cycloplegics: Dilate and paralyze pupil
    – Cholinergic blockers (anticholinergics): Inhibit parasympathetic nervous system, producing mydriasis (pupil dilation) and cycloplegia
    – Adrenergic agonists: Mimic action of sympathetic nervous system, causing mydriasis
- Mast cell stabilizers: Prevent release of histamine, thereby diminishing the allergic response
- Diuretics: Reduce aqueous humor production and decrease IOP
    – Carbonic anhydrase inhibitors: Decrease IOP by decreasing aqueous humor production
    – Osmotic agents: Decrease IOP by reducing the volume of vitreous humor

● Pharmacokinetics
- Absorption: Some drugs are systemically absorbed
- Distribution: Varies with drug; may penetrate the cornea, conjunctiva, and aqueous humor
- Metabolism: Varies with drug
- Excretion: Varies with drug; some anti-infectives are excreted through nasolacrimal duct

● Drug examples
- Anti-infectives
    – Antibacterial drugs: Bacitracin (AK-Tracin), chloramphenicol (Chloromycetin), ciprofloxacin (Ciloxan), erythromycin (Ilotycin), gatifloxacin (Zymar), gentamicin (Garamycin, Gentak), levofloxacin (Quixin), moxifloxacin (Vigamox), neomycin, ofloxacin (Ocuflox), polymyxin B sulfate, sulfacetamide (Bleph-10), sulfisoxazole (Gantrisin Ophthalmic), tobramycin (Tobrex), trimethoprim-polymyxin B sulfate (Polytrim)
    – Antifungals: Amphotericin B (Fungizone), natamycin (Natacyn)
    – Antivirals: Cidofovir (Vistide), fomivirsen (Vitravene), foscarnet (Foscavir), ganciclovir (Cytovene, DHPG), trifluridine (Viroptic), vidarabine
- Anti-inflammatories: Dexamethasone sodium phosphate (Decadron Phosphate), dexamethasone/neomycin/polymyxin B (Maxitrol), diclofenac (Voltaren Ophthalmic), fluorometholone (FML), flurbiprofen sodium (Ocufen), ketorolac (Acular), loteprednol (Lotemax), medrysone (HMS), prednisolone (Pred Forte), suprofen (Profenal)
- Anesthetics: Proparacaine (Ophthaine), tetracaine (Pontocaine)

- Lubricants: Hydroxypropyl methylcellulose (Lacrisert), petroleum-based ointment, polyvinyl alcohol for hard contact lenses (artificial tears [Liquifilm Tears, Tears Naturale])
- Miotics
    - Cholinergic agonists (direct-acting): Acetylcholine, carbachol (Carboptic), pilocarpine (Isopto Carpine)
    - Acetylcholinesterase inhibitors: Demecarium, latanoprost (Xalatan), physostigmine
- Beta-adrenergic blockers: Betaxolol (Betoptic), carteolol (Ocupress), levobetaxolol (Betaxon), levobunolol (Betagan), metipranolol (OptiPranolol), timolol (Timoptic)
- Mydriatics and cycloplegics
    - Cholinergic blockers: Atropine (Isopto Atropine), cyclopentolate (Cyclogyl), homatropine (Isopto Homatropine), scopolamine (Isopto Hyoscine), tropicamide (Mydriacyl)
    - Adrenergic agonists: Dipivefrin (Propine), epinephryl borate (Epinal), epinephrine hydrochloride, hydroxyamphetamine (Paredrine), phenylephrine (Neo-Aynephrine)
- Mast cell stabilizers: Cromolyn sodium (Crolom); histamine-1 receptor agonist antiallergy drugs (azelastine hydrochloride [Optivar], emedastine difumarate [Emadine], ketotifen [Zaditor], olopatadine [Patanol]); lodoxamide tromethamine (Alomide); nedocromil (Alocril); pemirolast (Alamast)
- Diuretics
    - Carbonic Anhydrase inhibitors: Acetazolamide, brinzolamide (Azopt), dorzolamide (Trusopt), methazolamide
    - Osmotic agents: Glycerin (Osmoglyn), isosorbide (Ismotic)

Indications

- Treat susceptible ocular bacterial infections (antibacterials)
- Treat susceptible ocular fungal infections (antifungals)
- Treat susceptible ocular viral infections (antivirals)
- Treat nonpyogenic inflammatory ocular conditions (anti-inflammatories)
- Anesthesia during eye examinations and eye surgery (anesthetics)
- Treat keratitis, moisten contact lenses or artificial eyes, replace tears, and protect eye during surgery or diagnostic procedures (lubricants)
- Treat chronic open-angle glaucoma and acute and chronic angle-closure glaucoma (miotics)
- Treat glaucoma (beta-adrenergic blockers)
    - Treat chronic open-angle glaucoma (betaxolol, levobunolol, and timolol)
    - Treat aphakic glaucoma (timolol)
- Treat inflammatory eye conditions, prevent adhesions, dilate pupils during eye examinations, and prepare patient for surgery (mydriatics and cycloplegics)

When to use ophthalmic drugs

- Susceptible ocular bacterial, fungal, or viral infections
- Nonpyogenic inflammatory ocular conditions
- Anesthesia
- Dilation and lubrication for eye examination or surgery
- Glaucoma
- Inflammatory eye conditions
- Adhesion prevention
- Allergic ocular disorders
- Allergic conjunctivitis and itching

When NOT to use ophthalmic drugs

- Acute eye infections
- Secondary glaucoma
- Acute iritis
- Inflammatory diseases
- Angle-closure glaucoma

Adverse reactions

- Superinfection, local irritation, cataracts, IOP, impaired healing, masking of signs and symptoms of infection, temporary stinging or burning, temporary loss of corneal reflex, discomfort, pain on instillation, myopia, decreased vision in poor light, eye ache, local irritation, headache, flushing, diaphoresis, GI upset, diarrhea, hypersensitivity, photophobia, tachycardia, hypertension, dry mouth, dizziness, lacrimation, paresthesia, lethargy, weakness, dehydration, hyperglycemia, glycosuria

Key nursing actions

- Assess patient for signs and symptoms of eye disorders and adverse effects.
- If patient is using more than one topical ophthalmic medication, wait at least 5 minutes before instilling second eye medication, as prescribed.
- Keep eye medications sterile; avoid skin or eye contact with applicator.
- Don't give ophthalmic anesthetics to patient for home use.
- After mydriatic or cycloplegic eyedrop administration, minimize systemic absorption by applying pressure to the lacrimal sac for 3 to 5 minutes.

- Treat allergic ocular disorders and symptomatic itching caused by allergic conjunctivitis (mast cell stabilizers)
- Treat glaucoma and prepare patient for surgery (diuretics)

● **Contraindications and precautions**
- Anti-inflammatories contraindicated in acute eye infections
- Miotics contraindicated in secondary glaucoma, acute iritis, and inflammatory diseases
- Mydriatics contraindicated in angle-closure glaucoma

● **Adverse reactions**
- Anti-infectives: Superinfection and local irritation
- Anti-inflammatories: Cataracts, increased IOP, impaired healing, and masking of signs and symptoms of infection
- Anesthetics: Temporary stinging or burning of the eye and temporary loss of corneal reflex
- Lubricants: Discomfort, burning, or pain on instillation
- Miotics: Ocular and systemic adverse effects
    - Ocular effects: Myopia, decreased vision in poor light, eye ache, and local irritation
    - Systemic effects: Headache, flushing, diaphoresis, GI upset, and diarrhea
- Beta-adrenergic blockers: Ocular irritation and vision disturbances
- Mydriatics and cycloplegics
    - Ocular effects: Increased IOP, eye ache, hypersensitivity, and photophobia
    - Systemic effects: Tachycardia, hypertension, headache, and dry mouth
- Mast cell stabilizers: Headache, dizziness, and lacrimation
- Diuretics: GI upset
    - Carbonic anhydrase inhibitors: Diarrhea, paresthesia, lethargy, and weakness
    - Osmotic diuretics: Dehydration, hyperglycemia, and glycosuria (glycerin)

● **Interactions**
- None significant

● **Nursing responsibilities**
- Assess the patient for signs and symptoms of eye disorders and adverse effects
- Wait at least 5 minutes before instilling a second medication, as prescribed, if the patient is using more than one topical ophthalmic drug
- Keep all eye medications sterile; avoid skin or eye contact with the applicator
- Teach the patient how to instill eye medications properly (see *Teaching about ophthalmic drugs*)
- Instruct the patient with glaucoma to carry identification describing disorder and drug therapy

- Keep in mind that ophthalmic anesthetics are used only for eye examinations and surgery; they shouldn't be given to the patient for home use
- Inform the patient receiving an eye anesthetic that an eye patch may be needed after administration to protect the eye from injury until the corneal reflex returns (about 1 hour)
- Inform the patient receiving either a mydriatic or a cycloplegic that dark glasses may be needed after eye examination to prevent photophobia
- Minimize systemic absorption after administering either mydriatic or cycloplegic eyedrops by applying pressure to lacrimal sac at inner canthus for 3 to 5 minutes; this prevents passage of eyedrops via nasolacrimal duct into areas of potential absorption (such as nasal and pharyngeal mucosa)

OTIC DRUGS

● **Mechanism of action**
- Anti-infectives: Kill or inhibit growth of susceptible bacteria
- Anti-inflammatories: Reduce redness and itching
- Antihistamines and decongestants: Stimulate adrenergic receptors of respiratory mucosa, thereby producing vasoconstriction and reducing respiratory tissue hyperemia to open obstructed eustachian tube
- Local anesthetics: Block nerve conduction at or near application site to control pain associated with ear infections
- Ceruminolytics: Emulsify and loosen cerumen (earwax) deposits

● **Pharmacokinetics**
- Absorption
  - Anti-inflammatories: May be systemically absorbed with long-term use
  - Local anesthetics and ceruminolytics: Not absorbed
- Distribution: Locally distributed
- Metabolism: Unknown
- Excretion: Unknown

● **Drug examples**
- Anti-infectives and anti-inflammatories: Boric acid

- Antihistamines and decongestants: Antihistamine-decongestant combinations (Actifed, Allerest, Chlor-Trimeton, Drixoral, Novahistine, Triaminic)
- Local anesthetics: Antipyrine and benzocaine combination (Auralgan Otic Solution), benzocaine (Tympagesic)
- Ceruminolytics: Carbamide peroxide (Debrox)

● **Indications**

- Dry the ear and kill susceptible bacteria (anti-infectives and anti-inflammatories)
- Adjunctive therapy for acute otitis media; treatment to reduce respiratory congestion or open obstructed eustachian tube (antihistamines and decongestants)
- Treat pain associated with ear infection (local anesthetics)
- Remove excess cerumen (ceruminolytics; efficacy questionable)

● **Contraindications and precautions**

- Contraindicated in patients with drug hypersensitivity or perforated eardrum

● **Adverse reactions**

- Hypersensitivity reactions (redness, burning, itching, stinging, urticaria, vesicular or maculopapular dermatitis, swelling, and mild irritation)
- Anti-infectives: Superinfection in patients with overgrowth of nonsusceptible organisms
- Local anesthetics: May mask symptoms of middle-ear infection

● **Interactions**

- None significant

● **Nursing responsibilities**

- Assess the patient for hearing loss, pain, and ear drainage
- Use the correct method to instill eardrops
  - For children younger than age 3: Pull the auricle down to straighten external canal
  - For an adult: Pull the auricle up and back to straighten external canal
- Teach the patient how to administer prescribed drug
  - Instruct him to keep his head tilted for 10 minutes to allow drug to be absorbed
  - If repositioning is necessary, advise him to use cotton ball or earplug to keep medication in ear canal
- Instruct the patient to contact the practitioner if ear pain and swelling persist
- Instruct the patient how to administer a ceruminolytic
  - Moisten a cotton ball with medication before insertion; don't use a swab because it may cause trauma to inner ear
  - Avoid touching ear with dropper
  - Flush ear gently with warm water, using a soft rubber bulb ear syringe within 30 minutes after instillation to remove cerumen
  - Keep container tightly closed and away from moisture

TIME-OUT FOR TEACHING

Teaching about otic drugs

Include these topics in your teaching plan for the patient receiving an otic drug:
- medication regimen, including the drug's name, dosage, frequency, duration, and possible adverse effects
- signs and symptoms to discuss with the practitioner

- proper procedure for administering the drug
- ear care after drug administration
- irrigation of ear, if indicated
- compliance with therapy for full course of treatment
- follow-up care, including practitioner visits.

- Warn the patient not to use ceruminolytic drops more often than prescribed (see *Teaching about otic drugs*)
- Advise the patient to call the practitioner if redness, pain, or swelling persists
- Keep in mind that the efficacy of ceruminolytics is questionable

NCLEX CHECKS

It's never too soon to begin your NCLEX® preparation. Now that you've reviewed this chapter, carefully read each of the following questions and choose the best answer. Then compare your responses with the correct answers.

1. A nurse is caring for a client with acute narrow-angle glaucoma. The nurse should expect to administer:
- ☐ **1.** acetazolamide (Diamox).
- ☐ **2.** atropine.
- ☐ **3.** furosemide (Lasix).
- ☐ **4.** urokinase (Abbokinase).

2. Which group of ophthalmic drugs is used to prepare a client's pupils for examination?
- ☐ **1.** Anti-inflammatories
- ☐ **2.** Cycloplegics
- ☐ **3.** Miotics
- ☐ **4.** Mydriatics

3. A client requires an eye examination to assess for the presence of a foreign body. In order to dilate the client's pupils, which drug would the nurse give?
- ☐ **1.** Carbachol (Carboptic)
- ☐ **2.** Cyclopentolate (Cyclogyl)
- ☐ **3.** Physostigmine
- ☐ **4.** Pilocarpine (Isopto Carpine)

Topics for patient discussion

- Medication regimen, including proper administration
- Signs and symptoms to discuss with the practitioner
- Importance of notifying the practitioner if redness, pain, or swelling persists
- Ear care after administration
- Irrigation of ear, if indicated
- Compliance with drug therapy for full course of treatment
- Follow-up care

TOP 7

Items to study for your next test on drugs and the sensory system

1. Mechanisms of action of ophthalmic and otic drugs
2. Rationales for using anti-infectives, anti-inflammatories, anesthetics, lubricants, miotics, beta-adrenergic blockers, mydriatics, and cycloplegics to treat eye disorders
3. Common adverse effects of ophthalmic and otic drugs
4. Correct techniques for instilling eardrops in children and adults
5. Proper administration of different types of eye medications
6. Nursing responsibilities when administering ophthalmic and otic drugs
7. Teaching for the patient who's receiving an ophthalmic or otic drug

4. A nurse expects the physician to order which type of diuretic to reduce IOP in a client with glaucoma?

- ☐ **1.** Loop diuretic
- ☐ **2.** Osmotic diuretic
- ☐ **3.** Potassium-sparing diuretic
- ☐ **4.** Thiazide and thiazide-like diuretic

5. A 76-year-old client is ordered boric acid. The nurse knows that boric acid is an example of which type of otic medication?

- ☐ **1.** Anti-infective
- ☐ **2.** Anti-inflammatory
- ☐ **3.** Ceruminolytic
- ☐ **4.** Local anesthetic

6. A client is ordered benzocaine (Tympagesic) to reduce ear pain. Which client statement demonstrates the need for additional teaching about this drug?

- ☐ **1.** "I'll have to stop using the drug if I get hives."
- ☐ **2.** "I'll report increased ear pain to the physician."
- ☐ **3.** "I'll insert an ear wick before taking the agent."
- ☐ **4.** "I'll report hearing loss or dizziness to the physician right away."

7. A client is ordered carbamide peroxide (Debrox) to treat impacted cerumen. Which nursing instruction is important to include in the client's teaching plan?

- ☐ **1.** Apply one drop to the affected ear canal.
- ☐ **2.** Flush your ears gently with warm water after using this product.
- ☐ **3.** Use this drug once, and return to the physician if you don't get results.
- ☐ **4.** Clean your ear canal with a cotton swab after using this product.

8. A client has been using timolol (Timoptic) and dorzolamide (Trusopt) eyedrops for glaucoma. In the clinic, the client reports wheezing after using the eyedrops. The nurse suspects that the most likely reason for this reaction is:

- ☐ **1.** systemic absorption of timolol.
- ☐ **2.** systemic absorption of dorzolamide.
- ☐ **3.** a condition unrelated to glaucoma treatment.
- ☐ **4.** a drug-drug interaction of timolol and dorzolamide.

9. A nurse is discharging a 10-month old infant with a prescription for eardrops. Which instruction about administering eardrops should the nurse give the parents?

- ☐ **1.** Pull the earlobe upward.
- ☐ **2.** Pull the earlobe up and back.
- ☐ **3.** Pull the earlobe down and back.
- ☐ **4.** Pull the earlobe down and forward.

10. A nurse is preparing to administer cycloplegic eyedrops. Indicate where the nurse should apply pressure after administering the eyedrops.

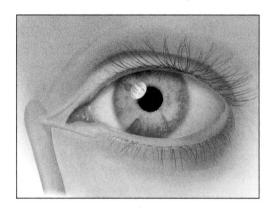

ANSWERS AND RATIONALES

1. CORRECT ANSWER: 1
The nurse should expect to administer acetazolamide because this drug decreases IOP by decreasing secretion from the aqueous humour. Atropine dilates the pupil and decreases the outflow of aqueous humour, increasing IOP. Furosemide is a loop diuretic, and urokinase is a thrombolytic; they aren't used to treat glaucoma.

2. CORRECT ANSWER: 4
Mydriatics dilate the pupils, thereby preparing them for examination. By contrast, miotics constrict the pupils. Anti-inflammatories are commonly used for allergic eye conditions. Cycloplegics are used to paralyze the ciliary muscles to perform eye refraction examinations or prepare for surgery, especially in children.

3. CORRECT ANSWER: 2
Cyclopentolate, an anticholinergic, dilates the pupils and paralyzes the ciliary muscles. Carbachol, physostigmine, and pilocarpine are cholinergics, which have the opposite effect and constrict the pupils.

4. CORRECT ANSWER: 2
Osmotic diuretics work by increasing plasma osmolarity, thereby pulling fluid into the vascular system and reducing IOP. Loop diuretics (such as furosemide [Lasix]), potassium-sparing diuretics (such as spironolactone [HydroDIURIL]), and thiazide and thiazide-like diuretics are best used for diuresis of edema.

5. CORRECT ANSWER: 1
Boric acid is an anti-infective that makes the ear canal a less suitable environment for bacteria and infection by changing the pH; it also helps dry out the ear. However, boric acid won't cure an infection when used as a sole treatment. An acid wouldn't be considered an anti-inflammatory. Boric acid doesn't have anesthetic or ceruminolytic properties.

6. CORRECT ANSWER: 3

The client requires additional teaching if he says he'll use an ear wick before taking the drug. Use of an ear wick isn't recommended with benzocaine. Presence of urticaria (hives) denotes a hypersensitivity to the drug, and the drug should be stopped. Hearing loss, dizziness, and increased pain are signs of a fulminating ear infection that should be investigated fully.

7. CORRECT ANSWER: 2

The client should be instructed to flush the ears gently with warm water because the drug softens cerumen and the water will gently flush out the cerumen. The correct dose is several drops to the affected ear. It may take several applications to achieve maximum results. A swab shouldn't be used because of the risk of trauma to the inner ear.

8. CORRECT ANSWER: 1

The client's complaints are most likely caused by systemic absorption of timolol, a beta-adrenergic blocker. Beta blockade causes bronchoconstriction and wheezing. The systemic absorption of timolol has been well described, so the nurse wouldn't necessarily suspect another condition unrelated to the glaucoma treatment. Dorzolamide doesn't cause pulmonary problems, nor does it interact with timolol.

9. CORRECT ANSWER: 3

The infant's parents should be told to gently pull the earlobe down and back to visualize the external auditory canal. For children older than age 3 and adults, the earlobe is gently pulled slightly up and back. Pulling upward only, or down and forward, wouldn't allow a visual of the external auditory canal.

10. CORRECT ANSWER:

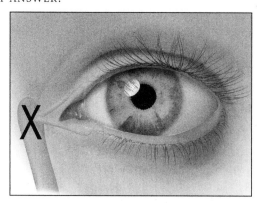

To minimize systemic absorption after administering a cycloplegic eyedrop, the nurse should apply pressure to the lacrimal sac at the inner canthus for 3 to 5 minutes. Doing so helps prevent passage of the drug into the nasolacrimal duct, thus preventing systemic absorption.

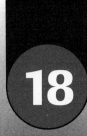

18

Nutritional agents and the body

1. Which electrolyte is found in higher concentrations in extracellular fluid than in intracellular fluid?

☐ 1. Calcium
☐ 2. Magnesium
☐ 3. Potassium
☐ 4. Sodium

CORRECT ANSWER: 4

2. A nurse knows that blood glucose levels increase as a result of total parenteral nutrition (TPN) administration because:

☐ 1. TPN solution has a high glucose concentration.
☐ 2. TPN solution has an increased concentration of amino acids.
☐ 3. most clients who require TPN have undiagnosed type 2 diabetes.
☐ 4. a client's liver responds poorly to increased glucose concentrations.

CORRECT ANSWER: 1

3. Which supplement should a nurse expect to be ordered for a client with chronic alcoholism and malabsorption?

☐ 1. Ascorbic acid
☐ 2. Manganese
☐ 3. Selenium
☐ 4. Thiamine

CORRECT ANSWER: 4

4. What's the maximum concentration of dextrose that should be infused through a peripheral vein?

☐ 1. Less than 5%

☐ 2. 15%

☐ 3. 20%

☐ 4. More than 50%

CORRECT ANSWER: 2

5. A nurse should question an order for which agent if a client has an allergy to shellfish?

☐ 1. Copper

☐ 2. Iodine

☐ 3. Molybdenum

☐ 4. Zinc

CORRECT ANSWER: 2

LEARNING OBJECTIVES

After studying this chapter, you should be able to:

● Discuss the mechanism of action and common uses of nutritional agents.

● List common adverse effects of various nutritional agents.

● Identify important nursing responsibilities when administering nutritional agents.

● Discuss patient teaching required for administering nutritional agents.

CHAPTER OVERVIEW

Nutritional agents—nutritional supplement solutions, electrolytes, vitamins, and minerals—are used to correct deficiencies in the patient's nutritional status. Enteral forms, preferred when the GI tract is functioning, are administered either orally or through a feeding tube. Parenteral forms are administered through a peripheral vein (peripheral parenteral nutrition [PPN]) or a central vein (total parenteral nutrition [TPN]).

ANATOMY AND PHYSIOLOGY

- **Anatomy**
  - Body fluid composition
    - Water constitutes more than 50% of average adult's body
    - Body water contains various dissolved substances (solutes) necessary for physiologic functioning, including electrolytes, glucose, amino acids, and other nutrients
  - Fluid compartments
    - Intracellular fluid (ICF) consists of fluid inside body's cells
    - Intravascular fluid consists of fluid in blood plasma and lymphatic system
    - Interstitial fluid consists of fluid distributed diffusely through loose tissues surrounding cells
    - Intravascular and interstitial fluids are separated by a capillary endothelium that's freely permeable to water, electrolytes, and other solutes
      - Intravascular and interstitial fluids are similar in composition
      - Intravascular and interstitial fluid compartments are commonly grouped as a single compartment, the extracellular fluid compartment (ECF)
  - Concentration of substances
    - ICF has higher concentrations of protein, potassium, magnesium, phosphate, and sulfate than does ECF
    - ECF has higher concentrations of sodium, calcium, chloride, and bicarbonate than does ICF
- **Physiology**
  - Fluid balance
    - Body gains and loses water daily through fluid intake and output
      - Water enters via the GI tract
      - Water leaves via skin, lungs, GI tract, and urinary tract
    - Two mechanisms help maintain fluid balance
      - Thirst regulates water intake
      - Countercurrent mechanism regulates urine concentration
        - Urine excretion is main route of water loss
        - Output is typically 1,000 to 1,500 ml daily

A&P highlights

- More than 50% of the average adult's body is water, which contains dissolved substances.
- Body fluid composition differs by compartment.
- These are three types of physiological balance: fluid balance, electrolyte balance, and acid-base balance.
- The body gains and loses water daily through fluid intake and output.
- Electrolytes dissociate into ions when dissolved into water.
- Acid-base balance results in a stable hydrogen ion concentration in body fluids.

Facts about fluid balance

- Water enters the GI tract and leaves via the skin, lungs, GI tract, and urinary tract.
- Thirst regulates water intake.
- Urine excretion is the main route of water loss.

Facts about electrolyte balance

- Ions may be positively charged cations or negatively charged anions.
- Electrical charges of cations and anions are balanced so that body fluids are electrically neutral.
- Kidneys and hormones regulate most of the electrolytes.

Facts about acid-base balance

- The body is an acid-producing organism.
- Hydrogen ion concentration of a fluid determines whether it's acidic or basic.
- Buffer systems and lungs and kidneys maintain the blood pH within a narrow range—7.38 to 7.42.

Key facts about enteral agents

- Use normal metabolic pathways and processes
- Metabolism unknown
- Excreted in feces

- Electrolyte balance
  - Electrolytes are substances that dissociate into ions (electronically charged particles) when dissolved in water
  - Ions may be positively charged cations or negatively charged anions
    - Major cations: sodium (Na^+), potassium (K^+), calcium (Ca^{++}), and magnesium (Mg^{++})
    - Major anions: chloride (Cl^+), bicarbonate (HCO_3^-), and phosphate (HPO_4^-)
  - Normally, electrical charges of cations and anions are balanced so that body fluids are electrically neutral
  - Body uses various mechanisms to maintain electrolyte balance; kidneys and hormones regulate most electrolytes
- Acid-base balance
  - Acid-base balance results in stable hydrogen ion (H^+) concentration in body fluids
    - Acid releases hydrogen ions in water
    - Base releases ions that can combine with hydrogen ions
  - Hydrogen ion concentration of a fluid determines whether it's acidic or basic (alkaline)
  - Human body is an acid-producing organism
  - Buffer systems and the lungs and kidneys maintain blood pH within a narrow range—7.38 to 7.42—by neutralizing and eliminating acids as rapidly as they're formed, thus helping maintain body's acid-base balance
  - Buffer systems minimize pH changes caused by excess acids or bases by reducing the effect of a sudden change in hydrogen ion concentration by converting a strong acid or base into a weak acid or base
    - Lungs affect acid-base balance by excreting carbon dioxide and regulating carbonic acid content of blood
    - Kidneys regulate acid-base balance by allowing tubular filtrate reabsorption of bicarbonate and by forming bicarbonate

● **Function**
- Homeostasis is achieved through complex interrelationship among fluid, electrolyte, and acid-base metabolism
- Water and fluid balance is essential to physiologic functioning
- Electrolyte balance and sufficient quantities of each major electrolyte are essential to normal metabolism and function
- Balance between acids and bases keeps hydrogen ion concentration stable and pH neutral (7.0)

ENTERAL AGENTS

● **Mechanism of action**
- Use normal metabolic pathways and processes

● **Pharmacokinetics**
- Absorption: Absorbed via GI tract

Enteral feeding routes

This table shows various enteral feeding routes and the indications for their use.

ACCESS	INDICATIONS
Nasogastric or orogastric	• Short-term use • No esophageal reflux • Gag reflex intact • Normal gastric and duodenum emptying
Nasoduodenal or nasojejunal	• Short-term use • Esophageal reflux • High risk of pulmonary aspiration • Delayed gastric emptying
Esophageal or pharyngostomy	• Long-term use • Head or neck tumors • Nasopharyngeal access contraindicated
Gastrostomy	• Long-term use • Swallowing dysfunction • Nasoenteric access contraindicated • Normal gastric and duodenum emptying • Esophageal stricture or neoplasm
Jejunostomy	• Long-term use • Esophageal reflux • High risk of pulmonary aspiration • Impaired gastric emptying • Failure to access upper GI tract • Postoperative feeding in trauma, malnourishment, or upper GI surgery

- Distribution: Well distributed
- Metabolism: Unknown
- Excretion: Excreted in feces

Drug examples
- Complete nutritional supplement feeding solutions (Amin-Aid, Arginaid, BCAD 2, Boost, Cyclinex-2, Ensure, Epulor, Glucerna, Glutarex-2, Hepatic-Aid II, Hominex-2, Immun-Aid, Isocal, I-Valex-2, Jevity, Ketonex-2, Nutrament, Osmolite, Peptamen, Peptinex, Phenex-2, Propimex-2, Pulmocare, Respalor, Suplena, Sustacal, TraumaCal, Tyrex-2, Vital, Vivonex)

Indications
- Supplement when oral intake is inadequate to meet nutritional needs
- Total or supplemental nutrition for patients who can't consume adequate calories because of physical impairments (dysphagia), GI tract problems (fistulas), psychological disturbances (dementia, depression), altered level of consciousness (delirium), or hypermetabolic states (burns, cancer, multiple trauma) (see *Enteral feeding routes*)
- Total or supplemental nutrition for patients with specific conditions
  - Renal failure (Amin-Aid and Respalor)

When to use enteral agents

- Nutritional needs
- Renal failure
- Liver impairment
- Pulmonary disease
- Glucose intolerance
- Hypermetabolic state

– Liver impairment (Hepatic-Aid II; contains branched-chain amino acids)
– Pulmonary disease (Pulmocare; higher in fat and lower in carbohydrates, yielding less carbon dioxide)
– Glucose intolerance (Glucerna)
– Hypermetabolic states (TraumaCal)

● Contraindications and precautions
- Contraindicated in patients with bowel obstruction, vomiting, or malabsorption syndrome

● Adverse reactions
- Diarrhea, nausea, aspiration, and hyperglycemia

● Interactions
- These agents may decrease phenytoin levels; give drug 2 hours before enteral therapy or stop enteral feeding for 2 hours before phenytoin administration

● Nursing responsibilities
- Assess nutritional status
  – Include dietary recall and anthropometric measurements
  – Make sure that the patient has an intact digestive system
- Obtain diagnostic test results to establish baseline values, identify deficiencies, and evaluate progress after supplementation
- Weigh the patient before initiating therapy to establish baseline; check daily weights to evaluate for changes
- Teach the patient about the nutritional agent to be used, and review any special modifications or procedures needed for administration
- Reinforce instructions on a well-balanced diet, with emphasis on food allowances and restrictions
- Know that enteral supplements may be given orally or via nasogastric tube, gastrostomy, or via needle-catheter jejunostomy
- Teach the patient how to prepare the supplement (for example, keep refrigerated, shake before using, mix powder with specified amount of water or fruit juice)
- Assist the patient with measures to enhance the taste of oral forms, such as serving supplement cold or poured over ice
- Verify the diet and fluid order and the formula to be used before administering a tube feeding
  – Check formula's expiration date, when it was opened, and how long it has been kept at room temperature
  – Verify whether feeding is to be intermittent (usually given every 3 to 4 hours) or continuous (usually given over 16 to 24 hours)
  – Check for possible agent-formula interactions
- Confirm tube placement and patency before an enteral feeding, and flush the tube with 30 to 50 ml of water every 4 hours or according to facility policy for continuous feedings; change the feeding solution every 8 hours and the administration set every 24 hours

TIME-OUT FOR TEACHING

Teaching about home enteral nutrition

Include these topics in your teaching plan for the patient requiring tube feedings at home:

- rationale for tube feeding
- type of feeding being used
- hand-washing and infection-control measures
- procedure for carrying out the feeding
- care of tube and equipment, including storage of solutions and temperatures for administration
- assessment of tube placement
- proper patient positioning for feeding
- tube flushing after medication administration
- environmental monitoring during feeding (making it as pleasant as possible)
- signs and symptoms to discuss with the practitioner, including intolerance or complications
- follow-up care, including practitioner visits.

Topics for patient discussion

- Tube feeding
- Care of tube and equipment
- Signs and symptoms

- Check gastric residual; notify the practitioner if residual is 100 ml or more (or according to facility policy)
- Position the patient upright or with the head of the bed elevated at least 45 degrees to prevent aspiration
- Provide oral care unless contraindicated
- Monitor intake and output and daily weight
- Slow the rate or reduce the concentration of the feeding if the patient complains of cramping or nausea, and notify the practitioner
- Stop the feeding immediately if the patient vomits
- Don't let feedings remain at room temperature for more than 8 hours (formulas provide an excellent media for bacterial growth)
- Don't add new formula to a feeding that has been hanging for more than 6 hours
- Provide tube insertion site care or dressing changes at least daily or when dressing is soiled
- Teach the patient and his family the tube feeding procedure if feedings are to continue at home (see *Teaching about home enteral nutrition*)

PARENTERAL AGENTS

Mechanism of action
- Absorb solution that's nutritionally complete except for essential fatty acids and provide the necessary calories, vitamins, electrolytes, minerals, and trace elements to the body

Pharmacokinetics
- Absorption: Administered I.V.
- Distribution: Well distributed
- Metabolism: Unknown

Key facts about parenteral agents

- Provide necessary calories, vitamins, electrolytes, minerals, and trace elements to the body
- Metabolism unknown
- Excreted in urine

- Excretion: Excreted in urine

● Drug examples

- Amino acid solutions (Aminosyn, FreAmine), dextrose solutions in water (D_5W, $D_{10}W$, $D_{20}W$, $D_{50}W$), lipid emulsions (Intralipid, Liposyn II, Liposyn III), specialized amino acid formulations (Aminess, Aminosyn-HBC, Aminosyn-RF, FreAmine HBC, HepatAmine, NephrAmine, RenAmin)

● Indications

- Provide nutrition when oral intake is inadequate to meet nutritional needs
- Treatment to achieve a zero or positive nitrogen balance when a negative balance is present and to provide enough protein to rebuild tissue
- Provide carbohydrates, protein, fat, water, electrolytes, vitamins, minerals, and trace elements when GI tract can't be used (PPN or TPN)
  - Preoperative or postoperative low-calorie nutrition supplementation; augment to enteral therapy as necessary (PPN)
  - Treatment to maintain or increase body weight, to achieve normal growth in infants and children, and to restore lean body mass and adequate tissue in emaciated patients (TPN)
- Short-term nutritional support for patients who don't need more than 2,500 calories/day (D_5W and $D_{10}W$)
- Total nutritional support; commonly used in admixtures with amino acid solutions ($D_{20}W$ and $D_{50}W$)
- High-calorie, low-protein formulation; used for patients with renal failure (Aminess, Aminosyn, Nephramine, and RenAmin)
- Nutritional support containing branched-chain amino acids and high protein levels; used for patients with liver disease (HepatAmine)
- Fat supplement that provides additional calories while sparing protein (Intralipid, Liposyn II, and Liposyn III)
- Stress formula used for hypermetabolic conditions (FreAmine HBC)

● Contraindications and precautions

- Contraindicated in patients with anuria; severe, uncontrolled electrolyte or acid-base imbalance; or decreased circulating blood volume

● Adverse reactions

- Pulmonary edema, fluid overload, hyperglycemia, glycosuria, electrolyte imbalances, catheter sepsis, rebound hypoglycemia, and pancreatitis (lipid formulations)

● Interactions

- None reported; see individual manufacturer's labeling

● Nursing responsibilities

- Assess nutritional status, including dietary recall and anthropometric measurements
- Obtain diagnostic test results to establish baseline values, identify deficiencies, and evaluate progress after supplementation

---

When to use parenteral agents

- Nutritional needs
- Body weight maintenance
- Normal growth in infants and children
- Lean body mass restoration
- Renal failure
- Liver disease
- Hypermetabolic conditions

When NOT to use parenteral agents

- Anuria
- Severe uncontrolled electrolyte or acid-base imbalance
- Decreasing circulating blood volume

Adverse reactions

- Pulmonary edema, fluid overload, hyperglycemia, glycosuria, electrolyte imbalances, catheter sepsis, rebound hypoglycemia, pancreatitis

- Weigh the patient before initiating therapy to establish baseline; check daily weights to evaluate for changes
- Teach the patient about the prescribed nutritional agent, and review any special modifications or procedures needed for administration
- Reinforce instructions on maintaining a well-balanced diet, with emphasis on food allowances and restrictions
- Verify the drug order to ensure the correct type and amount of solution to administer and the proper infusion rate
- Follow procedures for initiating and maintaining peripheral or central vein infusion therapy; concentrations of dextrose greater than 15% should be administered through a central vein only
- Monitor for signs and symptoms of fluid overload and electrolyte imbalance
- Monitor vital signs, intake and output, and daily weight
- Don't hang solutions for longer than 24 hours
- Assess the patient's response to therapy as evidenced by weight gain; obtain ongoing assessment of nutritional and metabolic status as evidenced by laboratory studies
  - Monitor serum electrolyte, glucose, and blood urea nitrogen levels and hepatic function, as ordered
  - Monitor serum calcium and phosphorus levels, as ordered
- Inspect the catheter insertion site at least every 8 hours, and change tubing, filters, and dressing according to facility protocol; maintain sterile technique during dressing changes
- Monitor the infusion rate and administration system every hour or according to facility protocol
- Monitor the patient receiving TPN for glycosuria and ketonuria every 4 to 6 hours; perform fingerstick blood glucose checks every 4 to 6 hours or as ordered to assess for hyperglycemia
- Know that insulin may be added to the TPN solution or otherwise administered based on the patient's blood glucose level
  - Begin TPN infusion at a slow rate to allow the body to adjust to increased glucose levels; starting TPN infusion too fast may cause hyperglycemia
  - Infuse $D_{10}W$ if TPN solution isn't available
- Never attempt to "catch up" a TPN solution by increasing the infusion rate
- Discontinue TPN gradually while increasing oral or enteral feedings
- Infuse lipid emulsions at a rate of 0.5 to 1 ml/hour initially, and observe for adverse effects; avoid rapid infusion, and use a pump to regulate rate
- Be aware that in-line filters with pores of 1.2 microns or larger are sometimes used to remove particulate matter
- Use only tubing supplied with the emulsion to prevent possible interaction with materials used to make plastic more flexible

Key nursing actions

- Assess the patient's nutritional status; include dietary recall and anthropometric measurements.
- Verify the order to ensure the correct type and amount of solution to administer and the proper infusion rate.
- Monitor for signs and symptoms of fluid overload and electrolyte imbalance.
- Never attempt to "catch up" a TPN solution by increasing the infusion rate.
- Be aware that lipid emulsions may be mixed with amino acid solution, dextrose, electrolytes, and vitamins in the same I.V. container; check with the pharmacist for acceptable proportions and compatibility information.
- Use lipid emulsion within 12 hours after starting the infusion; lipids support bacterial growth.

- Be aware that lipid emulsions may be mixed with amino acid solution, dextrose, electrolytes, and vitamins in the same I.V. container; check with the pharmacist for acceptable proportions and compatibility information
- Use lipid emulsion within 12 hours after starting infusion; lipids support bacterial growth
- Know that lipid solutions should initially be infused slowly to observe for adverse reactions
- Monitor serum lipid levels closely; elevated lipid levels must return to normal between doses

ELECTROLYTE REPLACEMENTS

● Mechanism of action
- Electrolyte agents: Replace and maintain electrolyte levels
- Sodium fluoride: Stabilizes apatite crystal of bone and teeth
- Sodium bicarbonate: Restores the body's buffering capacity and neutralizes excess acid
- Ammonium chloride: Increases free hydrogen ion concentration
- Tromethamine: Combines with hydrogen ions and associated acid anions with excretion of resulting salts; also produces osmotic diuretic effect

● Pharmacokinetics
- Varies with electrolyte

● Drug examples
- Ammonium chloride, calcium, magnesium oxide (Mag-Ox, Maox), magnesium sulfate, phosphorus, potassium chloride (Kaochlor, Kay Ciel, K-Dur, Micro-K Extencaps, Slow-K), potassium phosphate (Neutra-Phos-K), sodium bicarbonate, sodium fluoride (Fluoritab, Flura-Drops, Pediaflor), tromethamine (Tham)

● Indications
- Supplement when oral intake is inadequate to meet nutritional needs
- Treat potassium depletion (potassium)
    - Treat potassium deficiency from diuretics, vomiting, diarrhea, or fistulas (potassium chloride)
    - Treat hypokalemia (potassium phosphate)
- Supplement to harden tooth enamel and prevent dental caries when adequate fluoride isn't provided in drinking water (sodium fluoride)
- Correct metabolic acidosis secondary to cardiac arrest, shock, renal failure, or diabetic ketoacidosis (sodium bicarbonate)
    - May be used to neutralize gastric acid but isn't recommended because of high sodium load
    - May be applied topically for itching and minor burns
- Supplement used during parenteral nutrition or as an antacid (magnesium oxide)
- Systemic acidifier in metabolic alkalosis to correct chloride depletion (ammonium chloride)

Key facts about electrolyte replacements

- They replace and maintain electrolyte levels.
- Sodium fluoride stabilizes apatite crystal.
- Sodium bicarbonate restores the body's buffering capacity and neutralizes excess acid.
- Ammonium chloride increases free hydrogen ion concentration.
- Tromethamine combines with hydrogen ions and associated acid anions.
- Metabolism and excretion vary.

When to use electrolyte replacements

- Nutrition
- Potassium depletion
- Potassium deficiency
- Hypokalemia
- Dental caries prevention
- Metabolic acidosis correction
- Minor burns and itching
- Magnesium supplement
- Systemic acidifier in metabolic alkalosis to correct chloride depletion
- Acidosis secondary to cardiac arrest or cardiac bypass surgery
- Rapid calcium replacement needed
- Cardiac arrest

Signs and symptoms of hyperkalemia

With potassium replacement therapy, overcorrection of an electrolyte deficit can lead to hyperkalemia. To prevent the dangerous effects of this imbalance, closely monitor the patient for its signs and symptoms.

- Watch for neuromuscular effects, such as listlessness, confusion, flaccid paralysis, paresthesia, weakness, and limb heaviness.
- Observe for electrocardiogram changes, including prolonged PR interval; widened QRS complex; depressed ST segment; and tall, tented T waves.
- Be alert for other cardiovascular effects, such as peripheral vascular collapse with a fall in blood pressure, arrhythmias, heart block and, possibly, cardiac arrest.

- Correct acidosis secondary to cardiac arrest or cardiac bypass surgery (tromethamine)
- Treatment when rapid calcium replacement is necessary (calcium gluconate and calcium chloride)
- Treatment during cardiac arrest (calcium chloride)

● Contraindications and precautions
- Sodium fluoride contraindicated when fluoride intake from drinking water is greater than 0.7 ppm (parts per million)
- Sodium bicarbonate contraindicated in patients with metabolic or respiratory alkalosis; patients experiencing chloride losses through vomiting or continuous gastric suctioning; patients receiving diuretics known to produce hypochloremic alkalosis; and those with hypocalcemia in which alkalosis may produce tetany, hypertension, seizures, or heart failure
- Ammonium chloride contraindicated in patients with renal or hepatic insufficiency
- Tromethamine contraindicated in patients with renal failure or anuria
- Potassium preparations used cautiously in patients with renal impairment or renal failure and those receiving potassium-sparing diuretics
- Calcium preparations used cautiously in patients receiving cardiac glycoside preparations and those with ventricular fibrillation, hypercalcemia, hypophosphatemia, or renal calculi

● Adverse reactions
- Phlebitis, confusion, restlessness, paralysis, and cardiac arrest (potassium preparations) (see *Signs and symptoms of hyperkalemia*)
- Headache, weakness, GI distress, and brown discoloration of teeth (sodium fluoride overdose)
- Gastric distention, renal calculi, metabolic alkalosis, hypernatremia, and hyperkalemia (sodium bicarbonate overdose)
- Constipation (magnesium oxide)
- Headache, confusion, twitching, tetany, bradycardia, metabolic acidosis, hyperchloremia, hypokalemia, and gastric irritation (ammonium chloride)

When NOT to use electrolyte replacements
- Fluoride intake from drinking water that exceeds 0.7 ppm
- Metabolic or respiratory alkalosis
- Chloride loss by vomiting or continuous gastric suctioning
- Hypochloremic alkalosis from diuretics
- Hypocalcemia
- Renal or hepatic insufficiency
- Anuria

Adverse reactions
- Phlebitis, confusion, restlessness, paralysis, cardiac arrest, headache, weakness, GI distress, brown discoloration of teeth, gastric distention, renal calculi, metabolic alkalosis, hypernatremia, hyperkalemia, constipation, twitching, tetany, bradycardia, metabolic acidosis, hyperchloremia, gastric irritation, respiratory depression, hypoglycemia, I.V. thrombosis, tingling sensation, chalky taste, hypercalcemia, vein irritation, local reactions with I.M. use

- Respiratory depression, hypoglycemia, hyperkalemia, and I.V. thrombosis (tromethamine)
- Constipation, tingling sensation, chalky taste (after I.V. administration), hypercalcemia, vein irritation, and local reactions with I.M. use (calcium preparations)

Interactions
- None significant

Nursing responsibilities
- Assess nutritional status, including dietary recall and anthropometric measurements
- Obtain diagnostic test results to establish baseline values, identify deficiencies, and evaluate progress after supplementation
- Weigh the patient before initiating therapy to establish baseline; check daily weights to evaluate for changes
- Teach the patient about the prescribed nutritional agent, and review any special modifications or procedures needed for administration
- Reinforce instructions on maintaining a well-balanced diet, with emphasis on food allowances and restrictions
- Evaluate serum electrolyte levels and arterial blood gases, as ordered
- Monitor serum levels closely to prevent toxicity
- Administer potassium chloride orally or as an I.V. infusion
  - Know that oral tablets should never be chewed or sucked; however, they may be crushed and added to water or fruit juice or swallowed whole
  - Administer I.V. potassium by infusion only as a dilute solution to prevent potentially fatal hyperkalemia from a too-rapid infusion
  - Never give potassium by I.V. push or I.M. injection
- Inform the patient that sodium fluoride tablets may be chewed, swallowed whole, or dissolved in liquids other than dairy products; advise him not to take fluoride within 2 hours of ingesting a dairy product
- Be aware that sodium bicarbonate isn't routinely recommended for use in cardiac arrest because it may produce a paradoxical acidosis from carbon dioxide production
- Give oral forms of ammonium chloride after meals to minimize adverse GI effects
- Be aware that tromethamine shouldn't be used longer than 1 day except in life-threatening situations; be prepared to adjust dosage carefully according to blood pH
- Give calcium chloride by I.V. only, using an in-line filter; watch for possible precipitate if added to parenteral solutions containing other additives, such as phosphorus and phosphates
- Monitor electrocardiogram (ECG) closely for changes, especially when administering potassium and calcium preparations

Key nursing actions

- Assess nutritional status; include dietary recall and anthropometric measurements.
- Teach about the nutritional agent to be used, and review any special modifications or procedures needed for administration.
- Administer potassium chloride orally or as an I.V. infusion.
- Give oral forms of ammonium chloride after meals to minimize adverse GI effects.
- Be aware that tromethamine shouldn't be used longer than 1 day except in life-threatening situations; be prepared to adjust dosage carefully according to blood pH.
- Monitor ECG closely for changes, especially when administering potassium and calcium preparations.

- Know that calcium gluconate is the antidote for magnesium sulfate toxicity; keep it immediately available at all times during magnesium sulfate administration

VITAMINS

● **Mechanism of action**
  - Replace vitamins in deficiency states

● **Pharmacokinetics**
  - Varies with vitamin

● **Drug examples**
  - Water-soluble vitamins: Calcium pantothenate (B_5), cyanocobalamin (B_{12}), folic acid (B_9 [Folvite]), nicotinic acid (niacin [B_3]), pyridoxine (B_6), riboflavin (B_2), thiamine (B_1), vitamin C (ascorbic acid)
  - Fat-soluble vitamins: Ergocalciferol (D_2 [Calciferol]), phytonadione (K_1), vitamin A (Aquasol A), vitamin E (Vita-Plus E)

● **Indications**
  - Supplement when oral intake is inadequate to meet nutritional needs
  - Coenzyme in carbohydrate metabolism; treatment for beriberi and neuritis in pregnancy and alcoholism (thiamine)
  - Supplement to combat pellagra and beriberi (riboflavin)
  - Adjunct to isoniazid in treatment of alcoholic polyneuritis (pyridoxine)
  - Treat megaloblastic anemia (folic acid)
  - Treat pernicious anemia (cyanocobalamin)
  - Maintain collagen, blood vessels, and skin cartilage; heal wounds; and provide resistance to infections such as common cold (ascorbic acid)
  - Calcium supplement, although calcium is plentiful in most diets (calcium pantothenate)
  - Supplement in pregnancy, breast-feeding, gastrectomy, and psoriasis; also promotes bone growth and development, mucosal integrity, and night vision (vitamin A)
  - Treat hypoprothrombinemia secondary to vitamin K deficiency or hepatic failure; also used prophylactically for neonatal hemorrhagic disease (vitamin K)

● **Contraindications and precautions**
  - All vitamins contraindicated in patients with hypersensitivity to drug
  - Vitamin A contraindicated in patients with malabsorption syndrome or hypervitaminosis A

● **Adverse reactions**
  - Yellow discoloration of urine (riboflavin)
  - Hypervitaminosis (malaise, lethargy, abdominal pain, anorexia, nausea) (vitamin A)
  - Hypotension (after rapid I.V. administration) and angioedema (thiamine)
  - Epigastric distress and renal failure (vitamin C)

Key facts about vitamins

- Act as replacements in deficiency states
- Metabolism and excretion vary with each vitamin

When to use vitamins

- Nutrition
- Carbohydrate metabolism
- Neuritis in pregnancy and alcoholism
- Pellagra and beriberi
- Alcoholic polyneuritis
- Megaloblastic anemia
- Pernicious anemia
- Collagen, blood vessels, and skin cartilage maintenance
- Wound healing
- Infection resistance
- Pregnancy
- Breast-feeding
- Gastrectomy
- Psoriasis
- Bone growth and development
- Mucosal integrity
- Night vision
- Hypoprothrombinemia
- Neonatal hemorrhagic disease

When NOT to use vitamins

- Hypersensitivity
- Malabsorption syndrome
- Hypervitaminosis A

Adverse reactions

- Yellow discoloration of urine, hypervitaminosis, hypotension, angioedema, epigastric distress, renal failure

Key nursing actions

- Assess nutritional status; include dietary recall and anthropometric measurements.
- Administer I.V. thiamine infusion carefully because cardiovascular collapse and anaphylaxis have been reported.

Key facts about minerals

- They act as the component of many enzyme actions.
- Chromium potentiates the action of insulin and regulation of lipoprotein metabolism.
- Iron is an essential mineral that's a component of hemoglobin, myoglobin, and other enzymes.
- Metabolism and excretion vary.

When to use minerals

- Nutrition
- Long-term TPN
- Goiter
- Hypothyroidism
- Iron deficiency anemia
- Zinc deficiencies

● Interactions

- Varies by vitamin

● Nursing responsibilities

- Assess nutritional status, including dietary recall and anthropometric measurements
- Obtain diagnostic test results to establish baseline values, identify deficiencies, and evaluate progress after supplementation
- Weigh the patient before initiating therapy to establish baseline; check daily weights to evaluate for changes
- Teach the patient about the prescribed vitamin, and review any special modifications or procedures needed for administration
- Reinforce instructions on maintaining a well-balanced diet, with emphasis on food allowances and restrictions
- Know that oral, I.V., and I.M. preparations of thiamine are available
- **Administer I.V. thiamine infusion carefully; cardiovascular collapse and anaphylaxis have been reported**
- Advise the patient against self-dosing with megadoses of vitamins without specific indications to avoid toxicity
- Instruct the patient in food sources of vitamins
- Monitor prothrombin time to determine drug effectiveness if the patient is receiving vitamin K

MINERALS

● Mechanism of action

- Act as component of many enzyme actions
- Chromium: Potentiates action of insulin and regulation of lipoprotein metabolism
- Iron: Assists in oxygen transport; essential mineral component of hemoglobin, myoglobin, and other enzymes

● Pharmacokinetics

- Varies by mineral

● Drug examples

- Chromium (Chroma-Pak), copper, iodine (SSKI solution), iron sulfate (ferrous sulfate [Feosol]), manganese, molybdenum (Molypen), selenium (Sele-Pak), zinc (Orazinc)

● Indications

- Supplement when oral intake is inadequate to meet nutritional needs
- Supplement in patients receiving long-term TPN (chromium and molybdenum)
- Supplement in TPN (copper and selenium)
- Treat goiter and hypothyroidism caused by iodine deficiency (iodine)
- Correct iron deficiency anemia; also used as iron supplement (iron)
- Dietary supplement (manganese)
- Treat zinc deficiencies (zinc)

Contraindications and precautions

- Don't give preparations containing iodine to patients allergic to shellfish or iodine
- Take seizure precautions in patients receiving large doses of chromium

Adverse reactions

- Nausea, vomiting, gastric ulceration, rash, joint swelling, bronchospasms, seizure, coma, and kidney or liver damage (chromium)
- Diarrhea, lethargy, altered behavior, diminished reflexes, and photophobia (copper)
- Metallic taste, skin lesions, eyelid swelling, increased saliva production, goiter, bloody diarrhea, fever, depression, and mouth, gum, and salivary gland tenderness (iodine)
- Nausea, vomiting, GI irritation, constipation, diarrhea, dark or blackened stools, and stained teeth (liquid form of iron)
- Anorexia, diarrhea, headache, and parkinsonian symptoms (manganese)
- Goutlike symptoms (molybdenum)
- Alopecia, skin lesions, GI irritation, and garlic breath odor (selenium)
- Stomach irritation, gastric ulceration, diarrhea, vomiting, elevated serum amylase level, hypothermia, and hypotension (zinc)

Interactions

- None significant

Nursing responsibilities

- Assess the patient's nutritional status, including dietary recall and anthropometric measurements
- Obtain diagnostic test results to establish baseline values, identify deficiencies, and evaluate progress after supplementation
- Weigh the patient before initiating therapy to establish baseline; check daily weights to evaluate for changes
- Teach the patient about the prescribed mineral, and review any special modifications or procedures needed for administration
- Reinforce instructions on maintaining a well-balanced diet, with emphasis on food allowances and restrictions
- Dilute liquid preparations well before administration
- Monitor hydration if the patient experiences vomiting or diarrhea
- Dilute parenteral solution well and administer via a central venous line
- Monitor the patient closely for signs and symptoms of toxicity
- Institute seizure precautions for the patient receiving large doses of chromium
- **Assess the patient for allergies to iodine or shellfish before administering an iodine preparation**
- Consider the mineral content of the patient's diet in addition to mineral supplements to prevent possible toxicity
- Give iron on an empty stomach; however, if GI upset occurs, give after meals or with food

TOP 4

Items to study for your next test on nutritional agents and the body

1. Purpose of each nutritional agent
2. Common adverse effects of nutritional agents
3. Nursing responsibilities when administering nutritional agents
4. Patient teaching related to nutritional agents

- Don't give iron within 2 hours of antacids, tetracyclines, or fluoro-quinolones
- Give iron liquid preparations in water or juice and through a straw to prevent tooth staining
- Use Z-track method to prevent staining skin when giving iron parenterally

NCLEX CHECKS

It's never too soon to begin your NCLEX® preparation. Now that you've reviewed this chapter, carefully read each of the following questions and choose the best answer. Then compare your responses with the correct answers.

1. A 78-year-old female client weighing 94 lb (42.6 kg) is to receive 240 ml of Sustacal between meals as a nutritional supplement. Which factor is most important to consider before giving this product?
- [ ] **1.** It provides 20 cal/ml.
- [ ] **2.** It's a low-carbohydrate, high-protein supplement.
- [ ] **3.** The client must have an intact digestive system.
- [ ] **4.** When given by itself, it's nutritionally incomplete.

2. A client with intestinal cancer is started on TPN at 25 ml/hour for the first 12 hours. This rate was selected because it:
- [ ] **1.** helps prevent catheter-site infections.
- [ ] **2.** reverses fluid volume deficits caused by low oral intake of fluids.
- [ ] **3.** allows the body to adjust to the increased glucose levels.
- [ ] **4.** reverses the negative nitrogen balance caused by the client's cancer.

3. Magnesium sulfate is ordered for a client diagnosed with preeclampsia. Which statement about magnesium sulfate is correct?
- [ ] **1.** Calcium gluconate is the antidote for magnesium toxicity.
- [ ] **2.** Magnesium sulfate is incompatible with normal saline solution.
- [ ] **3.** Magnesium sulfate increases acetylcholine released by nerve impulses.
- [ ] **4.** Enhanced knee-jerk and patellar reflexes are signs of impending magnesium toxicity.

4. Which drug should a nurse expect to be ordered for a client diagnosed with pernicious anemia?
- [ ] **1.** Ferrous sulfate (Feosol)
- [ ] **2.** Iron dextran (INFeD)
- [ ] **3.** Thiamine (vitamin B$_1$)
- [ ] **4.** Cyanocobalamin (vitamin B$_{12}$)

5. A nurse is providing discharge instructions for a client taking ferrous sulfate (Feosol). Which statement by the client indicates that the nurse's teaching was successful?

☐ **1.** "If I miss a dose, I need to double the next dose."
☐ **2.** "I should eat extra fiber and whole-grain cereals."
☐ **3.** "I need to take it only when my stomach hurts bad."
☐ **4.** "Smoking won't harm the drug's effectiveness. It might even help."

6. A physician orders an I.V. infusion of dextrose 5% in quarter-normal saline solution to be infused at 7 ml/kg/hour for a 10-month-old infant. The infant weighs 22 lb. How many milliliters per hour should the nurse infuse the ordered solution? Record your answer as a whole number.

_____ ml/hour

7. A client is admitted to the medical-surgical unit from a nursing home with a potassium level of 2.2 mEq/L. One of the client's drug orders states to give potassium, 20 mEq in 50 ml of dextrose 5% in water, over 30 minutes. Which assessment finding is crucial when administering this drug?

☐ **1.** Pulse pressure of 54 mm Hg
☐ **2.** Serum glucose level of 320 mg/dl
☐ **3.** Urine output of 350 ml in 24 hours
☐ **4.** Respiratory rate of 28 breaths/minute

8. A 3-year-old child has just ingested a large amount of multivitamins with iron. What should the nurse instruct the mother to do?

☐ **1.** Do nothing because vitamins and iron aren't toxic.
☐ **2.** Offer the child a glass of milk to drink.
☐ **3.** Immediately take the child to the emergency department.
☐ **4.** Give the child salt and water until he vomits.

9. A nurse is caring for a client with a history of alcohol abuse. Which vitamin supplement would the nurse expect the physician to prescribe to help prevent Wernicke's encephalopathy?

☐ **1.** Vitamin B_1
☐ **2.** Vitamin B_6
☐ **3.** Vitamin B_{12}
☐ **4.** Vitamin D

10. A client is to receive 500 ml of fat emulsion (Liposyn) over 8 hours. At the time the administration is started, there are no I.V. pumps available. If the drop factor for the tubing is 10 gtt ml, how many drops per minute should the nurse set the I.V. infusion for?

☐ **1.** 10 gtt/minute
☐ **2.** 25 gtt/minute
☐ **3.** 38 gtt/minute
☐ **4.** 50 gtt/minute

ANSWERS AND RATIONALES

1. CORRECT ANSWER: 3

Sustacal, like many other supplements, is a milk-based product that requires an intact digestive system for breakdown and absorption of the supplement. Sustacal provides 1 cal/ml and is a nutritionally complete product. It's high in carbohydrates and fats but lower in proteins.

2. CORRECT ANSWER: 3

The high glucose content of TPN can cause hyperglycemia if TPN is started at too fast a rate, so TPN is started at a slow rate to allow the body to adjust to increased glucose levels. The rate of 25 ml/hour is considered slow for TPN and would be appropriate to infuse the TPN for the first 12 hours. Catheter-site infections are best prevented by good sterile technique. The rate would need to be faster to affect fluid volume deficit. The negative nitrogen balance would be reversed with faster rates of TPN.

3. CORRECT ANSWER: 1

Calcium gluconate reverses magnesium toxicity. Because magnesium toxicity is a danger with magnesium sulfate therapy, this antidote should be immediately available at all times during magnesium sulfate therapy. Magnesium sulfate is compatible with normal saline solution. Magnesium sulfate decreases (not increases) acetylcholine released by nerve impulses. The absence (not the presence) of knee-jerk and patellar reflexes is a sign of impending magnesium toxicity.

4. CORRECT ANSWER: 4

Pernicious anemia results from the lack of intrinsic factor, which is essential for vitamin B_{12} absorption. Lifelong vitamin B_{12} therapy is given to clients lacking intrinsic factor. Ferrous sulfate and iron dextran are indicated for treatment of iron deficiency anemia. Thiamine is indicated for anemia that results from thiamine deficiency.

5. CORRECT ANSWER: 2

Constipation is a common adverse reaction to ferrous sulfate therapy. Eating extra fiber and whole-grain cereals will help decrease the risk of constipation. Missed doses of ferrous sulfate should be taken as soon as possible, but doses should never be doubled. Ferrous sulfate should be taken on a scheduled basis, not in response to symptoms, for the full term of therapy. Smoking should always be avoided.

6. CORRECT ANSWER: 70

To perform this dosage calculation, the nurse should first convert the infant's weight to kilograms:

$$2.2 \text{ lb/kg} = 22 \text{ lb/X kg}$$
$$X = 22 \div 2.2$$
$$X = 10 \text{ kg}$$

Next, the nurse should multiply the infant's weight by the ordered rate:

$$10 \text{ kg} \times 7 \text{ ml/kg/hour} = 70 \text{ ml/hour}$$

7. CORRECT ANSWER: 3

The client's low urine output (less than 400 ml of urine in 24 hours, characterizing oliguria) indicates that he might be in renal failure. Because potassium is excreted by the kidneys, the client could very easily become hyperkalemic. A pulse pressure of 54 mm Hg is normal. The client's glucose level and respiratory rate aren't significant when giving potassium.

8. CORRECT ANSWER: 3

Vitamins and iron can be toxic in large amounts; therefore, the child requires immediate emergency medical attention. Milk will coat the stomach, but it won't prevent absorption of these drugs. Excessive amounts of salt and water can cause electrolyte disturbances and won't stop absorption.

9. CORRECT ANSWER: 1

Wernicke's encephalopathy results from a deficiency of thiamine (vitamin B_1) and is commonly related to chronic alcohol abuse. Preventing Wernicke's encephalopathy requires supplementing the client's diet with vitamin B_1. Vitamin B_6 is commonly given to prevent peripheral neuropathy in clients receiving isoniazid. Vitamin B_{12} replacement therapy is used to treat pernicious anemia. Vitamin D is needed for calcium regulation.

10. CORRECT ANSWER: 1

The correct formula to use is volume (milliliters) times drop factor: 500 ml $\times$ 10 gtt/minute. Next, divide the product by 480 minutes (or 8 hours). This yields 10.4 gtt/minute, or about 10 gtt/minute.

Herbal drugs

HERBAL MEDICINE	COMMON USES	SPECIAL CONSIDERATIONS
Aloe	*Oral* • Constipation • Bowel evacuation *Topical* • Minor burns • Skin irritation	• The laxative actions of aloe may take up to 10 hours after ingestion to be effective. • Monitor the patient for signs of dehydration; elderly patients are particularly at risk.
Chamomile	*Oral* • Anxiety or restlessness • Diarrhea • Motion sickness • Indigestion *Topical* • Inflammation • Wound healing • Cutaneous burns *Teas* • Sedation • Relaxation	• People sensitive to ragweed and chrysanthemums or others in the *Compositae* family may be more susceptible to contact allergies and anaphylaxis. • Patients with hay fever or bronchial asthma caused by pollens are more susceptible to anaphylactic reactions. • Pregnant women shouldn't use chamomile. • Chamomile may enhance anticoagulant's effect.
Cranberry	• Prophylaxis for urinary tract infection (UTI) • Treatment of UTI • Prevention of renal calculi	• Only the unsweetened form of cranberry prevents bacteria from adhering to the bladder wall, thereby preventing or treating UTIs.
Echinacea	• Supportive therapy to prevent and treat common cold and acute and chronic infections of the upper respiratory tract	• Echinacea is considered supportive therapy and shouldn't be used in place of antibiotic therapy.
Feverfew	• Prevention and treatment of migraines and headaches • Hot flashes • Rheumatoid arthritis • Asthma • Menstrual problems	• Avoid using in pregnant patients because feverfew is also an abortifacient. • Feverfew may increase the risk of abnormal bleeding when combined with an anticoagulant or antiplatelet. • Abruptly stopping feverfew may cause "postfeverfew syndrome" involving tension headaches, insomnia, joint stiffness and pain, and lethargy.
Garlic	• Decrease cholesterol and triglyceride levels • Prevent atherosclerosis • Age-related vascular changes • Prevent GI cancer • Coughs, colds, fevers, and sore throats	• Odor of garlic may be apparent on breath and skin. • Garlic may prolong bleeding time in patients receiving anticoagulants. • Excess raw garlic intake may increase the risk of adverse reactions. • Garlic shouldn't be used in patients with diabetes, insomnia, pemphigus, organ transplants, or rheumatoid arthritis or in those who have recently undergone surgery.
Ginger	• Nausea (antiemetic) • Motion sickness • Morning sickness • GI upset (colic, flatulence, indigestion) • Hypercholesteremia • Liver toxicity	• Ginger may increase the risk of bleeding, bruising, or nosebleeds. • Pregnant women should obtain medical advice before using ginger medicinally. • Ginger may interfere with the intended therapeutic effects of certain conventional drugs.

HERBAL MEDICINE	COMMON USES	SPECIAL CONSIDERATIONS
Ginger *(continued)*	• Burns • Ulcers • Depression	
Ginkgo biloba	• "Memory" agent • Alzheimer's disease • Multi-infarct dementia • Cerebral insufficiency • Intermittent claudication • Tinnitus • Headache	• Adverse effects occur in less than 1% of patients; the most common is GI upset. • Ginkgo biloba may potentiate anticoagulants and increase the risk of bleeding. • Ginkgo extracts are considered standardized if they contain 24% flavonoid glycosides and 6% terpene lactones. • Seizures have been reported in children after ingestion of more then 50 seeds. • Treatment should continue for 6 to 8 weeks but for no more than 3 months.
Ginseng	• Fatigue • Improve concentration • Treat atherosclerosis • Also believed to strengthen the body and increase resistance to disease after sickness or weakness	• Ginseng may cause severe adverse reactions when taken in large doses ($>$ 3 g per day for 2 years), such as increased motor and cognitive activity with significant diarrhea, nervousness, insomnia, hypertension, edema, and skin eruptions. • Ginseng may potentiate anticoagulants and increase the risk of bleeding.
Green tea	• Prevent cancer • Hyperlipidemia • Atherosclerosis • Dental caries • Headaches • Central nervous system (CNS) stimulant • Mild diuretic	• Green tea contains caffeine. • Avoid prolonged and high caffeine intake, which may cause restlessness, irritability, insomnia, palpitations, vertigo, headache, and adverse GI effects. • Adding milk may decrease adverse GI effects of green tea. • Green tea may potentiate anticoagulants and increase the risk of bleeding.
Kava	• Antianxiety • Stress • Restlessness • Sedation • Promote wound healing • Headache • Seizure disorders • Common cold • Respiratory infections	• Kava is contraindicated in pregnancy and lactation. • Kava shouldn't be used in combination with St. John's wort. • Kava shouldn't be taken with other CNS depressants, monoamine oxidase inhibitors, levodopa, antiplatelets, alcohol, or anxiolytics. • Kava can cause drowsiness and may impair motor reflexes and mental acuity; advise the patient to avoid hazardous activities. • Effects should appear within 2 days of initiation of therapy.
St. John's wort	• Mild to moderate depression • Anxiety • Psychovegetative disorders • Sciatica • Viral infections	• Effects may take several weeks; however, if no improvement occurs after 4 to 6 weeks, consider alternative therapy. • St. John's wort interacts with many different types of drugs. • St. John's wort shouldn't be used in combination with prescription antidepressants or antianxiety medications.
Vitex	• Premenstrual syndrome	• Vitex should be taken in the morning with water. • Vitex is a very slow-acting substance; it may take several cycles to see an effect.
Yohimbine	• Impotence (works as an aphrodisiac)	• Yohimbine may cause CNS excitation, including tremor, sleeplessness, anxiety, increased blood pressure, and tachycardia. • Don't use in patients with renal or hepatic insufficiency.

Commonly abused substances

SUBSTANCE	IMMEDIATE EFFECTS	WITHDRAWAL SYMPTOMS	ROUTE
Tobacco/nicotine	• Stimulant • Increased heart rate	Intense craving, tension, irritability, difficulty concentrating, drowsiness, weight gain, headache	• Chewing, smoking
Caffeine	• Stimulant • Increased alertness, sleep delay • May increase heart rate in sufficient quantities	Severe throbbing headaches, drowsiness or decreased sociability and anxiety, muscle stiffness, nausea, waves of hot or cold sensations sweeping the body	• Oral via drinks or over-the-counter products
Amphetamine ("Speed")	• Stimulant • Excitement, increased activity, decreased appetite, may delay sleep	Anxiety, agitation, fatigue, extended sleep, increased appetite, psychosis, suicidal thoughts	• Snorting • Injecting • Oral • Rectally
Cocaine	• Feeling of self-confidence and power • Increased energy • Decreased appetite	Agitation, depression, intense craving for the drug, extreme fatigue, anxiety, angry outbursts, lack of motivation, nausea and vomiting, shaking, irritability, muscle pain, disturbed sleep	• Snorting • Injecting • Oral • Smoking • Rectally
MDMA ("Ecstasy")	• Increased confidence • Feeling of closeness with others • Sensation of floating, anxiety, nausea, paranoia	Depression, anxiety, sleeplessness, depersonalization, derealization, paranoid delusions	• Oral • Injecting • Rectally
Alcohol	• Slurring of speech • Loss of inhibitions, relaxation, feeling of happiness and well-being • Large amounts can lead to unconsciousness	Tremors, nausea, anxiety, sweats, sleep disturbances, visual or tactile hallucinations, seizure, vomiting, diarrhea	• Oral
Benzodiazepines (lorazepam [Ativan], diazepam [Valium], alprazolam [Xanax], oxazepam [Serax])	• Calmness, relief of tension, drowsiness, muscle relaxation, blurred vision	Anxiety, sleep disturbances, hypersensitivity to light, noise, touch, perceptual disturbances, feelings of unreality, memory impairment, headache, depression, suicidal thoughts, agoraphobia, seizure	• Oral • Injecting • Rectally
Opioids (heroin, morphine, hydromorphone [Dilaudid], oxycodone, methadone)	• Pain relief and anxiety • Feeling of well-being • Diminished awareness of outside world • Drowsiness • Large doses may lead to unconsciousness and death	Lacrimation, rhinorrhea, perspiration, restlessness, insomnia, dilated pupils, anorexia, nausea, weakness, muscle aches, abdominal cramps, diarrhea, fatigue	• Oral • Injecting • Rectally • Smoking • Snorting

SUBSTANCE	IMMEDIATE EFFECTS	WITHDRAWAL SYMPTOMS	ROUTE
Marijuana	• Relaxation, increased appetite, slowing down of time • Poor coordination, blood shot eyes • May be hallucinogenic	Irritability, anxiety, physical tension, decreases in appetite and mood	• Oral • Smoking
Hydrocarbon (petrol, glue, aerosol cans, butane gas)	• Feeling of happiness, relaxation, drowsiness	Sweating, rapid pulse, hand tremors, insomnia, nausea or vomiting, hallucinations, and, in severe cases, generalized tonic-clonic seizures	• Inhalation
LSD ("Magic mushroom," "Trip")	• Hallucinations • Anxious feelings, panic • Nausea	Minimal physical withdrawal	• Oral
GHB (gamma hydroxybutyrate) ("Fantasy")	• Euphoria, happiness, sociability; with high doses, dizziness, sleepiness, vomiting, muscle spasms, loss of consciousness	Early symptoms: insomnia, tremor, anxiety, confusion, nausea and vomiting Later symptoms: agitation, vivid hallucinations, combative behavior, disorientation	• Oral
2CB ("Nexus," "Venus," "Brom")	• Hallucinations, heightened visual imagery, acute awareness of body, increased sensitivity to smells and tastes, sexual stimulation	Depression, anxiety, sleeplessness, depersonalization, derealization, paranoid delusions	• Primarily oral, but can be snorted or smoked
Rohypnol ("Date rape drug," "Rib," "Roofies," "R2," "Roachies")	• Tranquilization for brief period	Headache, muscle pain, confusion, hallucinations, seizures	• Oral

Glossary

abruptio placentae: premature detachment of the placenta

accommodation: adjustment of the eye by contraction of ciliary muscles and a change in the lens curvature that allows focusing at various distances; inhibited by cycloplegic drugs, which paralyze ciliary muscles

achalasia: failure to relax

acromegaly: a disorder marked by progressive enlargement of the head, face, hands, and feet, due to excessive somatotropin secretion

Adams-Stokes syndrome: a syndrome characterized by slow or absent pulse, vertigo, syncope, seizures and, sometimes, Cheyne-Stokes respirations; usually a result of advanced atrioventricular block or sick sinus syndrome

agranulocytosis: severe and acute decrease in granulocytes (basophils, eosinophils, and neutrophils) as an adverse reaction to a drug or radiation therapy resulting in high fever, exhaustion, and bleeding ulcers of the throat, mucous membranes, and GI tract

akathisia: syndrome characterized by the inability to remain in a sitting position, motor restlessness, and a feeling of muscular quivering; may appear as an adverse effect of antipsychotic and neuroleptic drugs

akinesia: complete or partial loss of movement

alopecia: loss of hair

anaphylaxis: immediate, transient allergic reaction characterized by the constriction of smooth muscle and dilation of capillaries due to the release of pharmacologically active substances

angiitis: inflammation of a blood vessel

angioedema: life-threatening reaction causing sudden swelling of tissues around the face, neck, lips, tongue, throat, hands, feet, genitals, or intestines

angioneurotic edema: see angioedema

anorgasmia: failure to experience an orgasm

antigen-antibody reaction: antibodies combining with an antigen of the type that stimulated the formation of the antibody, resulting in agglutination, precipitation, complement fixation, or the neutralization of the exotoxin

anuria: without urine

aphakic: without a lens

aplastic anemia: anemia characterized by a decrease in erythrocyte and hemoglobin levels, usually caused by bone marrow failure from neoplastic bone marrow disease or by destruction of the bone marrow by exposure to toxic chemicals, radiation, or certain medications; usually associated with granulocytopenia and thrombocytopenia; also known as *pancytopenia*

apnea: absence of spontaneous breathing

arthralgia: joint pain

ascites: accumulation of fluid (edema) in the peritoneal cavity

asthenia: weakness or debility

ataxia: incoordination of voluntary muscle action, particularly during such activities as walking and reaching for objects

atony: relaxation, flaccidity, or lack of tone or tension

bacteriocidal: causing death of bacteria

bacteriostatic: inhibiting or retarding bacterial growth

bipolar affective disorders: affective disorders characterized by mania and overactivity, depression and decreased activity, or a combination or alternation of the two

blood dyscrasias: diseases of the blood

bradykinesia: abnormally slow body movements

bronchospasm: narrowing of the bronchioles resulting from an increase in smooth-muscle tone; causes wheezing

cachexia: general weight loss and wasting that occurs in the course of a chronic disease

cardiac tamponade: heart compression caused by fluid accumulation in the pericardium

cholelithiasis: presence or formation of gallstones in the gallbladder or bile duct

cholinergic crisis: situation caused by overdose of an antimyasthenic drug, resulting in muscle weakness, dyspnea, and dysphagia (usually within 1 hour of drug administration); other symptoms may include increased respiratory secretions and saliva, nausea, vomiting, cramping, diarrhea, and diaphoresis

chorioamnionitis: infection that involves the chorion, amnion, and amniotic fluid

Churg-Strauss syndrome: an allergic reaction in the small- and medium-sized arteries characterized by fever, weight loss, joint pain, headache, and respiratory distress

Chvostek's sign: abnormal spasm of facial muscles elicited by light taps on the facial nerve; indicates hypocalcemic tetany

corneal reflex: closing of the eyelids on direct touch or irritation of the eye; disappears with application of corneal anesthetics

cretinism: congential hypothyroidism

Crohn's disease: disorder of the GI tract that involves deep ulcers, narrowing and thickening of the bowel, and lymphocytic infiltration. Symptoms include fever, diarrhea, cramping, abdominal pain, and weight loss

cryptorchidism: failure of one or both of the testes to descend

cycloplegia: loss of power in the ciliary muscle of the eye

diabetes insipidus: chronic excretion of large amounts of pale urine with a low specific gravity, that leads to dehydration and extreme thirst; most commonly caused by an inadequate output of antidiuretic hormone

diabetic ketoacidosis: buildup of ketones in the blood due to the breakdown of stored fats for use as energy; a complication of diabetes mellitus

digitalization: administration of a larger-than-maintenance dose (loading dose) of cardiac glycosides to attain a therapeutic serum level rapidly; necessitates close patient observation to detect toxicity

diplopia: the condition in which one object is perceived as two

diverticulitis: inflammation of a diverticulum, especially in the small wall of the colon

dysarthria: a speech disturbance due to paralysis, incoordination, or spasticity of the muscles used for speech

dyskinesia: difficulty in performing voluntary movements

dysphoria: feelings of unrest, restlessness, and anxiety

effector organs: a peripheral gland that receives nerve impulses and reacts by secreting a hormone

encephalopathy: any disorder of the brain

endometriosis: abnormal condition characterized by ectopic growth and function of the endometrium

enuresis: urinary incontinence, especially in bed at night (called *nocturnal enuresis*)

epididymitis: inflammation of the epididymis

epistaxis: nosebleed

erythema: redness of the skin caused by dilation and congestion of the capillaries; commonly signifies an inflammation or infection

erythropoiesis: formation of red blood cells

extrapyramidal symptoms: symptoms caused by an imbalance in the extrapyramidal portion of the nervous system; typically include pill-rolling motions, drooling, tremors, rigidity, and shuffling gait

extravasation: infiltration of I.V. fluid

galactorrhea: production of breast milk at a time other than during lactation

gastroparesis: a smaller degree of gastroparalysis

gate-control theory: a theory to explain the mechanism of pain; pain, a small-fiber afferent stimuli, can be modulated by large-fiber afferent stimuli and descending pathways so that their transmission to ascending spinal pathways is blocked (gated)

gingival hyperplasia: overgrowth of gum tissue

globus hystericus syndrome: difficulty swallowing; a sensation as of a ball in the throat or as if the throat were compressed

goiter: enlarged thyroid gland, usually manifested as a swelling in the neck

goitrogenesis: causing goiter

gout: disorder of purine metabolism that causes high serum uric acid levels; leads to joint pain and inflammation that usually begins in the knee or foot

granulocytopenia: less than the normal number of granular leukocytes in the blood

gynecomastia: excessive development of male mammary glands

hemochromatosis: rare disorder of iron storage characterized by excessive accumulation of iron

hemolytic anemia: anemia resulting from hemolysis, or premature destruction of red blood cells

hemosiderosis: see hemochromatosis

herpetic encephalitis: acute brain disease caused by herpes simplex virus, characterized by early repeated seizures and signs indicating temporal or frontal lobe involvement

hirsutism: excessive growth of dark and course body hair in a masculine distribution

hydatidiform mole: polycystic mass caused by the proliferation of a trophoblast

hyperaldosteronism: excessive excretion of aldosterone

hyperkinesia: excessive muscle activity

hyperosmolar hyperglycemic nonketotic syndrome: a complication of diabetes in which severe hyperglycemia occurs; causes a shift of the water in the brain cells and can result in a coma

hyperplasia: increased number of cells

hyperprolactinemia: elevated levels of prolactin; normal during lactation but abnormal otherwise

hyperpyrexia: extremely high fever

hypertensive crisis: medical emergency characterized by a sudden, severe increase in diastolic blood pressure to a level exceeding 120 mm Hg

hypertonia: extreme tension of the muscles or arteries

hypogonadism: inadequate gonad function

hypohidrosis: diminished perspiration

hyporeflexia: weakened deep tendon reflexes

hypoxemia: subnormal oxygenation of arterial blood

iritis: inflammation of the iris

irritable bowel syndrome: a GI condition characterized by constipation, diarrhea, and gas and bloating; usually associated with uncoordinated and inefficient contractions of the large intestine

Lennox-Gastaut syndrome: generalized, myoclonic epilepsy in children

leukopenia: abnormal decrease in white blood cells to fewer than 5,000 cells/μl

lipodystrophy: thickening of tissues and accumulation of fat at an injection site; results from too-frequent injection of insulin in the same site

long QT syndrome: a syndrome in which the QT interval is longer than the established measurement for age and sex; places an individual at risk for arrhythmias and sudden death

Lyme disease: inflammatory disorder that's mainly transmitted by ticks; characterized by skin lesions, fever, malaise, fatigue, headaches, and a stiff neck

malaise: general overall feeling of discomfort, uneasiness, or fatigue; commonly the first indication of an infection or other disease

malignant hyperthermia: potentially fatal reaction to an inhalation anesthetic; characterized by a marked increase in the rate of muscle metabolism, a rapid temperature rise, and muscular rigidity

mastitis: inflammation of the breast

megaloblastic anemia: anemia in which there's a predominant number of megaloblastic erythroblasts and few normoblasts

miosis: contraction of the pupil

myalgia: diffuse muscle pain, usually associated with malaise

myasthenia gravis: disease characterized by muscle weakness that may involve all skeletal muscle groups, including muscles responsible for swallowing and breathing

myasthenic crisis: situation caused by underdosage of or resistance to an antimyasthenic drug; signs and symptoms, such as muscle weakness, dyspnea, and dysphagia, usually occur 3 or more hours after drug administration

mydriasis: dilation of the pupil

myoclonus: one or a series of shocklike contractions of a group of muscles, or variable regularity, synchrony, and symmetry, generally due to a central nervous system lesion

myopathy: any abnormal condition or disease of the muscular tissue; commonly designates a disorder involving the skeletal muscle

myopia: vision defect in which objects can be seen distinctly only when held close to the eyes (also called *nearsightedness*)

myxedema: nonpitting waxy edema of the skin, mostly in the face and shins; due to subcutaneous deposits of mucoid material in hypothyroidism

narcolepsy: chronic ailment characterized by recurrent attacks of drowsiness and sleep; the patient can't control the spells but is easily awakened

nephrotic syndrome: abnormal kidney condition characterized by marked proteinuria, hypoalbuminemia, and edema

neurodermatitis: atopic dermatitis

neurogenic bladder: defective functioning of the bladder due to impaired innervation

neuroleptic malignant syndrome: life-threatening, rare syndrome caused by antipsychotic drugs, characterized by extreme diaphoresis, muscle rigidity, tachycardia, fever, and renal failure

neutropenia: neutrophil count in circulating blood below the normal percentage

nevi: circumscribed malformation of the skin with hyperpigmentation or increased vascularity, numbness, tingling, burning, or pain in extremities

nystagmus: constant involuntary eye movement

oligospermia: lower than normal sperm count

optic neuritis: inflammation, and usually degeneration, of the optic nerve

organic brain syndrome: a constellation of behavior and psychological signs and symptoms, including problems with attention, concentration, memory, confusion, anxiety, and depression; caused by transient or permanent dysfunction of the brain

orthostatic hypotension: abnormally low blood pressure that occurs when a person stands; also known as *postural hypotension*

osteomalacia: gradual softening and bending of the bones; usually due to a lack of vitamin D or renal tubular dysfunction

otitis media: infection or inflammation of the middle ear

Paget's disease: chronic progressive bone disorder characterized by excessive bone destruction and unorganized bone repair

pancytopenia: abnormal decrease in erythrocytes, white blood cells, and platelets; also known as *aplastic anemia*

paralytic ileus: obstruction of the bowel due to bowel wall paralysis

paresthesia: abnormal sensations (including numbness, prickling, and tingling) with no known cause

parkinsonism: neurologic disorder characterized by tremors, muscle rigidity and weakness, and hypokinesia

peripheral neuropathy: inflammation and degeneration of peripheral nerves; usually associated with numbness, tingling, burning, or pain in extremities

pernicious anemia: chronic anemia caused by failure of the stomach to secrete enough intrinsic factor to ensure intestinal absorption of vitamin B_{12}

pheochromocytoma: an abnormal collection of cells in the adrenal medulla which secretes catecholamines

phlebitis: inflammation of a vein

pinocytosis: the cellular process of actively engulfing liquid; resembles phagocytosis

pleural effusion: increased amount of fluid in the pleural cavity

pleuritis: inflammation of the pleura

polycystic ovary syndrome: the presence of an enlarged ovary with multiple cysts; causes masculinization, menstrual irregularities, and infertility

polycythemia vera: form of polycythemia characterized by bone marrow hyperplasia, skin redness or cyanosis, and splenomegaly

polydipsia: prolonged, excessive thirst

polyuria: excessive urination

porphyria: a group of disorders involving heme biosynthesis characterized by excessive excretion of porphyrins or their precursors

Prader-Willi syndrome: congential syndrome characterized by severe obesity, mental retardation, and small hands, feet, and genitalia

preeclampsia: hypertension with protein in the urine or edema that develops in or shortly after pregnancy

priapism: abnormal, painful, prolonged, or constant penile erection, usually without sexual desire

proteinuria: presence of an abnormally large amount of protein (usually albumin) in the urine

pruritus: itching

pseudomembranous colitis: complication of prolonged antibiotic therapy that causes severe inflammation of the colon, usually from *Clostridium difficile*; causes watery diarrhea, abdominal pain and cramping, and fever

psoriasis: inherited condition characterized by the eruption of reddish maculopapules on the elbows, knees, scalp, and trunk

pyelonephritis: inflammation of the renal parenchyma, calices, and pelvis, usually due to a local bacterial infection

Q fever: febrile disease caused by *Coxiella burnetii* that's characterized by headache, myalgia, and pneumonia or hepatitis; transmitted to humans when contaminated soil or dust is inhaled

Raynaud's disease: vasospastic disorder characterized by bilaterally symmetrical pallor and cyanosis of the fingers and precipitated by cold or emotional upset

Reye's syndrome: encephalopathy affecting children linked to use of aspirin and other salicylate-containing medications and other causes; syndrome may follow an upper respiratory infection or chicken pox; its onset is rapid, usually starting with irritable, combative behavior and vomiting, and progressing to unconsciousness, coma, seizures and, possibly, death

rhabdomyolysis: acute and potentially fatal skeletal muscle disease

rhinorrhea: discharge from the nasal mucous membranes

Rocky Mountain spotted fever: acute infectious disease characterized by headaches, lumbar pain, high fever, and a rash; caused by the organism *Rickettsia rickettsi* and is mainly transmitted by ticks in the Rocky Mountain regions.

seborrheic dermatitis: common scaly eruption that occurs in areas with a high concentration of sebaceous glands, such as the face and neck

serotonin syndrome: adverse reaction causing confusion, agitation, restlessness, tachycardia, muscle rigidity or twitching, tremors, and nausea; most commonly reported in patients taking two or more medications that increase central nervous system serotonin levels; most common drug combinations are monoamine oxidase inhibitors, selective serotonin reuptake inhibitors, and tricyclic antidepressants

serum sickness: an immune complex disease causing local and systemic reactions that appears 1 to 2 weeks after an injection with a foreign serum or serum protein

sick sinus syndrome: degeneration of the conductive tissue that maintains heart rhythm

sickle cell anemia: an autosomal dominant disease occurring almost exclusively in blacks; characterized by sickle-shaped red blood cells that block capillaries

Sjögren's syndrome: a syndrome commonly seen in menopausal women associated with rheumatoid arthritis that causes dryness of the mucous membranes, purpuric spots on the face, and bilateral parotid enlargement

Somogyi effect: rebound hyperglycemia caused by an excessive insulin dosage

spasticity: continuous resistance to muscle stretching that results from increased tension and muscle tone, usually caused by an upper motor neuron lesion; results in stiff, awkward movements

status asthmaticus: severe, prolonged asthma

status epilepticus: rapid succession of seizures without intervals of consciousness; constitutes a medical emergency

Stevens-Johnson syndrome: form of erythema involving the mucous membranes and large areas of the body that may be extensive; it may produce serious symptoms and can lead to death

stomatitis: inflammation and possible ulceration of the mucous membranes of the mouth

subaortic stenosis: congenital narrowing of the outflow tract of the left ventricle by a ring of tissue

syncope: brief loss of consciousness caused by lack of oxygen to the brain

systemic lupus erythematosus: inflammatory connective tissue disease; symptoms include fever, weakness and fatigue, joint pain, and skin lesions on the face, neck, or upper extremities

tardive dyskinesia: disorder characterized by involuntary repetitious movements of the muscles of the face, limbs, and trunk; most commonly results from extended periods of treatment with phenothiazine drugs

tetany: a neurologic syndrome characterized by muscle twitches, cramps, spasms; can cause laryngeal spasms when severe; usually the result of low ionized calcium or magnesium levels

thalassemia: inherited disorders of hemoglobin metabolism

thrombocytopenia: abnormal decrease in platelets, predisposing the patient to bleeding

thrombocytopenic purpura: bleeding disorder characterized by marked decrease in platelets, causing multiple bruises, petechiae, and tissue hemorrhage

thrombosis: formation of a thrombus in a blood vessel; may cause infarction of the tissue supplied by the vessel

thyrotoxic crisis: exacerbation of symptoms of thyrotoxicosis

thyrotoxicosis: toxic condition resulting from thyroid hyperactivity; causes thyroid enlargement, a rapid heart rate, tremors, increased basal metabolism, exophthalmos, nervousness, and weight loss

tinnitus: ringing, buzzing, or whistling in one or both ears occurring without external stimuli; may be caused by an ear infection, drugs, head trauma, or blocked ear canal

torsade de pointes: a form of ventricular tachycardia that's usually caused by medications; characterized by a long QT interval and a "short-long-short" sequence in the beat preceding its onset

Tourette syndrome: neurologic disorder characterized by multiple tics (such as blinking, grimacing, and shrugging) that progresses to grunting, shouting, barking, and in some cases compulsive swearing

toxic epidermal necrolysis: a syndrome in which a large portion of the skin becomes intensely erythematous with epidermal necrosis; results from drug sensitivity or unknown cause

toxic megacolon: acute nonobstructive dilation of the colon commonly seen in ulcerative colitis and Crohn's disease

transplant rejection: destruction of transplanted material at the cellular level by the host's immune response

trigeminal neuralgia: severe, paroxysmal bursts of pain in one or more branches of the trigeminal nerve; commonly induced by touching trigger points in or along the mouth

Trousseau's sign: carpal spasm elicited by applying pressure to the upper arm (for example, with a blood pressure cuff); usually indicates hypocalcemic tetany

Turner's syndrome: syndrome characterized by having only 45 chromosomes and only one X chromosome

ulcerative colitis: chronic disease characterized by ulceration of the colon and rectum, abdominal pain, and diarrhea

urticaria: itchy skin inflammation characterized by pale wheals with well-defined red edges; usually an allergic response to insect bites, food, or certain drugs

uveitis: inflammation of the uveal tract, which includes the iris, ciliary body, and the choroid

vaginitis: inflammation of the vagina

vasospastic angina: uncommon form of angina in which attacks occur during rest rather than activity (also called *Prinzmetal's angina*)

vitreitis: inflammation of the corpus vitreum (vitreous body)

von Willebrand's disease: inherited coagulation disorder caused by deficiency of factor VIII and characterized by prolonged bleeding time, spontaneous nosebleeds, and gingival bleeding; affects equal numbers of males and females

Zollinger-Ellison syndrome: peptic ulceration with gastric hypersecretion and non–beta cell tumor of the pancreatic islets

Selected references

"2005 American Heart Association Guidelines for Cardiopulmonary Resuscitation and Emergency Cardiovascular Care," *Circulation* 112(suppl I): IV1-IV211, November 2005.

Abrams, A.C. *Clinical Drug Therapy: Rationales for Nursing Practice,* 8th ed. Philadelphia: Lippincott Williams & Wilkins, 2006.

American Drug Index, 50th ed. Philadelphia: Facts and Comparisons, 2006.

American Hospital Formulary Service. *AHFS Drug Information 2007.* Bethesda, Md., 2007.

Aschenbrenner, D.S., et al. *Drug Therapy in Nursing,* 2nd ed. Philadelphia: Lippincott Williams & Wilkins, 2006.

Chobanian, A.V., et al. "The Seventh Report of the Joint National Committee on Prevention, Detection, Evaluation, and Treatment of High Blood Pressure," *JAMA* 289(19):2560-72, May 2003.

Chu, E. *Physicians' Cancer Chemotherapy Drug Manual 2007.* Sudbury, Mass.: Jones & Bartlett Pubs., Inc., 2007.

DiMaria-Ghalili, R.A., and Amella, E. "Nutrition in Older Adults: Intervention and Assessment Can Help Curb the Growing Threat of Malnutrition," *AJN* 105(3):40-50, March 2005.

Gever, M.P. "Combination Drugs…" *Nursing2006* 36(9):70, September 2006.

Karch, A.M. *2008 Lippincott's Nursing Drug Guide.* Philadelphia: Lippincott Williams & Wilkins, 2008.

Klieman, L., et al. "Cardiovascular Disease Risk Reduction in Older Adults," *Journal of Cardiovascular Nursing* 21(5 Suppl 1):S27-39, September-October 2006.

Lutz, C.A., and Przytulski, K.R. *Nutrition and Diet Therapy: Evidence Based Application,* 4th ed. Philadelphia: F.A. Davis Co., 2006.

Marangell, L.B., and Martinez, J.M. *Concise Guide to Psychopharmacology,* 2nd ed. Arlington, Va.: American Psychiatric Association, 2006.

Messina, B.A. "Herbal Supplements: Facts and Myths—Talking to Your Patients about Herbal Supplements," *Journal of Perianesthesia Nursing* 21(4):268-78, August 2006.

Nursing I.V. Drug Handbook, 9th ed. Philadelphia: Lippincott Williams & Wilkins, 2006.

Nursing Pharmacology Made Incredibly Easy. Philadelphia: Lippincott Williams & Wilkins, 2005.

Professional Guide to Pathophysiology, 2nd ed. Philadelphia: Lippincott Williams & Wilkins, 2007.

Sande, M.A., et al. *The Sanford Guide to HIV/AIDS Therapy,* 15th ed. Sperryville, Va.: Antimicrobial Therapy, Inc., 2006.

Springhouse Nurse's Drug Guide 2008. Philadelphia: Lippincott Williams & Wilkins, 2008.

Turner, A.M., and Jowett, N.I. "The Role of Statin Therapy in Preventing Recurrent Stroke," *Nursing Times* 102(38):25-26, September 2006.

Wilkes, G.M., and Burke, M.B. *2007 Oncology Nursing Drug Handbook.* Sudbury, Mass.: Jones & Bartlett Pubs., Inc., 2007.

Web resources

Drug Digest: *www.drugdigest.org/DD/Home*

E medicine: Instant Access to the Minds of Medicine: *www.emedicine.com*

Family Practice Notebook: A Family Medicine Resource: *www.fpnotebook.com*

U.S. Food and Drug Administration: *www.fda.gov*

Index

i refers to an illustration; t refers to a table.

i refers to an illustration; t refers to a table.

i refers to an illustration; t refers to a table.

i refers to an illustration; t refers to a table.

i refers to an illustration; t refers to a table.

i refers to an illustration; t refers to a table.

i refers to an illustration; t refers to a table.

Etoposide, 275-276
Eulexin, 274
Eurax, 336
Evaluation, drug administration
　　and, 10
Excretion, 4
　altered, 7
　in children, 17
Exelon, 28
Exemestane, 274-275
Expectorants, 123, 131-132
Extended insulin zinc suspension,
　　224-227, 225t
Eye medications, administering,
　　14, 16
Eyes, 344, 345
Ezetimibe, 170
Ezetimibe and simvastatin,
　　168-169

F

Factive, 248
Factor Xa inhibitors, 205-206
Famciclovir, 256-259, 335-338
Famotidine, 290-291
Famvir, 257, 336
"Fantasy," 377t
Fareston, 274
Faslodex, 274
5-FC, 253-255
Federal Food, Drug, and Cosmetic
　　Act of 1906, 8
Felbamate, 54-56
Felbatol, 55
Feldene, 72
Felodipine, 158-159
Female reproductive hormones,
　　309-310
Female reproductive system. *See*
　　Reproductive system.
Femara, 274
Femiron, 194
Fenofibrate, 167-168

Fenoprofen, 71-73
Fentanyl, 74-76
Feosol, 194, 368
Feostat, 194
Feratab, 194
Fer-Gen-Sol, 194
Fergon, 194
Fer-In-Sol, 194
Ferralyn, 194
Ferrlecit, 194
Ferrous fumarate, 194-196
Ferrous gluconate, 194-196
Ferrous sulfate, 194-196, 368-370
Fertility drugs, 320-322
Fertinex, 321
Feverfew, 374t
Fexofenadine, 237-238
Fiberall, 300
FiberCon, 298, 300
Fibric acid derivatives, 167-168
Fibrinolysis, 193
Fight-or-flight response, 216
Filgrastim, 199-200
Finasteride, 313-314
First pass effect, 4
Flagyl, 250
Flatulex, 295
Flecainide, 145-147
Fleet Mineral Oil Enema, 300
Fleet Phospho-soda, 300
Flexeril, 116
Flonase, 133
Florinef, 238
Flovent, 128
Floxuridine, 272-273
Fluconazole, 253-255
Flucytosine, 253-255
Fludara, 272
Fludarabine, 272-273
Fludrocortisone, 238-240
Fluid balance, 357
Fluid compartments, 357
Fluid transfer, 142

Flumadine, 257
Flunisolide, 127-128
Fluoritab, 364
Fluorometholone, 345-349
Fluoroquinolones, 248-249
Fluorouracil, 272-273
Fluothane, 79
Fluoxetine, 99-101
Fluoxymesterone, 311-313
Fluphenazine, 94-96
Flura-Drops, 364
Flurazepam, 92-93
Flurbiprofen, 71-73
Flurbiprofen sodium, 345-349
Flutamide, 274-275
Fluticasone, 133-134
Fluvastatin, 168-169
Fluvoxamine, 99-101
FML, 346
Focalin, 47
Folic acid, 197-198, 367-368
Folinic acid, 197-198
Follistim, 321
Follitropin alfa, 320-322
Follitropin beta, 320-322
Folvite, 197, 367
Fomivirsen, 256-259, 345-349
Fondaparinux, 205-206
Food, Drug, and Cosmetic Act—
　　Amendment of 1938, 8
Food, Drug, and Cosmetic Act—
　　Durham-Humphrey Amend-
　　ment of 1952, 8
Food, Drug, and Cosmetic Act—
　　Kefauver-Harris Amendment
　　of 1962, 8
Foradil, 125
Forane, 79
Formoterol, 124-125
Fortaz, 244
Forteo, 223
Fortovase, 257
Fosamax, 223

─────
i refers to an illustration; t refers to a table.

i refers to an illustration; t refers to a table.

i refers to an illustration; t refers to a table.

i refers to an illustration; t refers to a table.

i refers to an illustration; t refers to a table.

i refers to an illustration; t refers to a table.

i refers to an illustration; t refers to a table.

i refers to an illustration; t refers to a table.

i refers to an illustration; t refers to a table.

i refers to an illustration; t refers to a table.

i refers to an illustration; t refers to a table.

i refers to an illustration; t refers to a table.

i refers to an illustration; t refers to a table.

Z

i refers to an illustration; t refers to a table.

ABOUT THE CD-ROM

The enclosed CD-ROM is just one more reason why the *Straight A's* series is at the head of its class. The more than 250 additional NCLEX-style questions contained on the CD provide you with another opportunity to review the material and gauge your knowledge. The program allows you to:

- take tests of varying lengths on subject areas of your choice
- learn the rationales for correct and incorrect answers
- print the results of your tests to measure progress over time.

Minimum system requirements

To operate the *Straight A's* CD-ROM, we recommend that you have the following computer equipment:

- Windows XP-Home
- Pentium 4
- 512 MB RAM
- 10 MB of free hard-disk space
- SVGA monitor with high color (16-bit); display area set to 800 × 600
- CD-ROM drive and mouse.

Installation

Before installing the CD-ROM, make sure that your monitor is set to High Color (16-bit) and your display area is set to 800 × 600. If it isn't, consult your monitor's user's manual for instructions about changing the display settings. (The display settings are typically found in Start/Settings/Control Panel/Display/Settings tab.)

To run this program, you must install it onto the hard drive of your computer, following these three steps:

1. Start Windows XP-Home (minimum).
2. Place the CD in your CD-ROM drive. After a few moments, the install process will automatically begin. Note: If the install process doesn't automatically begin, click the Start menu and select Run. Type D:\setup.exe (where D: is the letter of your CD-ROM drive) and then click OK.
3. Follow the on-screen instructions for installation.

Technical support

For technical support, call toll-free 1-800-638-3030, Monday through Friday, 8:30 a.m. to 5 p.m. Eastern Time. You may also write to Lippincott Williams & Wilkins Technical Support, 351 W. Camden Street, Baltimore, MD 21201-2436, or e-mail us at *wkhealth-support@wolterskluwer.com*.
